# THE PLAGUE EPIC IN
# EARLY MODERN ENGLAND

*For Greg*

# The Plague Epic in Early Modern England

## Heroic Measures, 1603–1721

Edited by

**REBECCA TOTARO**

*Florida Gulf Coast University, USA*

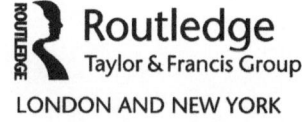

Routledge
Taylor & Francis Group

LONDON AND NEW YORK

First published 2012 by Ashgate Publishing

Published 2016 by Routledge
2 Park Square, Milton Park, Abingdon, Oxon OX14 4RN
711 Third Avenue, New York, NY 10017, USA

First issued in paperback 2017

*Routledge is an imprint of the Taylor & Francis Group, an informa business*

**British Library Cataloguing in Publication Data**
The plague epic in early modern England: heroic measures, 1603–1721.
1. Plague – Poetry. 2. Epic poetry, English. 3. Heroic verse, English. 4. English poetry –
Early modern, 1500–1700. 5. Plague in literature.
I. Totaro, Rebecca.
821.4'08'03561-dc23

**Library of Congress Cataloging-in-Publication Data**
The plague epic in early modern England: heroic measures, 1603–1721 / edited by Rebecca
    Totaro.
    p. cm.
Includes bibliographical references and index.
ISBN 978-1-4094-4171-7 (hardcover: alk. paper)
1. English poetry—Early modern, 1500–1700—History and criticism. 2. Plague—
Poetry. 3. Epic poetry, English. 4. Plague in literature. 5. Plague—England—History. I.
Totaro, Rebecca Carol Noel, 1968–
PR408.P62B75 2012
821'.4093561—dc23


ISBN 13: 978-1-138-10941-4 (pbk)
ISBN 13: 978-1-4094-4171-7 (hbk)

# Contents

# Acknowledgments

This book initially grew out of research conducted for *Suffering in Paradise: The Bubonic Plague in English Literature from More to Milton* (2005), an examination of the practical effects of hope that enabled and sustained literary responses to pandemic disease. Conversations deriving from a fortuitous seat assignment next to Linda McJannet, as we were both returning from the 2006 World Shakespeare Congress in Brisbane, Australia, led me to think in new ways about scholarly editions. With the assistance of knowledgeable, generous Folger Shakespeare Library librarians, the bulk of the research for this volume occurred while I was a member of the Folger Institute Year-Long Colloquium on "Vernacular Health and Healing" (2006–2007) and as a short term fellow on sabbatical there (2007–2008). The vast and largely untapped resources I discovered led me to produce two books: this one, on plague poetry in the seventeenth century, and *Plague in Print: Essential Elizabethan Sources, 1558–1603* (2010), a representative sample of genres of plague writing codified in the sixteenth century, showing the predominance of prose. I revised earlier versions of Part 1 of the current volume in response to research for the Introduction to *Representing the Plague in Early Modern England* (2011); for an essay, "Mother London and the Madonna Lactans," forthcoming in *Medieval and Renaissance Lactations: Images, Rhetorics, Practices*; and as a result of my participation in the Early Modern Studies Research Group at University of Miami's Center for the Humanities. I extend my gratitude, respectively, to Ernest B. Gilman; Jutta Sperling; and Mihoko Suzuki, Jeffrey Shoulson, Karl Gunter, Susanne Woods, and Mary Lindemann. Thanks also to members of the 2010 Renaissance Society of America session "The Bubonic Plague in Art and Literature: England, Spain, Italy," especially Sheila Barker. With great appreciation, I also acknowledge the generous efforts of my research writing group colleagues Kimberly Jackson and Delphine Gras, and Patricia Rice, each of whom read Part 1 in various forms during the last two years of its revision; their comments markedly enhanced its organization in particular. At final draft, Wendy Furman-Adams and Amy Tigner offered scrupulous, clarifying comments. University graduate student Dane Olsen provided diligent, insightful review of the majority of transcriptions; English major Jessie Carcamo read each of the current transcriptions for sentence-level comprehension with an eye toward the usefulness of the appendices and footnotes; independent researcher Evdoxia Kolydaki provided the translations of Greek passages in the poems; and the beautiful index is the work of Pat Rimmer. Last and certainly not least, I thank the Ashgate Publishing Company team: external reviewers for their invaluable comments, which they will see have improved the work immensely; editor Seth F. Hibbert, for his scrupulous and comforting attention to detail; and Erika Gaffney, Publishing Manager for Ashgate, who led the way with her warm support and essential advice, from proposal to cover image and title.

# ACKNOWLEDGMENTS

Part 1

# An Introduction to the Plague in Heroic Measures, 1603–1721

Between 1603 and 1611, England endured unrelenting visitations of bubonic plague. No other span of years saw the same persistence of the disease. It was as if the plague had taken up residence, testing the people's resolve, in many ways to an even greater extent than during what are currently the better known plague years of 1348-49 and 1665-66, what we have come to call the Black Death and the Great Plague of London, respectively. A rude awakening to the new century, the 1603–1611 series of outbreaks set something of a standard for the next fifty years. Between 1603 and 1666, a total of fourteen years were among the deadliest for plague in England's history: 1603–1604, 1609–10, 1625–26, 1630, 1636, 1638, 1643, 1657–58, 1665–66.[1] With a visitation every five years on average, England was sorely challenged, even before factoring in the effects of the civil war, the London fire of 1666, the Anglo-Dutch wars, and increased rates of maternal mortality. Decades later, in the summer of 1720, the plague struck Marseilles, France, where it ravaged the population for more than a year. The English had become accustomed to reports of plague on the Continent preceding its visitation to the island, and they feared the worst. The government mobilized, shoring up plague orders. Ready for what they feared was the beginning of yet another century of epidemic disease, England was spared. But it was years before the nation would know this, and in those early decades of the eighteenth century, the threat of another visitation was enough to revive an active writing campaign that included medical treatises, sermons, and disputations regarding quarantine law.[2]

---

[1]    These dates are compiled from Paul Slack, *The Impact of Plague in Tudor and Stuart England* (London and Boston: Routledge & Kegan Paul, 1985; reprinted with corrections, Oxford: Clarendon Press, 1985; New York: Oxford University Press, 2000), 146–47—currently the preeminent source on British historical analysis of the plague; Charles Creighton, *History of Epidemics in Britain: From AD 664 to the Extinction of the Plague,* 2 vols. (Cambridge: Cambridge University Press, 1891–94), 1:229–303, 575; Charles Mullett, *The Bubonic Plague and England: An Essay in the History of Preventative Medicine* (Lexington: University of Kentucky, 1956), 31–210; and *English Short Title Catalogue* listings under "England, Proclamations" for 1604–1609, 1625, 1636. Among the many gruesome causes of increased mortality in the seventeenth-century were childbirth-related injuries; see the award-winning study, *Milton and Maternal Mortality,* by Louis Schwartz (Cambridge and New York: Cambridge University Press, 2009), especially chapters 1–2.

[2]    On the written response to the threat of plague in England in the 1720s, see Paula R. Backscheider, ed., *Daniel Defoe, A Journal of the Plague Year,* A Norton Critical Reader (New York and London: W. W. Norton & Company, 1992), ix-xiii, 218-30.

In the early seventeenth century, as England felt the blows, one visitation after another, the plague epic emerged as a new literary genre. Showcasing unusual combinations of passion and restraint, heartrending lamentation and nation-building fervor, the plague epic functioned as a call to active faith and as a literary memorial for the fallen. Consisting primarily of brief epics, typically less than 1000 lines each, and written in the heroic prosody associated with the epic, the plague epic testifies powerfully to the need for shared but still flexible and complex discourse in times when individuals endure overwhelming affliction together. Although it may not speak to us in the form or in the words we would currently use to articulate catastrophic suffering, the early modern plague epic invites us to consider the ways that we give shape to our disaster narratives. In the plague epic, poets voice concerns regarding topics we now call medical malpractice, end-of-life care, economic recovery, national healthcare, homeland security, and individual liberty. Such large-scale and relevant issues find pronounced representation in scenes of visceral, solitary misery and, ironically at first glance, in the heroic measures of epic poetry. In the very same measures, poets invoke muses, pay tribute to the fallen, and express outrage as they describe London's plague-time transformation. They advance causes for the plague, track its course through the human body and the streets of London, and proclaim England's potential for immediate, complete, material recuperation. Standing as witness to scenes of personal physiological and psychological horror, the poets admit their own failings and the fears that afflict them as they write, at the same time providing didactic accounts of the plague's meaning within English, world, and Christian history. As they redefine heroism in post-Reformation plague-time, they also cry out against corrupt medical practitioners, prophets, and civic leaders, and they articulate an urgent theodicy. For over 100 years, the epic was the literary form comprehensive and serious enough to contain the many rhetorical modes needed to render in a single creation the complex experience of and views on the plague—the most physiologically alarming, historically recurring, and baffling cause of human agony England had ever known.

In *The Plague Epic in Early Modern England: Heroic Measures, 1603–1721*, I provide the first examination of this genre. In Part 1, I identify the specific features of the plague epic, consider the broad range of authors who took up this distinctly heroic form of plague writing, and offer the first scholarly examination of the genre's content, with special attention to the function of the poems in their post-Reformation, post-Elizabethan context. As a symptom of shifting needs arising over the course of more than a century of plague visitations, the plague epic emerged in response to the very same cultural conditions that led to war and that compelled John Milton to write his epics, *Paradise Lost* (1667) and *Paradise Regained* (1671).[3] In Part 2, I present ten of the most fascinating and representative

---

[3]    With respect to the research of other scholars on these subjects, my most direct debts are to Paul Slack; Barbara Kiefer Lewalski, especially for *Milton's Brief Epic: The Genre, Meaning, and Art of Paradise Regained* (Providence: Brown University Press, 1966); Raymond A. Anselment for *The Realms of Apollo: Literature and Healing in*

of these plague poems—each transcribed and edited with critical commentary and endnotes, including the original marginal notes. Preceding each poem are the record of its publication history, details regarding any relevant materials published in the same volume as the original poem, and the location of the poem now with respect to library holdings. The volume concludes with a General Glossary of Terms and an Index of Names, to expedite queries, as well as a Works Cited section that includes additional plague epics not transliterated here and an Index keyed to the entire volume, including the transcribed poetry.

## "Proper for an *Epic Poem*": A Consideration of Generic Form

Writers in the seventeenth century represented the plague as an unstoppable force that surprised its victims and exposed them to unfathomable hardship. In their accounts, all sources of security fail as mothers watch their infants die, grieving fathers bury their sons, friends avoid friends, religious and civic leaders neglect those in their care, even the best of physicians and other caretakers are unable to offer relief to those in their charge, and dishonest practitioners of physic prey on people who are desperate for aid. Adding to the misery, people die in flight from infected areas, refused lodging by those in the country who fear them; prayer fails; graves fill to overflowing; and those who survive face the concomitant challenges of famine, poverty, and the temptation of quick money offered by pawn brokers and usurers. Such events signal the end of an era of prosperity, at best. These are the stable elements of the plague visitation narrative, which appear in European plague literature as early as the fourteenth century.[4] The steady appropriation of these narrative elements derives from their observable relationship to real plague-time events, observable in written form from as early as the fifth century B.C.E., when Thucydides recorded details of the plague at Athens in his *History of the Peloponnesian War.*[5] As successive generations faced the disease without any

---

*Seventeenth-Century England* (Newark: University of Delaware Press and London: Associated University Presses, 1995), especially chapter three on the plague, which is the only other treatment in one place of most of the poems contained here; Ernest B. Gilman for *Plague Writing in Early Modern England* (Chicago: University of Chicago Press, 2009), especially on the concept of what he calls the "plague theodicy" of the seventeenth century (64–69); and Margaret Healy for her powerful yoking of *De Rerum Natura* and *Paradise Lost,* in the first pages of *Fictions of Disease in Early Modern England: Bodies, Plagues and Politics* (Houndmills, UK and New York: Palgrave, 2002, 1–2).

[4]   On plague literature from the fourteenth century, see Rosemary Horrox, *The Black Death,* Manchester Medieval Sources Series (Manchester and New York: Manchester University Press, 1994)—an ideal starting point, because among the many documents it includes are plague-specific passages from Boccaccio's *Decameron,* Chaucer's *Pardoner's Tale,* and letters by Petrarch, whose beloved Laura died of plague, thus inspiring Petrarch in his writing of sonnets.

[5]   Thucydides, *History of the Peloponnesian War, Volume I: Books 1–2,* trans. C. F. Smith, Loeb Classical Library (1919, 1921; Cambridge, MA: Harvard University Press, 1991). See especially book 2, pages 343ff.

marked change in its prevention or treatment, plague literature grew in volume, length, and complexity, but in its essential content, it changed by relatively small degrees.

In England, a marked increase in plague writing followed the coronation of Queen Elizabeth I. Her survival through a near-fatal battle with smallpox early in her reign suggested that England might finally have secured for itself a fit head of state and church—one more likely than her most recent predecessors to endure great hardship but live a long life, and even produce viable heirs. Under Elizabeth I, England again distanced itself from its Catholic past, eliminating prayer to saints, processions, and pilgrimages from their arsenal of defenses against the plague, and investing in nationwide schedules for special common prayer and plague orders, the latter based on Continental practices. The English imagined they might join their European colleagues as leaders in healthcare—this, the early hope of humanists Thomas Linacre, Thomas More, and John Colet, who had helped found the Royal College of Physicians under Elizabeth's father in 1518. Plague writing flourished, with the printing press placing medical regimens, sermons, prose pamphlets, plague bills, and prayers—all in the vernacular—in the hands of readers, who were eager to do what they could to help themselves through the next visitation.[6]

By 1603, with the death of the queen, decades of plague visitations, and regular reissue of plague prayers and orders, there had been no noticeable reduction in plague-related deaths or improvement of other conditions during visitations. As a comparison of plague writing from the beginning and the end of Elizabeth I's reign suggests, hope diminished. By way of brief example, physician and writer William Bullein (c. 1515-1576) appears far more certain in 1563 of the salubrious effects of his plague literature than Thomas Dekker (1572–1632) does of his in 1603. Although both of their works—Bullein's *A Dialogue of the Fever Pestilence* and Dekker's *The Wonderful Year*—have been classified as Elizabethan prose satire, their conclusions alone illustrate the gap between them. After a lengthy narrative that includes medical and theological advice, as well as humorous husband-wife banter and animal fables, Bullein provides a morality tale ending in which the protagonist's soul is secured passage to heaven. His tone is hopeful, he has drawn his medical and moral instruction from the latest manuals, and his conclusion is certain and positive. In contrast, Dekker closes anti-climactically (if he can be said to close at all), offering only a string of absurd, grotesque stories uttered

---

6   On plague in Tudor literature and culture, see Rebecca Totaro, *Suffering in Paradise: The Bubonic Plague in English Literature from More to Milton,* Medieval & Renaissance Literary Studies (Pittsburgh: Duquesne University Press, 2005), especially chapters 1–3, and 5; Rebecca Totaro, *The Plague in Print: Essential Elizabethan Sources, 1558–1603,* Medieval & Renaissance Literary Studies (Pittsburgh: Duquesne University Press, 2010), especially the Introduction; and Rebecca Totaro and Ernest B. Gilman, editors, *Representing the Plague in Early Modern England,* Routledge Studies in Literature and Culture (New York: Routledge, 2011), especially the Introduction.

in exasperation.[7] By its end, Dekker's entertainment contains enough bile to diminish even his early promise to help the reader secure mirthful distraction from plague-time sorrow and fear. Dekker offers a brutal form of entertainment, not consumable in large quantities. It would not sustain readers over the next century of plague visitations—a fact Dekker himself may have admitted by way of his later choice to partner with fellow playwright Thomas Middleton (1580–1627) in the writing of a plague epic.

Few at the close of the sixteenth century could have anticipated the many changes that would lead men like John Milton to turn to epic poetry to "justify the ways of God to men."[8] The need for theodicy grew in urgency beginning in 1603 with the death of Elizabeth, the long-ruling, self-styled mother to her people. This alone was enough to send tremors through the nation, but making matters worse, the plague had struck so soon after her death that King James VI of Scotland had not yet been crowned King James I of England, and this exacerbated anxieties. This visitation would kill an estimated 25,000 in London alone—20 percent of the population. And plague would linger, outbreak after outbreak, through the first full third of James' reign.[9] Almost as soon as it began to recede, it would return, and in 1625, it again followed the death of a monarch, killing another 20 percent of London's population. Slightly more than ten years later, in 1636, the plague returned once more, leaving the population reduced by an additional 10,000. In 1665, its full force was felt, as it killed an estimated 55,750. As Paul Slack notes, "in terms of the gross number of deaths" this last plague was the most deadly (*Impact of Plague,* 151). In many other ways, however, including the percentage of the population that died and the number of towns within England that were affected in any given visitation, other years were just as deadly (including 1630, 1638, 1643, and 1657–58 as mentioned earlier). In addition, in between each major, London-based visitation, the plague was often endemic in human and epizootic in

---

[7]    On Bullein's satire, especially in relationship to Dekker's *Wonderful Year*, see William Kerwin, "Writing the Plague in English Prose Satire," in Totaro and Gilman, 37–53; R. W. Maslen "The Healing Dialogues of Doctor Bullein, *The Yearbook of English Studies* 38.1 (2008): 119–135; see also Lawrence Manley *Literature and Culture in Early Modern London* (Cambridge and New York: Cambridge University Press, 2000), 118–122, 352–66; Totaro, *The Plague in Print,* especially the introduction and chapters 1 and 6; and Healy's chapters 2 and 3 on "The Plaguy Body." On the reputed health value of mirth, especially in plague-time, see Nichole DeWall, "'Sweet recreation barred': The Case for Playgoing in Plague-Time" in Totaro and Gilman, 133-40.

[8]    John Milton, *Paradise Lost,* in *John Milton: The Complete Poems and Essential Prose,* ed. William Kerrigan, John Rumrich, and Stephen M. Fallon (New York: Random House, 2007), 1.26.

[9]    Slack 151, 13, 62. On mortality rates and the perception of monarchs in these years, see also Richelle Munkhoff, "Contagious Figurations: Plague and the Impenetrable Nation after the Death of Elizabeth" in Totaro and Gilman, 99 and 109 n.12; and James D. Mardock, "Thinking to pass unknown": *Measure for Measure,* the Plague, and the Accession of King James I, in Totaro and Gilman, 113–130. On the concept of the "great years of plague," see Totaro, *Suffering in Paradise,* 32–5.

animal populations elsewhere in England, making its reemergence at any point a possibility. It also traveled in figurative form by rumor and in rhetoric, increasing fear as regularly as it increased mortality rates.

In response to these and many other mounting concerns, and desperate to assert meaning where little common understanding existed, people pondered the meaning of the plague, and they considered the nation's future. Giving voice to these discussions in 1625, Richard Milton (n.d.) explains in his plague epic,

> We study now and often cast about
> And call to mind what heretofore fell out
> Upon the Death of any Sovereign Prince,
> Or in Successor's reign hath hapned since.
> There's many of us do remember yet
> It was so late, we can it not forget,
> When first King *James*, came here this Crown to sway,
> How many by the plague were caught away (124)

Remembering the nationally debilitating 1603 visitation, and having suffered through many smaller visitations in the intervening years, Milton places himself among the "we" who "study" the past to try to make sense of the present. The outcome of this reasoning is not a positive one. The conclusion can only be that England had not learned from its prior mistakes. As Milton reviews the plague bills, seeing the death toll continue to rise, he fears that, finally, this time, in 1625, conditions might reach apocalyptic pitch: in fact, "now we think the sickness will not cease / Because we find it weekly doth increase" (124).

In the same year, John Taylor (1578–1653) confirms this general rationale for the plague's return and speculates further. Known as the Water Poet, Taylor was a waterman who plied the Thames, taking passengers to and from their destinations. Some suspect that it was in conversation with his patrons that he found his literary calling and a vast audience, leading him to achieve greater notoriety than is currently appreciated.[10] In *The Fearful Summer* (1625), he suggests that visitations coinciding with the deaths of Elizabeth and James function as a form of national purgation:

> The ways of God are intricate, no doubt
> Unsearchable and past man's finding out.
> He at his pleasure worketh wondrous things
> And in his hand doth hold the hearts of kings,
> And for the love, which to our *King* he bears,
> By sickness, he our sinful country clears,
> That he may be a patron and a guide
> Unto a people purg'd and purifi'd:
> This by a precedent is manifest,

---

[10]    As James Mardock makes clear, "Taylor was one of the most prolific popular writers of the seventeenth century" and he would go on to become "the most popular and prolific royalist propagandist in England" ("*The Spirit and the Muse*: The Anxiety of Religious Positioning in John *Taylor's* Prewar Polemics," *The Seventeenth Century* 14 [1999]: 1, 11).

> When famous late *Elizabeth* deceast:
> Before our gracious *James* put on the crown
> God's hand did cut superfluous branches down. (153)

In something approaching a Malthusian argument for the natural reduction by disease of populations that exceed their bounds, Taylor advances an oddly positive interpretation of the disease: God has brought the plague "for the love, which to our *King* he bears." In 1625, Taylor imagines, God has "purg'd and purify'd" England for Charles I just, he explains later, "As *He* did for his Father formerly / A sinful nation cleanse and purify" (153). Each death of a monarch is an opportunity to "cut superfluous branches down," and give the new king a better chance to govern effectively.

This etiology for plague is inherently dissatisfying, of course, because it fails to account for plague visitations that cause high mortality in years when a sovereign does not die, and it suggests that England deserves each time to feel again the wrath of God. It does nothing to help relieve anxieties or to account for the deaths of the innocent, faithful, or otherwise beyond reproach. Such thinking likely instead helped to fuel discontent and a lack of trust in England's religious and civic leadership. Citing the loss of the "exclusive control of the cultivation of memory," that had allowed former kings and queens (and at one time the Catholic church) to maintain support for the versions of history that legitimized their own power, David Cressy explains that in just these years, "English history became contested among competing religious and political groups."[11] As the Stuart government sought to hold on more and more tightly to its power over the people, the result was less control and increasing factionalism that would lead the nation to the religious and political identity crisis of civil war.

In the absence of trust in the kind of medical, religious, and governmental security offered early in the reign of Elizabeth I, people filled in the gaps with revised beliefs and rituals that helped them account for the past, endure the present, and anticipate the future. Seventeenth-century poets did so by appropriating the epic form to suit what they imagined was their own "epochal change," which Van Kelly explains in this way: "For Tolkien, *Beowulf* bears resemblance to the *Aeneid* because the respective heroes witness major epochal changes, from the Hellenic to the Roman world in one case, from the pagan to the Christian world in the other."[12] The poets of England's plague epic saw their own stories bearing this very resemblance to the *Odyssey* and the *Aeneid.* Unlike the *Beowulf* poet or Virgil, however, these poets found themselves living through the epochal change about which they wrote. As John Davies of Hereford (1565?–1618) exclaims in 1609, "Never came there like Mortality, / Since Death from Adam to his Children

---

[11] David Cressy, "National Memory in Early Modern England," in *Commemorations: The Politics of National Identity* (Princeton: Princeton University Press, 1994), 66.

[12] Van Kelly, "Introduction: Criteria for the Epic: Borders, Diversity, and Expansion," in *Epic and Epoch: Essays on the Interpretation and History of a Genre*, eds. Steven M. Oberhelman, Van Kelly, and Richard J. Golsan, *Studies in Comparative Literature* 24 (Lubbock, Texas: Texas Tech University Press, 1994), 20 n. 14

came"; and still almost three decades later, George Wither (1588–1667) claims with all seriousness, "A braver Subject, *Muses never* had."[13]

In concert with this opportunity for poets to write about epochal change from a first-hand perspective, the century saw a new primacy placed on the authentic experience of the plague-time author. Readers stuck in London did not want to hear about the plague from pampered poets who had afforded escape to the country, and those in the country likewise wanted news they could believe, coming from within the infected city. The increase in literacy and in the number of printed texts available in the vernacular supported this call. As London poets participated in an epic discourse that extended the story of England's great trial beyond the boundaries of their cultural moment, they rooted their accounts distinctively in local detail that would speak to their seventeenth-century English readers. The poets describe the streets of London, abandoned but for those who pass through quickly, their noses stuffed with tarred rope and other agents thought to prevent them from inhaling plague-tainted vapors. In as much detail, poets turn their attention to their own afflicted bodies, overcharged with grief and fear, as they witness and record the catastrophic alterations wrought by plague.

In the seventeenth-century plague visitation experience, as in the literary epic, the marvelous and mundane appear side by side in ways poignant and problematic, creating tensions between classical and Christian thinking about the purpose of disease as well as between public expressions of faith and the solitary, unique experience of extreme suffering and bearing witness to it. To give correspondingly sublime voice this set of tensions, poets of the seventeenth century turned consistently to the epic—the genre trusted to direct their tragedy and lamentation toward a heroic, hopeful conclusion.[14] The many epic markers in these plague

---

[13]    John Davies, *The Triumph of Death* (1609), 93. George Wither, *Britain's Remembrancer* (1638), 214. Wither also wrote, 'History of the pestilence' (MS 1999, Pepys Library, Magdalene College, Cambridge) and a revised version of the *Remembrancer* entitled, *A memorandum to London* (1665; Wing [CD-Rom, 1996], W3170). On the *Remembrancer* in its plague-time context, especially with respect to memory and Reformation politics, see Gilman, *Plague Writing,* 101–109. On Wither's life, see Michelle O'Callaghan, 'Wither, George (1588–1667)', *Oxford Dictionary of National Biography*, Oxford University Press, 2004 [http://www.oxforddnb.com/view/article/29804, accessed 16 March 2010].

[14]    As Sir Philip Sidney argues in *The Apology for Poetry,* the epic was considered "not only a kind, but the best and most accomplished kind of poetry," ed. R. W. Maslen (Manchester: Manchester University Press, 2002), 99. With respect to "why Milton incorporated so complete a spectrum of literary forms and genres in *Paradise Lost,*" for example, Lewalski explains, "a partial answer must be that much Renaissance critical theory supports the notion of the epic as a heterocosm or a compendium of subjects, forms, and styles" ("The Genres of *Paradise Lost*: Literary Genre as a Means of Accommodation," *Milton Studies* [Pittsburgh, PA: University of Pittsburgh Press, 1983], 77). See also her *Paradise Lost and the Rhetoric of Literary Forms* (Princeton: Princeton University Press, 1985). One might say, as S. Clark Hulse has for the Elizabethan minor epic, that the plague epic "is by nature metamorphic verse" ("Elizabethan Minor Epic: Toward a Definition of

poems in particular—from *praepositio*, invocation, and epic simile to martial and navel themes, digression, moral exempla, and allusion to other epics—offered layers of assurance that the narrative would not slip too far into the fear-producing realm of tragedy or the grief-inducing territory of lamentation. By these methods, inscribed in the heroic measures of their metrical form, the poets forcefully appropriated their gravest enemy, Death, making him serve their turns.

In heroic measures, the metrical feet and rhyme scheme of their poems, these seventeenth-century poets approximated the dactylic hexameter verse form of those they considered the world's master poets, the classical authors of martial and didactic verse, including Homer, Hesiod, Aratus, Lucretius, Virgil, Manilius, Ovid, and Lucan. Through iambic pentameter and rhyming couplets, they demonstrated their own literary kinship and fitness. The plague epic, like its biblical and secular siblings in the same century, deviated little from this form, particularly as the century advanced and brief epics grew in popularity. Even those few poets who did adopt a slightly altered verse form appear to have done so to call attention to their choices, thereby highlighting the heroic purpose and content of their poems. William Muggins' (n.d.) *London's Mourning Garment* (1603), for example, appears in rhyme royal, the standard meter in Chaucer's time, which Chaucer used for *Troilus and Criseyde* (c. 1385) and Shakespeare used for *The Rape of Lucrece* (1594)—poems since identified as "brief" or "minor" epics.[15] John Davies wrote

---

Genre" *Studies in Philology* 73.3 [Jul., 1976], 279). On mixed modes in early modern literature, see Sir Philip Sidney, *The Apology for Poetry,* 97; Rosalie Colie, *The Resources of Kind: Genre-Theory in the Renaissance* (Berkeley, London, and New York: University of California Press, 1973), 20–31; John M. Steadman, *Epic and Tragic Structure in* Paradise Lost (Chicago: University of Chicago, 1976); Kenneth Borris, *Allegory and Epic in English Renaissance Literature: Heroic Form in Sidney, Spenser, and Milton* (Cambridge and New York: Cambridge University Press, 2000), especially 57–8; John T. Shawcross, "Milton and Epic Revisionism" in Oberhelman, Kelly, and Golsan, 186–207; Jennifer O'Meara, *Alchemists, Epics, and Heroes: The Rhetorical Construction of the Seventeenth Century Experimental Philosopher* (Diss. University of Illinois at Urbana-Champaign, 2007), 11. As a starting place for consideration of the epic sublime in this period, see David Quint, *Epic and Empire: Politics and Generic Form from Virgil to Milton* (Princeton, NJ: Princeton University Press, 1993), 140, 208, 304.

[15]   On the brief epics of Chaucer, Shakespeare, and others, see Elizabeth Story Donno, *Elizabethan Minor Epics* (New York: Columbia University Press, 1963); Hulse, "Elizabethan Minor Epic," pp. 302–319; and Paul W. Miller, "The Elizabethan Minor Epic," *Studies in Philology*, Vol. 55, No. 1 (Jan., 1958), pp. 31–8. For a list of common characteristics of minor and brief epics, see Paul W. Miller, *Seven Minor Epics of the English Renaissance (1596–1624)* (Gainesville: Scholars' Facsimiles and Reprints, 1967), xvi. On the popularity of the brief epic among poets, see especially Hulse: "Except for Sidney, every major Elizabethan poet, and most of the minor ones, wrote minor epics" in *The Metamorphic Verse: The Elizabethan Minor Epic* (Princeton: Princeton University Press, 1983). On Chaucer's poem as a five act "minor" epic, see Richard H. Perkinson, "The Epic in Five Acts," *Studies in Philology* 43.3 (1946), 465–81. On the dating of Chaucer's poem, see Larry Dean Benson, *The Riverside Chaucer* (Oxford and New York: Oxford University Press, 2008), 1020.

his plague epic, The *Triumph of Death* (1609), in iambic pentameter with heroic quatrains rather than couplets—a form of English heroic verse that John Dryden and William Davenant, among others, utilized for their epics.[16] And although *News from Graves-end* (1604) by Thomas Dekker and Thomas Middleton appears in the ballad form of iambic tetrameter with heroic couplets, their choice of meter creates an undoubtedly intentional contrast between the poem's common prosody and its many other overtly heroic markings.[17]

As these poets crafted their plague epics, they contributed to an international discourse that was increasing in popularity in those years. Abraham Cowley, John Dryden, and John Milton were among the many involved in debates over what constituted an epic. These debates grew in part, as Barbara K. Lewalski has shown, because of the century's preference for Christian over classical subject matter, and because such content created what Judith Kates has called "the problem of Christian epic."[18] As Tobias Gregory most recently explains, the problem faced by Christian poets who attempt to write epics is exactly the problem of theodicy: "How can the poet generate tension within the epic plot when one omnipotent character holds all the cards? How does the violence the poem relates reflect on the ostensibly benevolent deity who orders all?"[19] Classical poets had not faced quite the same dilemma: "The motives of the Olympian gods are perspicuous to the reader; we know the reasons for Neptune's ire, or Juno's" (7). Like Kates, Gregory addresses the problem of a Christian God in the martial epic, and, when applied to the plague epic in particular, the questions are all the more salient. Moreover, in the early modern martial Christian epic, violence comes to God's chosen and to their adversaries, but we know the ending: the Christians will win, due to a "Mosaic distinction" that is "ubiquitous" in the Renaissance epic (13). That distinction exists in *The Faerie Queene*, *Paradise Lost*, and in the seventeenth century's biblical epic, a popular close cousin to the plague epic.[20] The

---

[16] On the relationship between the seventeenth-century heroic quatrain used for epics and the very same form called the elegiac quatrain in the eighteenth century and used more often for elegies, see Henry Weinfield, *The Poet Without a Name: Gray's Elegy and the Problem of History* (Carbondale: Southern Illinois University Press, 1991), 93; Peter Thorpe, *Eighteenth Century English Poetry* (Chicago: Nelson-Hall, 1975), 161–62; and Paula R. Backscheider, *Eighteenth-Century Women Poets and their Poetry: Inventing Agency, Inventing Genre* (Baltimore: The Johns Hopkins University Press, 2007), 271–72.

[17] The Dekker and Middleton blending of epic and ballad elements is in keeping with the contrasting but linked modes of satirical correction and saturnalia that Lawrence Manley finds in Dekker's early plague pamphlets (352–66).

[18] See Lewalski, *Milton's Brief Epic*, and Judith Kates, *Tasso and Milton: The Problem of Christian Epic* (Lewisburg: Bucknell University Press, 1983).

[19] Tobias Gregory, *From Many Gods to One: Divine Action in Renaissance Epic* (Chicago: University of Chicago Press, 2006), 9. See also Gregory Machacek, *Milton and Homer: "Written to Aftertimes,"* Medieval & Renaissance Literary Studies (Pittsburgh: Duquesne University Press, 2001), 76–81.

[20] See Lewalski, *Milton's Brief Epic,* and, in this volume, notes 53 and 55.

Mosaic distinction does not, however, appear in the plague epic. All who suffer in these plague epics are Christians, and plague is the only clear victor. In fact, poets regularly employ the saying that a Londoner, regardless of his or her particular faith, was more feared in plague-time than any Spaniard, Jew, or pagan.[21] The chosen people in the plague epic appear at times to be their own worst enemies, a plague upon themselves.

How, then, might one depict the plague in an epic for Christian readers? Certainly, the plague appears at the heart of classical epics, plainly available for appropriation. Homer's Greeks in *The Iliad* experience Apollo's anger as a plague, a sign of disapproval they cannot ignore or circumvent.[22] Their decisions regarding how best to appease Apollo, and thereby lift the plague, exacerbate the conflict between Achilles and Agamemnon and set the stage for protracted battle with the Trojans, who would otherwise have had little chance against the Greeks. In the *Aeneid*, Apollo sends a plague to prevent Aeneas from settling in Crete, forcing the hero to move on, eventually founding Rome. Even in *The Metamorphoses*, the jealousy Hera experiences when she learns of yet another of Zeus' dalliances results in a plague on one of his favorite towns. These representations of plague could not be appropriated by seventeenth-century Christian poets without serious adjustment; their readers knew a very different plague, which came to many more people in an array of forms and with far less warning or (satisfying) explanation, and these readers were also raising questions regarding God's involvement.

To account for suffering wrought by this unique adversary, without diminishing the epic quality of their poems or stumbling over how to depict God's role in the action, poets of the century appropriated additional depictions of the plague from another form of classical heroic verse, the didactic.[23] As in martial epic poems,

---

[21]   For instances in plague writing that show Londoners more feared or hated than the historical enemies or groups perceived to threaten Christianity, see in this volume Dekker and Middleton, who write that one "does a Jew or Turk prefer, / Before that name of Londoner" (82); and Taylor, "to be thought a *Londoner* is worse / Than one that breaks a house or takes a Purse"; moreover, "in his house (to harbor) he'll prefer / An Infidel before a *Londoner* (145).

[22]   On early modern conceptions of anger and plague as related to the bodily humor of choler, externalized during the act of cursing, see Rebecca Totaro, "'Revolving This Will Teach Thee How to Curse': Lessons in Sublunary Exhalation," *Rhetorics of Bodily Disease and Health in Medieval and Early Modern England*, ed. Jennifer C. Vaught (Aldershot and Burlington: Ashgate, 2010), 135–51. See also in this volume notes 43 and 56. War and plague were considered symptoms of fiery, overheated humoral and meteorological systems, as Homer had related centuries earlier in *The Iliad*. On the infectious nature of wrath and plague in Homer's epic, see Daniel R. Blickman, "The Role of the Plague in the *Iliad*," *Classical Antiquity* 6.1 (1987): 1–10. See in this volume's poems the many representations of plague as spreading like fire: for example, Dekker and Middleton (76); Austin (232), and Davies (108–9).

[23]   For current discussion regarding genres of epic and didactic verse, see Volk, *The Poetics of Latin Didactic*; Monica Gale, ed., *Latin Epic and Didactic Poetry: Genre, Tradition and Individuality* (Swansea: The Classical Press of Wales, 2004); Monica Gale,

written likewise in dactylic hexameter, didactic poets invoke muses and mention gods, but the plague does not emanate from these gods, nor is it associated with emotion. In the didactic account, the narrator reports the plague as a matter of fact, to be understood as part of life experience and considered in the way that the farmer studies the thundercloud and the positions of the sun and moon. The didactic plague is not associated with individual characters, such as Agamemnon or Apollo, and it is not concerned with the merits of those it smites. In the didactic arena, the plague comes on the air to all people and often to all animals and other forms of life. In *De Rerum Natura*, for example, Lucretius closes his treatment of the natural world with a description of the great plague of Athens, the bringer of dissolution to all matter that ensures that new life may combine out of the newly released atoms.[24] These representations of plague informed the writing of poets and natural philosophers from the period who were eager to teach their readers what they believed were the most compelling truths about the plague they were experiencing.[25]

---

*Lucretius and the Didactic Epic* (London: Bristol Classical Press, 2001); Monica Gale, *Virgil on the Nature of Things: The Georgics, Lucretius and the Didactic Tradition* (Cambridge: Cambridge University Press, 2000); Philip Hardie, *Lucretian Receptions: History, the Sublime, Knowledge* (Cambridge and New York: Cambridge University Press, 2009), especially page 2 and chapters 4, 5, 7, and 8; Peter Toohey, *Epic Lessons and Introduction to Ancient Didactic Poetry* (New York: Routledge, 1996); Alexander Dalzell, *The Criticism of Didactic Poetry: Essays on Lucretius, Virgil, and Ovid* (Toronto: University of Toronto Press, 1996); and M. Owen Lee, *Virgil as Orpheus: A Study of the Georgics* (Albany: State University of New York Press, 1996).

[24] See the end of book six of Lucretius' *De Rerum Natura* (*Lucretius: De Rerum Natura*, tr. W.H.D. Rouse, rev. M.F. Smith, The Loeb Classical Library [Cambridge, Mass. and London, Harvard University Press, 1975], 576–91). See also Virgil's *Georgics,* the end of book three in (*Virgil in Two Volumes: I, Eclogues Georgics Aenied I–VI*, ed. H. Rushton Fairclough, The Loeb Classical Library [Cambridge and London: Harvard University Press, 1942], especially pages 192–95); and see Manilius' *Astronimica,* the end of book one (Manilius, *Astronomica,* trans. G.P. Goold, The Loeb Classical Library [Cambridge and London: Harvard University Press, 1977], especially pages 74–7). According to Ian Green, *De Rerum Natura* was available in English translation by Abraham Fleming as early as 1589. It had been available as early as the 1550s in Latin, common enough to be used for sample passages in Thomas Cooper's Latin-English dictionary of 1565 (*Humanism and Protestantism in Early Modern English Education* [Farnham : Ashgate Publishing Ltd, 2009], 1). Grammar school boys read Virgil's *Georgics* in Latin in their fourth year (Margaret Tudeau-Clayton, *Jonson, Shakespeare and Early Modern Virgil* [Cambridge and New York: Cambridge University Press, 1998], 44).

[25] On the relationship between depictions of the plague in Lucretius' *De Rerum Natura* and in Virgil's *Georgics,* see Gerard Passannante, "The Art of Reading Earthquakes: On Harvey's Wit, Ramus's Method, and the Renaissance of Lucretius," *Renaissance Quarterly* 61 (2008): 820–821; David West, "Two Plagues: Virgil, *Georgics* 3.478–566 and Lucretius 6.1090–1286, in *Creative Imitation and Latin Literature,* ed. David West and Tony Woodman (Cambridge: Cambridge University Press, 1979), 71–88; Richard F. Thomas, "Prose into Poetry: Tradition and Meaning in Virgil's *Georgics,*" in *Oxford Readings in*

When appropriating representations of the plague from classical, didactic verse, seventeenth-century poets altered what they found, suiting it to a Christian paradigm for creation.[26] In this teleological model, the didactic cycle of life in which plague is naturally recurring gives way to something more like path that begins in a sin- and disease-free Eden, leads to a postlapsarian world of hardship, and ends with apocalyptic purification. Whereas in the classical didactic poem the

---

*Vergil's Georgics,* ed. Katharina Volk (Oxford and New York: Oxford University Press, 2008), 65. On the relationship between the depictions of plague in *De Rerum Natura* and in Lucretius' source, Thucydides' description of the plague of Athens within his *History of the Peloponnesian War*, see E. J. Kenney, "Lucretian Texture: Style, Metre and Rhetoric in the *De rerum natura,*" *The Cambridge Companion to Lucretius,* ed. Stuart Gillespie and Philip Hardie (Cambridge and New York: Cambridge University Press, 2007), 108–110. On the interpretation of plague by natural philosophers of the seventeenth century, with special attention to the role of Lucretius' writings in their interpretations, see Jonathan Gil Harris, *Sick Economies: Drama, Mercantilism, and Disease in Shakespeare's England* (Philadelphia: University of Pennsylvania, 2003), 16; and Totaro, *Suffering in Paradise,* 115–16. On the blending of cosmological and national themes in classical didactic verse, see Philip Hardie, "Cosmology and National Epic in the *Georgics* 2.458–3.48," in Volk, 161–81.

[26]   In *Of Education,* John Milton includes the didactic poems of Lucretius, Manilius, and Virgil in his list of required reading for all English students (cited in Kerrigan, Rumrich, and Fallon, 976); see Richard J. DuRocher, who adopts the term "didactic epic" for these works by Lucretius, Manilius, and Virgil, as Milton would have done (*Milton Among the Romans: The Pedagogy and Influence of Milton's Latin Curriculum,* Medieval & Renaissance Literary Studies [Pittsburgh: Duquesne University Press, 2001], 1–34. See also John Dryden's discussion of epics in "Letter to Sir Robert Howard," in the prefatory material to *Annus mirabilis, The year of wonders* (1667), sig. A1r–A8v. Dryden's poem is something of a plague epic, but because it equally takes up war and fire as subjects with the plague, I have chosen not to transliterate it for this volume. The same applies for John Tabor's *Seasonable Thoughts in Sad Times* (1667). On Bede's classification of the epic and the history of this criticism in England, see Lewalski, *Milton's Brief Epic,* 15–16. Guillaume de Salluste Du Bartas' enormously popular *Divine Weeks* (1605)—an hexameral biblical epic translated into English heroic couplets by Joshua Sylvester (1563–1618) and championed by John Milton and King James I and VI—is an important example of a Christianized didactic presentation of plague. Du Bartas takes his readers through the six days of creation and then forward in time to show that although God created a bountiful earth, humans have quickly forgotten to whom they owed thanks and obedience. The latter portion of his hexameral epic is what Marie Loretto Lilly might call a "town georgic," describing a depleted, non-rural, and in many ways post-georgic environment (*The Georgic: A Contribution to the Study of the Vergilian Type of Didactic Poetry* [Baltimore: The Johns Hopkins Press, 1919], 43). In the English translation, as Joshua Scodel notes, Du Bartas' translator, Sylvester, emphasizes the especially poisonous excesses of the city (*Excess and the Mean in Early Modern English Literature* [Princeton: Princeton University Press, 2002], 91). On the role that Du Bartas' works played in the securing interest in Lucretius in this period, see Stuart Gillespie, "Lucretius in the English Renaissance," Gillespie and Hardie, 247–49. See also Anne Lake Prescott, "The Reception of Du Bartas in England," *Studies in the Renaissance* 15 (1968): 144–73.

plague is constitutive of the created world, in the Christian version the plague is a feature only of the postlapsarian version of the created world. Plague had not existed before Adam and Eve fell, and it only came into being with their sin. In the postlapsarian world, the plague is recurs not because it is inherent in nature itself but because it is the result of sin that will accompany humankind until the world's literal end. The plague might then be seen as sewn into the fabric of human life. Furthermore, Protestants generally believed that this plague visited humans by working its way through nature. It was not sent directly from God to humans but seemed to arise out of miasma, travel through the air, or spread person to person by breath—versions of natural transmission similarly representation in the didactic poetry of Lucretius, Virgil, Manilius, and others.

By turning to Lucretius in particular, early moderns reinforced a relatively new turn toward rational accounts of material conditions and causes and away from what they considered the superstitious fictions that claimed magic where none existed. In *The Seeds of Things: Theorizing Sexuality and Materialism in Renaissance Representations*, Jonathan Goldberg calls this turn to Lucretius a "turning to the world" and finds ample evidence of Lucretian materialism in paintings of the period—evidence of a belief that all matter, in all forms large and small, enduring and transient, derives from a common material substance and warrants attention.[27] This Lucretian turn, some have recently argued, would eventually help pave the way for the scientific revolution and for the novel.[28] In the meantime, in their serious, elevated measures, seventeenth-century poets made room for the viewpoint of the material witness, a plague that more closely resembled their own, and a God that was far less involved. Their plague was a metamorphic monster that stalked them in dreams, made their bodies quake (or

---

[27]   Jonathan Goldberg, *The Seeds of Things: Theorizing Sexuality and Materiality in Renaissance Representations* (New York: Fordham University Press, 2009), 7–31. On this Lucretian turn in the writings of Edmund Spenser, Margaret Cavendish, and John Milton, see also his chapters 3–5.

[28]   On the Renaissance appropriation of Lucretius, paving the way toward a new materialism, the scientific revolution, and challenging the concept of tradition itself, see especially Gerard Passannante, *The Lucretian Renaissance: The Philology and the Afterlife of Tradition* (Chicago: University of Chicago Press, 2011); Gerard Passannante, "The Art of Reading Earthquakes," 792–832; and Gerard Passannante, "Homer Atomized: Francis Bacon and the Matter of Tradition," *English Literary History* 76.4 (2009): 1015–1047. See also John Rogers, *The Matter of Revolution: Science, Poetry, and Politics in the Age of Milton* (Ithaca: Cornell University Press, 1998); Anthony Low, "New Science and the Georgic Revolution in Seventeenth Century English Literature," *English Literary Renaissance* 13 (1983): 231–59; Anthony Low, *The Georgic Revolution* (Princeton: Princeton University Press, 1985); and also recently, Stephen Greenblatt, *The Swerve: How the World Became Modern* (New York: W. W. Norton, 2011). On early modern didactic literature in general, see Natasha Glaisyer and Sara Pennell, Introduction to *Didactic Literature in England, 1500-1800: Expertise Constructed*, ed. Glaisyer and Pennell (Aldershot, England; Ashgate, 2003), 4–18.

worse), sent even their kings on the run, and threatened to upturn civilization itself. It demanded correspondingly vast, complex, and close-up treatment. As classical poets had attested to the plague's essential presence in world history, seventeenth-century poets demonstrated why the epic form was still the cage most fit to hold their own century's plague.

### "Grim Death, Hold not my pen": Plague-Time Poets

By writing of the plague in heroic measures, poets in the century distinguished themselves from their peers, contributing to what was considered the most serious and comprehensive of literary forms. Taking the plague as their subject, they distinguished themselves further by the degree of experience, knowledge, attestation of faith, or special insight they provided on the subject. Some of these poets were tradesmen, some remain anonymous but for their single poetic contribution, and others were already or fast becoming well-known poets, dramatists, and pamphlet writers. A short sketch of some of their lives and works delineates many differences among them as well as the degree to which their poems and purposes are of a kind. Given the range of poets who wrote plague epics, the coherence among the poems is all the more striking.

William Muggins wrote one of the first brief plague epics in English, and, as is the case for Richard Milton and Thomas Clark, we would know nothing of certainty about him were it not for his poetry. Some scholars believe he was a weaver, perhaps imprisoned with Thomas Deloney in 1595 for circulating a protest on behalf of the Company of Weavers.[29] What is more certain is that while many Londoners evacuated the city during plague outbreaks, many more, like William Muggins, stayed and became witness to London's transformation. In *London's Mourning Garment* (1603), Muggins takes London's plight to heart, personifying the city as an abandoned mother who speaks to her citizen-children of her grief at their departures and deaths during this visitation. This specific trope of mothers,

---

[29] Scott Oldenburg speculated in *"London's Mourning Garment*: An Epidemiology of Class," a paper delivered as part of the 2006 Renaissance Society of America conference (25 March 2006), that Muggins was a weaver and sometime cellmate of Thomas Deloney—imprisoned for their parts "in a 1595 petition to bring French immigrant weavers into line with guild ordinances. The petition was signed by three weavers who described themselves and the weavers they represented as the 'Yeomanry of the Company of distressed Weavers.'" On Deloney, with special examination of his depiction of women in his own writings, see Mihoko Suzuki, *Subordinate Subjects: Gender, the Political Nation, and Literary Form, 1588-1688, Women and Gender in the Early Modern World* (Aldershot and Burlington: Ashgate, 2003), 27–74. On Muggins, see also Patricia Phillippy's chapter "London's Mourning Garment: Maternity, Mourning and Succession in Shakespeare's *Richard III*," in *Women, Death, and Literature in Post-Reformation England* (Cambridge and New York: Cambridge University Press, 2002), 109–138; and Totaro, "Mother London and the *Madonna Lactans* in England's Plague Epic," in *Medieval and Renaissance Lactations— Images, Rhetorics, and Practices,* ed. Jutta Sperling (forthcoming from Ashgate).

fathers, and infants separated from one another appears in plague writing that dates to at least as early as Lucretius' account of the plague in Athens, and here it is all the more compelling when delivered in London's voice and, later in the poem, in the voices of London mothers who step forward to tell their own stories.[30] Initially, London describes herself as all but fully human, suffering the slings and arrows of outrageous fortune that result in overt, physiological signs of grief:

> With heavy heart and sighs of inward Cares,
> With wringing hands, explaining sorrow's woe,
> With blubbered cheeks, bedewed with trickling tears,
> With mind opprest, lamenting griefs that flow—
> London, lament, and all thy losses show. (54)

"Opprest" with "griefs" that affect her mind and body, London wrings her hands and cries out alone in a lament that, she will show, is the product of child loss. Muggins has given his London a voice, heart, lungs, hands, cheeks, and copious tears. She is London and a London mother; she is also his *alma mater*. In the next lines, he then adds epic content to this scene of maternal loss, as London challenges her own claim that she might "*all* thy losses show" (my emphasis): "What all? Nay, some. All were too much to tell; / The learned Homer could not pen it well" (54). At once, London plays the part of poet, muse, and Christian hero. She is the grieving every-mother who recalls the details of birth and nursing, *and* she keeps the company of Homer, Agamemnon, Jupiter, Caesar, Venus, Icarus, and King David. By the end, mother London also recasts her didactic role, moving from teacher of London's mothers to teacher of London's civic leaders, instructing them in the art of compassionate governance that will ensure their mutual return to glory.

Writing from outside of London, and in many ways from the opposite side of the proverbial track, John Davies of Hereford, author of *The Triumph of Death* (1609), trained at Oxford where he became a writing master with an unquestionable reputation. As P.J. Finkelpearl explains, "Thomas Fuller in his *Worthies of England* called Davies 'the greatest master of the pen that England in her age beheld' (Fuller, *Worthies*, 2.79), and his renown reached as far as Germany according to a commendatory poem in Davies's *Microcosmos*."[31] He taught at Magdalen College at Oxford, tutoring the elite and moving within circles that included John Donne, William Shakespeare, Inigo Jones, Lady Mary Wroth and many of England's most prominent families. Among his students, for example, was Elizabeth Cary (1585–1639), the first woman to write a full-length play (*The Tragedy of Miriam* [1613])

---

[30]    From Lucretius: "Sometimes you might see the lifeless bodies of parents lying upon their lifeless children, and contrariwise children yielding up their life upon the bodies of mother and father" (Lucretius, *De Rerum Natura*, in Rouse, 587).

[31]    P.J. Finkelpearl, 'Davies, John (1564/5–1618)', *Oxford Dictionary of National Biography*, Oxford University Press, 2004 [http://www.oxforddnb.com/view/article/7244, accessed 13 March 2010].

and a political history in English (*The History of the Life, Reign and Death of Edward II* [published in 1680]). Davies is also familiar to those who now believe that he, and not Shakespeare, wrote "A Lover's Complaint."[32]

Davies wanted to be a great poet, and in the years leading up to his writing of *The Triumph of Death,* he wrote many poems in high style, with lengthy dedications, heroic prosody, invocations, and ponderous marginal reference notes. None of these poems gained him the notoriety he sought, but he persisted and found perhaps his greatest success with his didactic epic mentioned above, the full title of which is *Microcosmos, The discovery of the little world* (1603). In this poem, which was published several times through 1631, Davies begins by invocation and sings of England's fortunes and failures, all delivered in heroic quatrains. In *The Triumph of Death,* he uses the very same heroic elements and prosody to offer a close-up of such failures, showing plague as a hungry tyrant who justly brings prideful London to her knees, such that, in the height of the catastrophe, "The *London* Lanes (themselves thereby to save) / Did vomit out their undigested dead, / Who by cartloads are carried to the Grave, / For all those Lanes with folk were overfed" (101). London is sick on her own inhabitants, made violently ill by their swarming prosperity. In the ensuing narrative, family members betray or otherwise abandon each other in death, and it appears that God's wrath will lead to utter destruction of the nation. Davies also likens London to Troy with the name "Troynovant" (112), employs epic similes, and uniquely supplies the personified antagonist, Death, with a lengthy monologue recommending a number of unappealing methods for spreading the plague more quickly: among them, "Beblaine the bosom of each Mistress / That bares her Breasts (lust's signs) guests to allure; / With a plague, kiss her (that plagues with a kiss)" (97). Davies also uses marginalia heavily to cite biblical passages; call attention to epic similes on autumn leaves and ships at sea (each marked "similitude" [109]); and offer the occasional plague fact. In the margin beside a reference to plague as "like a Jerffe" (103), for example, he explains that the exotic Jerffe (giraffe) is "A Beast never but feeding, and when he hath eaten as much as his paunch hold, goes to a forked tree, and there strains out his food undigested between the twist of the tree, and so again presently falls to feed, and being full, again to the tree, and so eftsoons to feed" (103n33). Now known to be a ruminant animal (thus accounting in part for Davies' depiction), the giraffe was only just becoming the kind of beast one might hear about in a tall tale of travel or see in a royal menagerie. Its penchant for eating here represents the strangely bulimic behavior of an ever gorging and purging, ever-hungry, plague. In another marginal note, Davies offers an early modern medical aphorism: "If the botch break not the Patient liveth not. It kills others with breaking" (107). This note highlights the belief that the plague acted like a poison that the body was

---

[32]   For more on Davies and his work, see Finkelpearl and Brian Vickers, *Shakespeare, 'A Lover's Complaint', and John Davies of Hereford* (Cambridge and New York: Cambridge University Press, 2007).

trying desperately to expel by the pushing out of buboes.[33] Lancing and draining of buboes ("botch"es) was thought to help the process along, but the treatment itself could expose the victim to another lethal threat, recovering from plague only to die from an infected wound; thus, the saying makes plain the danger in either case. Even when Davies cites the Bible, his choices are memorable, as in his associating the oft-repeated observation that many in flight out of London die on the highways, with a marginal note citing Lamentations 4.5: "They that feed delicately perish in the streets; they that were brought up in scarlet, embrace the dung" (107n42). These are some of the many reasons to return to the writings of Davies.

The plague epic of Thomas Clark is equally engaging for many different reasons, among them that Clark's personal experience with the plague is enormously compelling. The only record we have of Clark is the poem in this volume, but its title alone offers more of a record of the man than the full poems do for other poets: *Meditations in my confinement, when my house was visited with the sickness: in April, May and June, 1666. In which time I buried two children, and had three more of my family sick* (1666). This is a rare account; few if any people other than Clark were quarantined, witnessed the deaths of their children, and then were able and willing to write about it, let alone in heroic couplets. No other account like this exists in print, and perhaps it is the title of the poem that has prevented scholars from considering Clark's intention to contribute formally to a body of heroic literature. In dedicatory verses to his "much Honored Friends, whose kindness and Affection hast been Expressed to me in my late Affliction," Clark explains his serious, scripted purpose:

> *Give ear* (my courteous friends) *and lend your vote,*
> *To this my doleful and* Swan-like *note;*
> *Though not so sweet (as that is said), more true,*
> *Which causeth me my cheeks with tears bedew:*
> That, *is a* Poet's fiction *of the* Swan;
> This, *sobs and groans of an* afflicted man,
> *One that with sorrows* God *doth* castigate,
> *That he may fit him for a better state.*
> *Expect not now in these lines* Melody,
> *Nor shall I promise any* Harmony.
> *Where grief predominates, it is a rein,*
> *To check the* Fancy *and* Invention's *strain.*
> *This* Piece *at best is rough and impolite,*
> *Not burnish'd o're with* art *to make it bright* (258)

By calling attention to the poem as song, Clark places his poem among other epics, which "claim at the outset," as Alison Higgins explains for Carolinian heroic

---

[33] On the belief that plague acted as a poison, see Totaro, "Chicken Soup (and Orange Juice) for the Plague-Time Soul?: Francis Bacon's Utopian Prescription." *English Language Notes* 47.2 (Fall/Winter 2009): 25–33. On the Medici giraffe, for example, see Belozerskaya, Marina. *The Medici Giraffe*. New York: Little, Brown, and Company, 2006.

verse, "that the subject of the poem shall be 'sung.'"[34] Distinguishing himself from the other epic poets of the century, however, Clark claims that his song will not contain *"Melody"* or *"Harmony,"* because it is composed of *"sobs and groans of an* afflicted man." His epic will be *"at best . . . rough and impolite."*

This representation of his own work is inaccurate, of course; so much of his content, and his heroic measures themselves, testify to a poetic polishing of experience to "make it bright." Hardly the product of anguish alone, Clark's representation of the plague here, for example, reinforces the place of his song among epics:

> This Sickness also, after Death, doth seem
> To trample o're the dead with disesteem,
> And (Victor-like, o're Captives) with despite,
> Denies such Obsequies and fun'ral rite,
> Which in a solemn manner is most due,
> As we have seen in this late time, not few. (262–3)

The plague's denial of funeral rites for the dead recalls the many famous classical episodes in which heroes and the sons of kings are refused burial by the enemy— the most egregious, final, and enduring form of military aggression, an act that makes clear there will be no mercy, forgetting, or forgiveness. The plague is this ruthless enemy of epic scale. This is also the enemy that challenged Clark physically, spiritually, and emotionally as an individual, forcing him to rethink roles as father, husband, friend, and citizen. In *Meditations in my Confinement,* Clark inscribes his own account into English and world history while anchoring the epic in the specific, private trauma experienced within his home.[35]

Unlike Clark, Abraham Holland was a noted poet by the time his plague epic, *A Description of the Great, Fearful, and Prodigious Plague, 1625* (1626), was published. He was the son of Philemon Holland (1552–1637), who had translated into English the essential Galenic medical distillation, *Regimen sanitatis Salerni,* as well as Pliny's *The History of the World* and the works of Livy—the *Regimen* and Pliny being especially important texts for natural philosophers and physicians of the time.[36] Abraham Holland might have seen his reputation flourish had he outlived his father, or at least survived the plague. He died in the year his plague epic was published. His brother Henry, a publisher, paid to bring Abraham's poem

---

[34]     Alison I. T. Higgins, *Secular Heroic Epic Poetry of the Caroline Period,* Schweizer Anglistische Arbeiten 31. (Bern: A. Francke, 1953), 13.

[35]     In his treatment of his own house as the space of suffering, Clark adds to the many accounts of the home turned pest-house in the period; see especially Barbara Traister, "'A plague on both your houses': Sites of Comfort and Terror in Early Modern Drama" in Totaro and Gilman 169–82.

[36]     Abraham Holland, *Regimen sanitatis Salerni* (1617); *The history of the world* (1601). On Philemon Holland's reputation in his lifetime, see William Winstanley, *The lives of the most famous English poets* (1687), 146–7.

to press as part of *Hollandi post-huma,* the posthumous works that include "The author's epitaph, made by himself." Reprinted by Henry during the next two London plague visitations of 1630 and 1636, Abraham's *A Description* was retitled *London look-back: a description or representation of the great and memorable mortality.* Part of its appeal, according to the new full title, derives from its "*heroic matchless lines.*" In these later editions, Henry combined his brother's poem with medical prescriptions translated from French sources by physician Thomas Phayer and a set of meditative exercises written by the now unidentified "I.D. Preacher of God's Word." In this combination of texts, Henry offers a compendium intended as suitable recreation to assuage fears and thereby improve health through the creation of mirth. Abraham Holland's *A Description* (later, *London look-back*) functions in this way itself, offering a variety of literary diversions for the reader, including a digression on the "age of gold" that was "happy" because free of disease (162); a catalog of animals and their plague-time behaviors (166–7); and epic similes on the court, war, falling autumn leaves, and the plague in *The Iliad* (157, 159, 162, 165).

In the last of England's plague epics on record, Christopher Pitt (1699–1748) articulates many of the concerns expressed in previous plague epics, despite the fact he could not have witnessed firsthand an English plague visitation. Pitt's father, also named Christopher (1662–1723), was a physician who may have introduced his son to accounts of plague recalled from his own childhood or from medical regimens of the day, most of which included a chapter on plague prevention. He may also have aided Thomas Creech in the translation of Lucretius' account of the plague in *De Rerum Natura* (*T. Lucretius Carus the Epicurean philosopher, his six books De natura rerum done into English verse, with notes,* 1682). The younger Pitt certainly encountered the plague in literature, while a student at Oxford. An early university exercise resulted in his translation of all of Lucan's *Pharsalia,* and after he had completed *The Plague of Marseilles* (1721), he translated the works of Virgil, including the *Aeneid* in heroic couplets (1740), which was received with great acclaim and often compared to Dryden's translation of 1697.[37]

---

[37]    On Pitt and his father, see Anna Chahoud, "Pitt, Christopher (1699–1748)," *Oxford Dictionary of National Biography*, Oxford University Press, 2004 [http://www.oxforddnb. com/view/article/22327, accessed 24 Feb 2011; and Theophilus Cibber, *The Lives of the Poets of Great Britain and Ireland* (1753) Volume V. Interest in epics and medicine seemed to run in the family: brother Robert Pitt (1693–1730) was a physician who translated part of *Paradise Lost* into Latin and wrote five medical tracts on illness, among them *The craft and frauds of physic expos'd.* (1703; first printed in 1702 with a shorter title). On other contributions from the Pitt brothers, see William Bridges Hodges, *A Milton Encyclopedia*, vol. 8. (New York: Associated University Presses, 1979), 79; and John T. Shawcross, *John Milton: The Critical Heritage Volume 2 1732-1801* (New York: Routledge, 1995), 5. On Pitt's *Aenied,* see the original complete text in Joseph Warton, ed., *The Works of Virgil in Latin and English,* (1753), and see Mark Thackeray, "Christopher Pitt, Joseph Warton, and Virgil," *The Review of English Studies* 43.171 (1992): 329–46. For the English translation of Lucan's *Pharsalia* available at the time, see *Lucan's Pharsalia: containing the civil wars between Cæsar and Pompey. Written in Latin heroical verse by M. Annæus Lucanus. Translated into English verse by Sir Arthur Gorges Knight* (1614).

The last great plague in England's history had struck in 1666, more than three decades prior to Pitt's birth, but Pitt was surely reading more than epic literature when reports of plague began to come to the island from France in 1720. He seized the opportunity to place into circulation an epic of his own, on what many feared would be the worst large-scale visitation yet. In Pitt's heroic measures, Marseilles is the "Queen of Nations fall'n from high" (279) due to that "Insatiate Tyrant" plague, "whose unbounded Will, / [is] Not yet contented with the Pow'r to kill" (279). Pitt's narrator endures verbalized struggle to give words to the horror he witnesses, including the murder of whole families who embrace as they die. Early on in the poem, then, it is clear that Pitt has taken upon himself the mantle of the plague-time poet, expressing full astonishment and rage at what he reports. In addition, although the poem is about the plague in Marseilles, France, as the poem closes, the plague approaches England's shores, and Pitt's narrator acts in desperation to call for aid:

> Genius of *Britain*, with Indulgence hear,
> The sighs of *Albion* and the Poet's Prayer:
> Exert thy utmost tutelary care,
> To curb this purple Tyrant's lawless Pow'r.
> Stretch thy auspicious Wings from Shore to Shore.
> To guard her Natives from the dire Disease,
> Oppose the watery Bulwark of her Seas.
> Screen all her Kingdoms from the fierce Attack.
> Bid the kind Tempests blow her Poisons back.
> Bid the devouring Plague this Island spare,
> Nor stretch her Circle of Destruction here.
> Or if thy delegated Pow'r is gone,
> Fall low before Heav'n's everlasting Throne,
> And make the Cause of *Britain's* Realm thy own.
> To stay the Vengeance of thy God, appear
> Armed with the sacred Violence of Pray'r.
> Present the Incense of thy Britain's Vows.
> Weigh down eternal Justice with her Woes,
> Till her Repentance wrests away the Rod,
> And sheath the Sword of an offended God. (282)

Pitt implores Britain's animating spirit to take action against the plague and to protect the island: to "exert," "curb," "stretch," "guard," "oppose," and "screen." Then he requests that Britain strike an equally active, militarized pose that is nevertheless a prayerful one: "To stay the vengeance of thy God, appear / armed with sacred violence of prayer." The Genius of Britain is invoked not as a muse but as the generalized heroic spirit of the British people—a figure we might misread by associating it with an eighteenth-century detachment made possible only after decades of plague-free living, were it not for the tyrant plague that throughout the poem has menaced France and is poised to destroy Britain. Joining his seventeenth-century predecessors, Pitt also puts into motion the tension between faith and doubt, explicitly rendered as a monster disease that is both part of God's plan of "Vengeance" and, more disturbingly, the result of "this purple Tyrant's *lawless* Pow'r" (emphasis mine).

The poets writing England's plague epics were clearly not of a kind by class, education, profession, political position, or religious persuasion. In their poems, they speak distinctively with voices marked by unique sets of local circumstances. What they share is the plague, a unique subject for appropriation which cut across most lines of demarcation and entirely frustrated definition. They also share a compulsion to capture the rage, grief, exasperation, doubt, faith, and hope of their moment—all in heroic verse. The result is a body of literature that uniquely expresses what no other artistic, literary, or cultural form could at the time. These epics are the nation's monuments and elegies to the Protestant plague-time dead.[38] They are the collective burial stones for those nameless, faceless scores in the plague pits. And they are a call to action, to do whatever it takes to return England to glory after so very many brutal defeats.

---

[38]  For a discussion of the vexed issue of funerary monument building in post-Reformation England, see especially chapter four in Peter Sherlock's illuminating study, *Monuments and Memory in Early Modern England* (Aldershot and Burlington: Ashgate, 2008); and Nigel Llewellyn, *Funeral Monuments in Post-Reformation England* (Cambridge and New York: Cambridge University Press, 2000), chapter four. See also Wither's position on the subject in this volume (220–23**).** Although elegies for those who died of smallpox were popular in the period, no set of plague elegies exists—the poems here are the closest equivalent. On the seventeenth-century smallpox elegy and the art of memory, see especially chapter three of David E. Shuttleton's *Smallpox and the Literary Imagination, 1660-1820* (Cambridge and New York: Cambridge University Press, 2007), and chapter five of Anselment's *The Realms of Apollo.* On elegies, memorials, and grief management in the period, see Peter Marshall, *Beliefs and the Dead in Reformation England* (New York and Oxford: Oxford University Press, 2002); Jeffrey A. Hammond, *The American Puritan Elegy,* Cambridge Studies in American Literature and Culture (Cambridge and New York: Cambridge University Press, 2000); Jameela Lares, *Milton and the Preaching Arts*, Medieval & Renaissance Literary Studies Series (Pittsburgh: Duquesne University Press, 2001), 80–90, 147–50; P.G. Stanwood, "Consolatory Grief in the Funeral Sermons of Donne and Taylor," *Speaking Grief in English Literary Culture: Shakespeare to Milton,* ed. Margo Swiss and David A. Kent, Medieval & Renaissance Literary Studies (Pittsburgh: Duquesne University Press, 2002), 197–216; G.W. Pigman III, *Grief and English Renaissance Elegy* (Cambridge and New York: Cambridge University Press, 1985); Ralph Houlebrook, *Death, Religion, and the Family in England, 1480–1750,* Oxford Studies in Social History (Oxford and New York: Oxford University Press, 1998), 220–254; W. Scott Howard, "'Mine Own Breaking': Resistance, Gender, and Temporality in Seventeenth-Century English Elegies and Jonson's 'Eupheme,'" in *Grief and Gender, 700-1700,* ed. Jennifer C. Vaught and Lynne Dickson Bruckner (New York: Palgrave Macmillan Ltd., 2003), 215–30.

### "Fair *London* that did late abound in bliss": London's Metamorphosis

In a quest for bodies to consume, the ever-hungry plague always seemed to begin with London. There it would feed unchecked, and once it had run its course through that population, it could expand its assault into the country. In Lawrence Manley's words, London was "the center of a complex network of changing relationships" due in large part to the printing press, and the plague made use of the very same routes for communication and trade that had allowed London to flourish (*Literature and Culture,* 2). In other words, London was the epicenter of plague and of print, and, as such, it figured as an essential setting in all early modern plague literature in England. After years of unremitting plague, for example, John Davies of Hereford chooses London as the setting for his plague epic and lays the blame for England's illness at London's feet:

> At *London* (sink of Sin) as at the Fount,
> This all-confounding Pestilence began,
> According to that Plague's most woeful wont,
> From whence it (flowing) all the realm o'reran (100)

It is an internal condition of sin in London that leads to the plague "flowing" over the entire realm. Given that the *Oxford English Dictionary* records "sink" in this period as meaning a cesspool pit, the metaphor turns the nation into an ill attended sewer system that spreads rather than clears away corruption, infecting itself from within.[39] This thinking about contagion also suited the dominant humoral theory that, as Margaret Healy has noted, led most people to imagine that England's own condition of internal imbalance was to blame for visitations, rather than foreigners from the Continent, for example (*Fictions of Disease,* 122). A number of the writers of plague epics blame London in similarly strong terms, but we might in part account for Davies' particularly vehement tone by considering that, as a Hereford man, he could not quite claim London as his *alma mater* in the way that other poets could and proudly did.

Among the majority of London poets who describe the capital's Ovidian metamorphosis in more empathetic terms is John Taylor the Water Poet.[40] In *The Fearful Summer* (1625), he assesses London's current woes by comparing them to her former glory: "Fair *London* that did late abound in bliss, / And wast our Kingdom's great *Metropolis*" has become "dejected, low in state, / Disconsolate, and almost desolate" (144–5). Once, his personified "Fair London" had been,

---

[39]   OED *s.v.* sink, noun, AI.1. As Ernest B. Gilman explains, some writers acknowledged the relationship between the press and the plague by representing the press as an agent of the disease, spring sinful ideas that in turn brought plague to bodies and the nation ("Afterword: Plague and Metaphor" in Totaro and Gilman, 221–223, 230–231).

[40]   On John Taylor, the Water Poet, see Bernard Capp, 'Taylor, John (1578–1653)', *Oxford Dictionary of National Biography*, Oxford University Press, 2004 [http://www.oxforddnb.com/view/article/27044, accessed 13 March 2010].

> . . . the Queen of Cities nam'd,
> Throughout the world admir'd, renown'd, and fam'd;
> Thou that hadst all things at command and will,
> To whom all *England* was a Handmaid still.
> For raiment, fuel, fish, fowl, beasts, for food,
> For fruits, for all our Kingdom counted good.
> Both near and far remote, all did agree
> To bring their best of blessings unto *thee*.
> Thus in conceit thou seem'dst to rule the *Fates*,
> Whilst *peace* and *plenty* flourish'd in thy Gates. (145)

As mentioned above, Taylor was a waterman, earning his living as a product of London's prosperity, and this placed him in a credible position to assess the city's condition before, during, and after the plague. London's positive reputation prior to the visitation was proclaimed widely, he asserts. All materials and blessings for the island passed through London. Yet, she only "seem'dst to rule the *Fates*," because, of course, Taylor is writing about the fearful summer of her terrible transformation. As Taylor and others announce in some despair, Fortune's wheel has spun London, "Queen of Cities," down from on high, making her case all the more pitiable.

Although earlier in the poem Taylor cites London's "pride of Heart and deeds unjust" as reason for God "justly" correcting her (145), he is short in such statements and long in his expression of concern for London's wellbeing. It seems to pain him to see London in her dejected state, and he speaks to her in lines that seek to provide her with comfort:

> Could I relieve thy miseries as well
> As part I can thy woes and sorrows tell,
> Then should my Cares be eas'd with thy Relief,
> And all my study, how to end thy grief. (145)

London becomes Taylor's "thy" for whom he respectfully, devotedly wishes relief. He wants to help her in her affliction, wishing he could tell at least a part of her story and thereby lighten her burdens, her heavy "woes and sorrows." Moreover, if he could help her, then his own burden would be "eas'd." Poetically, this is a moving image: poet and London/beloved, hero and damsel in distress. Her rescue is his. From a material perspective this image is apt as well, because London had given Taylor his livelihood. But he can only tell those woes and sorrows in "part." Her burden is so great he cannot even articulate her sorrows fully, let alone relieve her of them.

In 1603, William Muggins had already gone more than one step further, with his full personification of London, who performs Muggins' song in first person. Beginning with a retrospective look at herself during what had only recently been the very height of her fortune, London cries out,

> Ay me poor London, which of late did flourish,
> With springing MARCH, the tidings of a King,

And APRIL showers, my blossoms so did nourish,
That I in MAY was called a famous thing.
Yea, Towns and Cities did my glory ring.
Nay, through the world my golden fame so grew
That Princes high crost Seas, my seat to view.
    And like to AGAMEMNON'S gallant train,
Throughout my streets, with stately steps did go,
Where them with welcomes, I did entertain,
Pleasing their liking, with each several show,
Where they in me, much treasure did bestow,
Honoring the Church with Prayers, the Change with gold,
Where Princes bought, and beauteous Virgins sold. (54)

London relishes her former, "golden fame" that "through the world" made her the desired destination of the princes of all nations. But she does so by opening with "Ay me poor London," because this glory has been entirely compromised. Like Taylor and others, Muggins takes readers from London's fall to her remembered glory, then through the fall again before lingering in the horrors of metamorphosis. Here, in recounting the conditions of the fall, Muggins shows a plague that is disquietingly invasive, as London explains, recounting something of a flashback:

But oh, a sudden qualm doth cross my heart.
Twixt cup and lip are dangers oft we see.
Unwelcome death approacheth with his dart,
Yelping, "Oh, LONDON, thou must yield to me.
I must have roots and branches for my fee.
The fruits full ripe and blossoms that might grow
Are mine, not thine; the Fates decreed it so." (55)

Muggins has London recall the words of "Unwelcome death," who comes to her not only "with his dart" but also as a male tyrant demanding that she "yield" to him because the "Fates decree'd it so." This is a scene of tragic *peripeteia*, bringing about London's reversal of fortune, and all without clear cause.[41] God does not appear in these lines as the prime or otherwise justified mover of events. Moreover, although Muggins makes London's Christian faith apparent elsewhere in the poem, here she is on her own, subject to an alteration of state so profound that little can account for it.

In an effort to assess London's metamorphosis in 1625, Richard Milton likens England's capital to her sister cities in world history:

. . . let us call to mind
What mighty City we in writings find,
That heretofore for glory bare the bell,

---

[41] On Aristotelian elements of tragedy embedded in the early modern epic, see John M. Steadman, *Epic and Tragic Structure in Paradise Lost* (Chicago: University of Chicago Press, 1976).

> And through the world did far and near excel
> The Famous *Nineveh, Jerusalem,*
> *Troy, Carthage, Rome,* and many more with them,
> Which for their sins were wholly overthrown,
> Their standing places hardly to be known. (140)

Blending Christian and classical history, Milton places London in the grandest of company. In fact, her "glory . . . did far and near excel" them, these most "Famous" of sister cities of the world. But so too, he cautions, were these sister cites "wholly overthrown." If London persists on course, she will become like them in their fatal errors, "their standing places hardly to be known," their glories remembered only through literary memorials—like the one Milton imagines he is writing.

For John Taylor, London's overthrow is graphically rendered, occurring viscerally around him: "grieved London, fill'd with moans and groans," he explains, "Is like a *Golgotha* of dead men's bones" (150). London has become "the field where death his bloody fray doth fight / And kills eight hundred in a day and night" (151). Taylor had been the one earlier to remind his readers that "Fair London" it was that "did late abound in bliss" (144). She is nothing like that later in his poem, reduced to a place of bones—Golgotha, one massive plague pit, one *danse macabre*, one "field" of unidentified, unburied corpses, just as they appeared in the plague bills. As Michael Neill explains in his magisterial study, *Issues of Death: Mortality and Identity in English Renaissance Tragedy*, "The death most to be feared ... is the mass death because of its extravagant multiplication of disfigured bodies"—all of these bodies without faces or names. [42]

### "Too much Matter for my Muse to form": Seeking Inspiration

These epic poets give voice to the psychophysiological burden that it is to witness the suffering that comes with a plague visitation. In the first line of his poem, for example, William Muggins explains that London herself is weighed down "With heavy heart and sighs of inward Cares"— a weightiness reinforced by the use of anaphora to describe her "with heavy heart," "with wringing hands," "with blubbered cheeks," and "with mind opprest" (54). This is the kind of emotion that in a Galenic paradigm must be purged, or it will only make the body more susceptible to illness. [43] In lines soon after, London comes forth to ask for help in

---

[42]   Michael Neill, *Issues of Death: Mortality and Identity in English Renaissance Tragedy* (New York: Oxford University Press, 1997), 15.

[43]   On humoralism and its psychophysiological basis, see as a starting place, Gail Kern Paster, *Humoring the Body: Emotions and the Shakespearean Stage* (Chicago: University of Chicago Press, 2004). On the glutted body, unpurged and pestilent, see Healy, chapter 6. On the belief in the health value of disgorging harmful bodily heat through speech, see Totaro, "'Revolving this will teach thee how to curse"; and Stephen Pender, "Rhetoric, Grief, and the Imagination in Early Modern England, *Philosophy and Rhetorica* 43.1 (2000): 54–81—

the discharging of her grief, asking her "children," Londoners, to join her. She gets no response and then implores those children, who are also the readers of Muggins' poem,

> Is there none, then, that will take London's part
> And help to sing a welcome unto woe?
> Is there none found that feels a present smart?
> Nor none alive that can cause Tears to flow?
> If any be, then freely them bestow.
> Two mourn together, 'suage each other's grief.
> Weep on a while, and I will be the chief. (56)

London takes the lead role in seeking a means to "'swage" grief, employing the word in both of its early modern senses: to relieve emotional and bodily suffering.[44] She then calls forward some of her citizens, those mothers who also lost children, to do the same for her. In this way, Muggins doubles the call for increased empathy during times when pain is at once too potent to express or to keep to oneself.

In the tradition of seeking aid to tell the ineffable tale in order to unburden the heart that otherwise will break, invoking a muse makes sense. It provides another way to support oneself in the difficult but crucial disgorging of horror. In *London's Misery* (1625), Richard Milton begins to recount the spectacle of London's change, but he stops short, exclaiming, "My flesh do tremble .../ My hand do quake and eke my joints do shiver." Unable to go on alone, he turns to a muse for aid:

> Go on my muse now, and right sadly tell,
> The doleful sound that every Parish bell
> Within this poor afflicted City make
> That we may from our sinful lives awake.
> Our daily sorrows and continual fears
> Our loss of dear friends and our daily tears
> That we for them do shed the sundry moans,
> Deep hearted sighings and the grievous groans,
> That many a husband for his tender wife
> Sends forth for her that is bereav'd of life. (120)

---

both referring to the practice of vociferation discussed by Sir Thomas Elyot, (*The castle of health* [1539], sig. 52v). See also Thomas Cogan, *The haven of health* (1584), 1. See also notes 22 and 56 in this volume.

[44]    Like Muggins, Thomas Brewer—author of one of the shortest of brief plague epics, *The Weeping Lady* (1625)—has London explain for herself the horrors of her plague-time condition. As Brewer explains in the verse preface, "Nor if I Had such a Will, had I the power to speak / My Grief; for Hers (too strong) makes me too weak" and "what's in Sorrows breast, / The Bearer of it, can decipher best" (sig. A1v). Like John Taylor, Brewer claims that London's grief has increased his own to such a degree that he is too weak to sustain the burden of the telling. See also Brewer's verse dialogue, *A dialogue betwixt a citizen, and a poor country-man and his wife, in the country, where the citizen remaineth now in this time of sickness* (1636).

Without the muse to aid in the song, it seems the narrator would have no voice or ability to write, his fear and trembling increasingly enlarged by the unremitting "sorrows," "fears," "tears," "moans," "sighings," and "groans," augmented by the relentless reckoning of "how many ... how many" (120) mothers, brothers, sisters, and fathers grieve as they lose each other. In this horror, a muse gives voice for and, thereby, relief to the poet. As Philip Edward Phillips explains, in a way that is all the more apt in plague-time, "Indeed, the Muse *is* the beginning" (8), because the muse can offer a start to a story in which the beginning is either less than certain (as in pinpointing the origins of this horrifying, enigmatic disease) or too painful to initiate (the teller suffering so). The story itself may start *in media res* or in an emotional mire, but the invoking of the muse begins the poet's heroic quest for meaning.

In the plague epic, however, this heroic quest becomes as much of a struggle for the muse as for the poet. Like Muggins' London, these muses suffer along with their trembling poets and require an equal amount of consolatory empathy if they can hope to move forward at all. In *News from Graves-end* (1604), dramatists Thomas Dekker and John Middleton offer an extended example of the struggles faced by muse and poet alike. They begin by invoking *"Physic"* as their muse:

> Thou nearest to a God (for none
> Can work it (but a God alone),
> O grave *Enchantress*, deign to breath
> Thy Spells into us and bequeath
> Thy sacred fires, that they may shine
> In quick and virtual medicine.
> Arm us to convince this Foe,
> This King of dead men, conquering so,
> This hungry Plague, Cater to death,
> Who eats up all, yet famisheth.
> Teach us how we may repair
> These Ruins of the rotten Air (72)

Invoking one "nearest to a God," whose breath might help teach readers how to "repair / These Ruins of the rotten air," the authors suggest that the poem itself will be "crown[ed]" with "sovereign cures." This is an epic hope indeed—the very largest Apollonian wish plague-time poets might construct, that their very verse might be infused with Physic's healing properties. If any poetic form might seem to have that potential, it would be the heroic, and if any muse might successfully teach repair in plague-time, Physic seems a particularly apt choice.

The burden, however, is soon overwhelming for Physic, who sees "Th'infection flying above [her] art" and "whose numb'd sprite" the playwright-poets tell us, "Now quakes, and nothing dare or can" (73). In a scholarly introduction to Dekker and Middleton's poem, Robert Maslen explains that after Physic is exhausted, "the poem effectively begins again" with the muse of Tragedy. [45] Perhaps she—"thou

---

[45]   R.W. Maslen, Introduction to *News from Gravesend: Sent to Nobody* (London, 1603), in Taylor and Lavagnino, 130.

the best of Nine" (73)—can perform well in the absence of Physic, guiding the poet and reader through the horrors that cannot be remedied. Yet, even Tragedy cannot entirely avoid being compromised, and soon Dekker and Middleton find they have a "panting Muse" on their hands. They decide to give her leave to "take breath" (78) with a retrospective digression on the welcome arrival into London of England's new king, James I of Scotland. This breathing room buys time for Tragedy, and for the reader, to prepare for what will come next in the section labeled "The Horror of the Plague" (79). There, and with some exasperation, the poets exclaim,

> O Thou, my Country:
> . . . . . . . . . . . . . . . . .
> O Dearest! say, how can we choose
> But have a sad and drooping Muse,
> When Corpses do so choke thy way
> That now thou lookst like Golgotha. (79–80)

The image is powerful, with corpses choking the nation so that the muse is "sad and drooping," unable to sing, as if she herself were choked as well, perhaps with tears of empathy or at least with exhaustion. What recourse then is left if one's strongest ally—one's immortal champion, the muse who serves well in other ventures of the tragic and epic form—is bested? This is a question addressed by nearly all who attempt to invoke a muse in plague-time. Like the women who step forward to aid Muggins' London, these muses cannot do much more than be companion witnesses, and their struggle highlights the hardships faced by those poets who remain in London. Attesting to atrocities, these poets tremble and sputter. Desperately seeking relief from what threatens to silence them, the poets invoke the muse—the aid for all high poetic inspiration—only to find that the proximity to suffering necessary to sing of plague is exactly what makes the song all but impossible. The muse for a plague-time poet in London cannot fly far enough above the plague for comfortable objectivity without compromising the details of the account. Yet by flying close enough to view the scene, these muses risk an alteration evident in their trembling, choking, and growing hoarse. It is as if they begin to grow bodies, or at least throats, that are subject to the plague as mortal bodies are.

With Apollo's lyre seemingly at rest in the plague epic, poets experimented with alternative sources of inspirational support. In *The Triumph of Death* (1609), John Davies powerfully justifies the invocation of another kind of muse:

> A shiv'ring cold (I sensibly do feel)
> Glides through my veins and shakes my heart and hand
> When they do prove their virtue to reveal
> This plague of plagues that overlays this Land!
> Horror stands gaping to devour my Sense
> When it but offers but to mention it.
> And Will, abandon'd by Intelligence,

> Is drown'd in Doubt, without her Pilot Wit!
> But thou, O thou great giver of all grace,
> Inspire my Wit so to direct my Will,
> That notwithstanding either's wretched case,
> They may paint out thy Plagues with grace, with skill,
> That so these Lines may reach to future times (92)

Like other poets of plague epics, Davies looks for support as he endeavors to write about "This plague of plagues that overlays this Land!" In dire need of aid, Davies invokes none other than the Holy Spirit, "great giver of all grace." Only with "her" help in this particularly daunting task might his "lines reach to future times," as Homer's and Virgil's had and as John Milton's would. Certainly, Davies chooses wisely, bringing in for support the highest form of inspiration, sure to succeed on his behalf.

Dekker and Middleton show a weary Physic and a wilting Tragedy, muses unable to perform on call, but these are secular muses; surely, the Christian Holy Spirit will do better for Davies. Only lines after the invocation, however, Davies exclaims,

> But too much Matter for my Muse to form.
> Her want (though she had words at will) is words,
> T'express this Plague's unutterable Storm!
> Fancy, thou needst not forge false Images
> To furnish Wit t'express a truth so true.
> Pictures of Death stop up all Passages,
> That Sense must needs those obvious objects view. (93)

Even Davies' divine muse does not have the words to express the ineffable, "a truth so true." The sensory experience is too great, "stop[ping] up all Passages"; yet it is "sense" that "must needs those obvious objects view." The truth in a plague visitation is no vision, nor does it require effort to achieve verisimilitude in its representation, because it is too terribly, tangibly expressed all around. It is truth, written not so directly on the soul or on the mind as on the body and in the alteration of every daily activity.[46] In keeping with the title of his poem, Davies describes Death's many triumphs, attending with precision to sensory data, going so far as to note "Feeling," "Tasting," and so forth, in his margins [148n2, 149n3–4].

Several poets opt not to invoke a muse in the first place, but this does not mean they are free from exploring the need for one. In his plague epic, *Epiloimia epē or The Anatomy of the Pestilence* (1666), the learned poet and barrister at Gray's Inn, William Austin (b. 1627/8, d. in or before 1677), wrestles with whether or not invoking a muse makes sense under the circumstances. Perhaps even writing verse is questionable:

---

[46]   For more on the concept of plague sores as God's legible marks on the body, see Gilman, *Plague Writing in Early Modern England*, especially pages 3, 53, 94–6.

In this *sad gloomy* state, what *cheering* ray
Hath *East* in *splendid* bosom to display?
Where shall we find that kind, *Elysian* vale
Will *echo* to us *joy* while we *bewail*?
Can any sweet *content of heart* distill
From consolatrix *Pitho's* sugar quill?
Will *smart* and *rage* of our disease disband
At *soft* and *gentle* touch of *Muse's* hand?[47]

Is it possible, he wonders, for a muse to do any good in plague-time? Can "consolatrix *Pitho's* sugar quill" cheer England in plague-time ("consolatrix" being "A female consoler" [OED, noun, rare] and Pitho daughter of Aphrodite, invoked for her aid in the art of seduction by persuasion)? Can a "*soft* and *gentle* touch," even of a Muse, relieve "*smart* and *rage*"? Perhaps Austin is keeping company with those in the century who argued that a classical muse is unfit for some tasks and that when the nation and souls are at stake, a Christian muse is required. He does not call upon greater aid, however, as he settles fully into an alternative method for assuaging grief:

When nothing else will do, *complaint* prevails,
While pain with vapor from the mouth exhales.
*Confession oft saves life*; when we endure
The smartest sores, our *crying* turns the *cure*. (229)

Austin will not import the song of a muse, in spite of his familiarity with its high value, demonstrated in his heroic panegyrics from preceding years.[48] He instead seeks to expel his grief and his sin by proclaiming them. This is a form of confession that links suffering with hope and closes off the possibility of despair. By Galenic standards, it also purges the body of harmful air and passions, and, biblically, it recalls a steadfast Job, whose speaking similarly allowed him to "exhale[]" the "pain with vapor," the anger and frustration from his overcharged system—the only method he had for enduring repeated assaults. William Austin gives expression to just these efforts at endurance, rendered poetically and taken seriously as an opportunity to help relieve some of the pressure on and within his own body and England's body politic.

---

[47] This passage is from part 2 of Austin's poem (part 2, p. 70). I have transcribed only part 1 in this volume. On Austin, see Sidney Lee, 'Austin, William (*b.* 1627/8, *d.* in or before 1677)', rev. Sarah Ross, *Oxford Dictionary of National Biography*, Oxford University Press, 2004; online edn, Jan 2008. [http://www.oxforddnb.com/view/article/918, accessed 24 Feb 2011]

[48] In the years preceding Austin's plague epic, he had written heroic poems demonstrating his knowledge of classical texts and his willingness to make a muse serve his turn: see for example *A joyous welcome to the most serene, and most illustrious queen of brides Catherine* (1662); *Triumphus Hymenaeus, a panegyric to the king and queen's most sacred majesties* (1662); and *Atlas under Olympus, or, The heroic poems of William Austin of Grays-Inn, Esq.* (1664).

Abraham Holland also thinks in extended verse passages about the vexed role any muse might play in plague-time. In fact, the writing of poetry itself is a questionable activity in such times. In prefatory verses of heroic measures that I treat as part of his poem proper, Holland first asks the question he assumes his readers will:

> Do you not wonder that in this sad time
> I still have leisure to compose a rhyme,
> When, as a Christian, care forbids me now
> The help of Poetry, that my hot brow
> Should sweat with active Wine, or that my heart
> Should be so free from passion to use Art
> Unto my wild expressions? The mirth
> That entertains a Muse and gives a Birth
> To happy lines is far more fit for you,
> Who in your Country's happiness do view
> Our slaughters from afar, as men in sight
> That stand remote from spectators of a Fight. (156)

Holland challenges those who are safely in the country to put themselves in his place and thereby marvel all the more at his ability to write at all, given that he is in the midst of this calamity. Then Holland supplies the reason behind his choice to remain in London: how could he possibly write about the plague any other way, from such a remove as to be "as men, in sight / That stand remote spectators of a Fight"? He will not be like his friends in the country. He will enlist with England in her battle against the plague, reporting from the frontlines.

Holland's story will be told firsthand. Before he begins, however, he again preempts readers' questions by persisting in his rationale for offering a museless heroic verse:

> In what a case poor London stands! To show
> Would ask a Pen and Muse that only know
> How to write grief. Alas, it is become
> A Theatre of Tragedies, where some
> Dy'd i'th' first acts, and, many slaughters pass'd,
> God knows what murder shall be in the last! (158)

Only a muse of Tragedy will suffice, but, then, she will only speak of "slaughters," And we recall what becomes of Dekker and Middleton's muse of Tragedy. Holland spares her, asking once more, quite directly, "What Muse shall I invoke t'indite a rhyme / That may express our miserable time" (159). His only answer is implied, as he commences with his full description of London, beginning with "The Wormwood Nosegays and the trembling Pace / Of them that pass, though they have Herb of Grace" (159) and other sights common on the streets in plague-time. It is worth recalling that Holland recorded these observations in the year he personally most needed not a muse but a champion—one that might have helped him beat his adversary.

## "Champions fell and stout": The Quest for Hero

The plague epic lacks a certain, trusted muse, and for many of the same reasons, the plague epic also lacks a martial hero. Who can stand against such disease if a muse cannot even sing of it? Who can face off against Nature herself when she undergoes an Ovidian metamorphosis capable of halting Hercules in his tracks? However fit they may be to combat other humans or monsters, the standard heroes of epic literature will not suffice. To depict battles against unpredictable, unrelenting forces operating within a decidedly Protestant universe, poets, like their readers, turned to accounts of the plague in the Bible. There they found models for how to endure scourges sent by God. Established leaders, like King David and Nineveh's king, had helped their people survive the plague, and common individuals, like the people of Nineveh and Job had also learned how to endure, the stronger for having been tested. Early modern plague writing of the period is full of references to both types, but in order to render extended treatment of individual suffering in their narratives, seventeenth-century poets found most compelling the story of the individual who had so very much to lose.

In the Book of Jonah, for example, readers encountered the citizens of Nineveh, who join together successfully as a whole to save themselves from God's threatened destruction. In the story, recounted here from the King James Bible, God determines that Nineveh in "forty days shall be overthrown" (Jonah 3.3–4), and he tells Jonah to warn the people. The narrative does not linger on details leading up to this judgment but rather focuses on the remedy: the people, "from the greatest of them even to the least of them" (3.5) heed Jonah's warning. Even their king joins with the people, "laid his robe from him, and covered him with sackcloth, and sat in ashes" (3.6) All together, "man and beast ... covered with sackcloth" (3.8), they repent. All equal, the inhabitants work to appease their angry God, and they succeed. God had said they would be "overthrown" (3.4), but once they repent together, God "saw their works, that they turned from their evil way; and God repented of the evil, that he had said that he would do unto them; and he did it not" (3.10). According to the Bible, such is the power of a people acting individually and together to prevent God from issuing forth a plague.

Preachers in the seventeenth century found this story of communal work toward common healing powerful, and they shared it frequently in sermons, in spite of the fact that all efforts at such unification failed time after time. Quarantine and prayer orders were ignored by some, overly enforced by others, and there were no measurable differences between the two behaviors with respect to survival rates.[49]

---

[49]     Examples of plague-time appropriation of the story of Nineveh in sermons of this period include that in The Church of England, *A Form to be used in Common Prayer* (1563), which was distributed to all churches in England to substitute in plague-time for the regular schedule of prayers (in Totaro, *The Plague in Print,* 32); Thomas Fuller (1608–1661), *A sermon intended for Paul's Crosse ... Upon the late decrease and withdrawing of God's heavy visitation of the plague of pestilence from the said city* (1626), 33–5; and Sampson Price, *London's Remembrancer for the staying of the contagious sickness of the plague* (1626), 4–5.

Special services for common prayer, requiring fast days and additional church attendance, were no more successful. Perhaps for these reasons, when writers of the plague epic appropriated the story of Nineveh, they did so primarily to cry out against London for failing to take Nineveh's story seriously enough as a model for their behavior.[50] Writing after the 1625 visitation, for example, George Wither explains the problem:

> …some the nature of this *Plague* beli'd;
> The number of the dead, some strove to hide.
> On groundless hopes, God's Judgments some deferred.
> Some scoffed others when they were deterred.
> Some rais'd a profit from it. Yea, so few
> Conceived what was likely to ensue,
> That when we should like *Nineveh* have fared,
> For sports and causeless *Triumphs* we prepared.
> Of pleasure, in excessive wise, we tasted.
> *We feasted*, when we rather should have *fasted*.
> And when in sack-cloth we should loud have cry'd,
> Ev'n then, we ruffled in our greatest pride. (208)

London has been unable to prepare herself as Nineveh had. Moreover, when the plague arrives, "some" attempt to "profit from it" rather than amend their ways. Others feast instead of fast and "ruffle" with pride instead of cry out in self-recrimination. Wither may see himself as the Jonah here, but whatever role he plays, London does not heed, and her failure to do so is not simply because her citizens are a prideful lot. At the very least, Londoners were by this time divided regarding whether or not to attend church during plague visitations. The government ordered theaters and markets closed during outbreaks, parliament was prorogued, and the idea of coming together, even for worship, ran counter to contagion theory, which was gaining traction.[51]

Nineveh's story served in sermons to fuel short-lived exhortations to better behavior, placing responsibility on all individuals rather than squarely on the secular or religious leadership, but the individual biblical figure all the more

---

[50]  See Thomas Brewer's *The Weeping Lady: Or London Like Nineveh in Sack-Cloth* (1625), the title of which makes plain the perceived relationship between the cities.

[51]  It should be noted as well that the kind of plague dominant at the time—the bubonic as opposed to the rarer pneumonic—was *not* communicated person to person but rather by flea-transmitted *Y. pestis* bacteria, flea to human. Early modern fears of contagion were reasonable given what was observable in many cases, as family members appeared to catch plague from each other, but in retrospect, we know that the proximity of most importance was that between to infected insect and human. On the vexed issue of church attendance, even for priests, see the 1603 pamphlet debate between Lancelot Andrews and Henoch Clapham, starting with an overview in Totaro, *Suffering in Paradise,* 42-7.

realistically resembling the person afflicted in plague-time was Job.[52] In *Milton's Brief Epic: The Genre, Meaning and Art of Paradise Regained*, Lewalski recounts the seventeenth-century preference for biblical stories as the basis for heroic writing and for biblical heroes able to surpass Achilles, Odysseus, and Aeneas in faith, courage, hope, repentance, and purity.[53] For its antiquity, verse form, and the merits of its hero, the Book of Job took its place as foremost among other options in this category, as demonstrated by the titles of two of the most popular biblical epics from the period: Francis Quarles' *Job Militant* (1624) and Henry Oxinden's *Jobus Triumphans* (1651). The former is of particular interest here given that Quarles' son John (1625–65) wrote a number of minor epics as well as a devotional plague epic, and he died of the plague in 1665, the very year his epic was published.[54] In *Paraphrase on the Book of Job* (1700), in a passage cited by Lewalski and here reproduced from the original, famous physician and writer Sir Richard Blackmore (d. 1729) explains why Job is as fit a hero as any martial type:

> *Job* then is a *Hero* proper for an *Epic Poem,* an Illustrious Person fit to support the *Dignity* of that *Character:* He is by the *Instigation* of *Satan* brought into miserable *Straights* and unparalell'd *Sufferings,* to try his *Constancy* and *Integrity.* He appears brave in *Distress,* and valiant in *Affliction,* maintains his *Virtue,* and with that his *Character,* under the most powerful *Temptations,* and exasperating *Provocations* that the Malice of *Hell* could invent, and

---

[52]   What follows are a few examples of the many plague-related sermons using Job as a model for behavior: John Dod (1549? –1645), *Four godly and fruitful sermons* (1611), 20, 25, passim; Thomas Fuller, 31, 43, 53; Josiah Hunter, *The dreadfulness of the plague* (1666), 21–2; Edward Reynolds, *A sermon preached before the peers in the Abby Church at Westminster* (1666), 42. Please also see in this volume George Wither's citation of lines from the Book of Job on his title page (172)—lines, interestingly, spoken by Elihu rather than by Job, and which have a good deal in common with Job's words at 13.19, cited in this volume by William Austin (229).

[53]   See Lewalski, *Milton's Brief Epic* in its entirety, and see John T. Shawcross, "Milton and Epic Revisionsism," 186–90. As Lewalski reminds us, John Milton cites the biblical Book of Job as "a brief model" of the epic. See Lewalski, *Milton's Brief Epic* and Milton's lines in context, in *Reason of Church Government,* in Kerrigan, Rumrich, and Fallon, 840.

[54]   John Quarles, *The Citizen's Flight* (1665). Quarles had already contributed to the canon of minor epics by expanding on one of Shakespeare's to give it an ending in which a perpetrator gets his due: *The rape of Lucrece, committed by Tarquin the Sixth; and the remarkable judgments that befell him for it* (1655). In the year of his death, Quarles' shorter poem, *London's disease, and cure* (1665), was also published. On Quarles senior's *Job Militant* (1624) and Oxinden's *Jobus Triumphans* (1656), see Lewalski, *Milton's Brief Epic,* 28, 31–2. In the appendix to *Milton and Christian Heroism: Biblical Epic Themes and Forms in Seventeenth-Century England,* Burton O. Kurth lists several of Francis Quarles' poems in the category of "brief epic," which he further distinguishes by "classical heroic" versus "allegorical" and "discursive" kinds.

thereby gives a most noble Example of *passive Fortitude,* a *Character* no
way *inferior* to that of the *active Hero.*[55]

Job is not a warrior in literal military battles but in battles of faith, standing firm
as Satan tests him, blow after excruciating, humiliating blow. He demonstrates
bravery by "maintain[ing] his Virtue" rather than by acting out. He wins the battle
over humanity's greatest adversary by remaining internally consistent "under the
most powerful *Temptations,* and exasperating *Provocations.*" He need not have
special protection or abilities, because his protection is his "passive fortitude," and
this is exactly what makes Job a relatively accessible model of heroic behavior in
times of irremediable trial.

   As one "brave in *Distress,* and valiant in *Affliction,*" and as one whose testing
comes in part by way of acute physiological suffering, Job was especially fit to
represent the plague-stricken. The association was not lost on epic poets, who
imagined Job suffering from the pestilence. In Francis Quarles in *Job Militant*
(1624), for example, Job's plague begins with the breath of "thankless Satan":

> Forth from the furnace of his Nostril, flies
> A sulfurous Vapor, which (by the envious eyes
> Of this foul Fiend inflam'd) possest the fair,
> And sweet complexion of th'abused Air
> With Pestilence, and (having power so far)
> Took the advantage of his worser Star,
> Smote him with Ulcers (such as once befell
> Th' Egyptian Wizards), Ulcers hot and fell,
> Which like a searching Tetter uncorrected,
> Left no part of his body unaffected.
> From head to foot, no empty place was found
> That could b'afflicted with another wound.
> So noisome was the nature of his Grief,
> That (left by Friends and Wife, that should be chief
> Assister) he (poor he) alone remain'd,
> Groveling in Ashes, being (himself) constrain'd,
> With Potsherds, to scrape off those rip'ned Cores,
> (Which Dogs disdain'd to lick) from out his sores. (sig. E2r–v)

Job is the plague victim who suffers under the air itself—"th'Abused Air" that
"With Pestilence" has become "possest." The vapor that abuses the air comes

---

[55]   Sir Richard Blackmore, *A Paraphrase on the Book of Job* (1700), sig. D1r. See
also Blackmore's *Creation: A Philosophical Poem in Seven Books* that begins "No more
of Courts, or Triumphs, or of Arms" (first published in 1712, this citation is from the 1797
*Poetical Works* [37]). In this volume, compare the opening of Richard Milton's *London's
Misery:* "No far fetcht Story brought from Foreign land / Or such like matters do I take
in hand;... Nor do I write the deeds of Martial men" (116). For more on Blackmore, who
also wrote a plague treatise, *A discourse upon the plague, with a preparatory account of
malignant fevers* (1721), see Lewalski, *Milton's Brief Epic* (36).

straight from the nostrils of his assailant, Satan, who carries within him an internal inferno, the choleric expression of a pride thought to cause sin and many of humanity's infectious diseases. Satan releases his hellish toxins into the air, the effect being a full physiological affront on Job, who essentially crusts over, top to toe in wounds that scab, becoming "ripe'ned Cores." Satan has the physical advantage in the battle, but the measure for glory used by God is not a material one; it is Job's patience that allows him to defeat the world's greatest adversary.

Regardless of how the story ends, this scene is the stuff of nightmares, and it resembles the plague experience, in which one loses all of one's external forms of support and comfort ("left by Friends and Wife, that should be chief Assister"); the integrity of one's body is compromised; and it is impossible to discern the enemy's strategy. No god or goddess of the pantheon or saints of the Catholic Church wait in the wings in these tales to rescue or otherwise advocate for their champions. The victim-hero undergoes trial alone. In his plague epic, *Epiloimia epē or The Anatomy of the Pestilence* (1666), William Austin marks "Job 13.19" in the margin, explicitly calling readers to look to Job, "The *Oracle* of tacit *patience*" (229). In its larger context, the biblical passage Austin recommends supplies a demonstration of Job's patience and of his integrity, in his own words:

> Though he slay me, yet will I trust in him: but I will maintain mine own ways before him. ... Hear diligently my speech, and my declaration with your ears. Behold now, I have ordered my cause; I know that I shall be justified. Who is he that will plead with me? for now, if I hold my tongue, I shall give up the ghost. (King James Bible, Job 13.15–19)

Job speaks out against those who would argue that he has been abandoned by God. In the midst of his suffering, he proclaims his faith. Austin recommends Job's faithful patience, and he offers an interesting qualification for the particularly outspoken form of this patience, stating that Job's "victory o're death, / Lay in the vocal virtue of his breath /...No other choice to him, but *speech* or *grave*" (229). Austin turns Job into an "Oracle" who in order to survive speaks out of his solitary affliction against the entire community that has turned on him. His speaking is spiritually and psychophysiologically purgative, the manifestation of a sound Christianized Galenic regimen of the kind described by Thomas Elyot and others in health regimens in the period.[56]

The allusion to an approximate tale of suffering such as this might not always have resulted in consolation for the reader, however. The comparison between old and new, biblical and current events, calls attention to the gap created where the fit is not exact. Just such a strain is palpable in a reading of Thomas Clark's *Meditations in my Confinement* (1666). In his introduction, and again, here, in his conclusion, Clark joins the ranks of those who compare themselves to Job:

---

[56] For Elyot's prescription of vociferation to expel bodily heat and improve health, see Thomas Elyot, *The castle of health* (1539), sig. 53r. See also notes 22 and 43 in this volume.

> Think not that where *affliction's* rod is sent,
> There always is deserv'd most *punishment*.
> (This was *Job's* friends' fault, and it is related
> To be avoided, and not imitated)
> God hath his sev'ral *ends*, past finding out,
> In all his *Dispensations*, without doubt,
> As for *trials*, some *examples* made
> That others may look on and be afraid,
> And when a public *Judgment's* on a Land,
> His precious ones do feel his angry *hand*
> As well as others . . . (272)

According to the poem's full title, Clark's entire family endured this dreadful experience together, and they were irreparably damaged by it. Perhaps making matters more difficult to bear, the quarantine imposed on them was voluntarily undertaken, and nothing had been able to prevent the deaths of his children. Clark had good reason to cry out against God, outraged at his many losses. But Clark casts himself poetically as the passive hero of active faith; he turns to song and faith rather than to aggression and despair. And he tries in the lines quoted above to make sense of the situation. This is not easy to do; it is the problem with the Christian plague epic. Clark poignantly struggles to explain that the afflicted are not always those deserving of the blow. Job's friends got it wrong, because even "[God's] precious ones"—even Clark's own children—"do feel his angry *hand.*"

Responses to reading Clark's poem might include a renewal of faith, a decision to increase one's almsgiving, or some alteration in one's thinking about those who undergo quarantine, but they also might include bafflement, sorrow, and outrage—responses common to a reading of the Book of Job. Because of this potentially mixed response to Clark's eager proclamation of God's goodness, in spite of Clark's unfathomable afflictions, the reading is all the more fascinating: here, one who had such cause to grieve, to despair, and to cry out against God in plague-time, sings. How? Why? In fact, Clark might be said to out-patience Job. Clark offers a compelling and lengthy case for why one's friends should *not* be blamed if they abandon one in plague-time. In brief,

> These cannot more than *others* quit their fear.
> They love *friends* well, but their own life is dear,
> Or should they dare, 'twould charg'd be in effect,
> As foolhardy fam'ly disrespect;
> Therefore *friends*, *friends* must pardon, when 'tis so. (268)

It is completely natural for friends to stay away from each other, he explains, because fear compels them to do so; essentially, to visit a plague-sick friend might be perceived as choosing friendship over family. Clark also assures readers that once the plague is over, true friends will come back around, and, of course, they should be forgiven for their absence and embraced. This is a view on plague-time friendship that is unique to Clark's account. Other poets record only the unnatural, and even uncharitable and sinful, behavior of friends in plague-time. What Clark supplies, then, is Christian charity that goes beyond what is possible in the Old Testament and in most of the plague epics written in his own day. Clark, the seventeenth-century Job, forgives those who abandon him, and then he pleads their case. The poem is unique in that this additional layer of Christian compassion, not for plague victims but for those who turn away from them, also functions to increase the gap between the experience of affliction and the expression of faith offered in its accommodation.

Richard Milton's appropriation of the figure of Jacob is equally fascinating. In his view, the plague visitation becomes a wrestling match between God and the faithful. Addressing the preachers of London who did not abandon their posts in plague-time, he commends them:

> ... I would my pen
> Had all the art that might be to give praise
> Unto your worthy actions; many ways
> You did declare yourselves like Champions stout,
> And were the only men that held us out
> From fainting; ....
> . . . . . . . . . . . . . . . . . . . . . . . . . . . . . .
> And let not the Almighty yet take rest,
> Until that by his mercies we do find
> God's wrath appeasd and he of other mind.
> And next on earth then you shall have the praise:
> Men, wives, and children, shall with pleasing lays,
> Have cause to sing your Victories about,
> And say you were their Champions fell and stout,
> That *Jacob*-like did wrestle with the Lord,
> And held him fast until he did afford
> To hold his hand, and this great sickness stay;
> This may be said of you another day. (128–9)

Imagining God as engaged in a full bodied confrontation with his people, Richard Milton makes the suffering personal. His extended metaphor turns all of the faithful preachers of London into Jacob, individually wrestling with God in a situation where they are "like Champions stout." Ironically, God is the one they hope to best—another illustration of the problem with the Christian epic. In lines that follow in his poem, Milton offers several other strategies for accounting for and providing mirth during the plague, including a Spenserian-style tall tale of "that hard Squire Sir *Henry* hight / A valiant, doughty, and courageous sprite" (134), and a plague bill, preceded by a prose section in which he compares the plague dead to bodies on a battlefield (135). These other forms of reckoning with the plague call attention to the extreme nature of the times, when poets, like everyone else, struggled to give voice to what they were witnessing, trying on many options for size, and none of them fitting quite right.

In this effort, William Austin opts by Part 3 of his epic to offer a string of consolations to his readers, who have likely grown weary from the preceding review of the plague's many forms of assault—each one, as discussed above, creating a situation that warrants a purgative, Job-like crying out. Beginning with "*Let's comfort take,*" each of the statements of consolation draw from natural and biblical imagery to provide evidence for the idea that the scourges sent by God are intended to better humankind. The best way to manage oneself during such smiting, then, is to be patient but also to draw comfort from the knowledge of future reward:

> *Let's comfort take.* For like as Jonas, he
> Courageously oppos'd tempestuous sea,
> And *Jacob* wrestling with the *Angel* found
> Best rise, as ball when hardest *thrown to ground.*
> So now may our intrepid spirits be
> Pompous rich *victors* o're *calamity.* (part 3, p. 80)

Austin appropriates the stories of Jonas (Jonah) and Jacob, both, as models for those who feel that in plague-time *they* are the bark on "tempestuous seat" or "ball when hardest *thrown to ground.*" These biblical heroes—enduring hardships alone, tested in situations that might easily have led to their deaths—survived, and they were better for the trial. Their stories offer hope in a positive metamorphosis caused by hardship—the very hope desperately needed in plague-time. But the reality before the eyes of Londoners was quite different: their "*calamity*" was known to repeat rather than ending in decided victory. The threat they faced also menaced their loved ones, which was not quite so for for the biblical Jonah, Jacob, or even Job, leaving at least some readers surely hard pressed to take full "comfort" from similes such as those Austin provides here. Austin's "ball" must for some have called to mind not souls bouncing by means of successful trial but the many thousands of bodies "hardest *thrown to ground*" that absolutely did not "rise."

### "But what I can, I utter": The Eyewitness and Authority

In the wake of the plague, gaps widened between inherited stories of suffering and triumph and the newly occurring personal stories of affliction and endurance. In the space opened up, writers experimented with narrative voice. Some appointed mother London as the narrator of her own tale, others invoked muses, and many more placed themselves as didactic poet, narrator, eyewitness, and teacher directly within the plague city's quotidian scenes. John Taylor the Water Poet is particularly keen to offer first-hand accounts of such on-the-ground sights, as here, describing some of the ways Londoners tried to avoid inhaling plague vapors:

> One with a piece of tasseld, well-*tarr'd* Rope
> Doth with that nosegay keep himself in hope.
> Another doth a wisp of wormwood pull

And with great Judgment crams his nostrils full.
A third takes of his socks from's sweating feet,
And makes them his perfume alongst the street. (149)

Humorous as this image is, coming from a poet known as much for light verse
as for serious, the description captures in detail the types of practices performed
by common people who could not afford more expensive preventative measures.
Those unable to flee from London did what they could to fortify their minds, souls,
and bodies against infection so that they might survive in town, surrounded by
infection. Practices such as those Davies describes made sense within the context
of seventeenth-century beliefs that plague came as a vapor through the air and
could be blocked by other smells—tar and foot odor sure to achieve this end.[57]
While painting a scene of desperation among those like himself, living through
the visitation rather than fleeing from it, Taylor establishes his credibility as an
eyewitness and his legitimacy as a loyal Londoner, thereby aiming to earn his
readership.

Taylor reinforces the importance of his special testimony by relaying an
account of his own sickness during the visitation of 1625. In doing so, he also
provides a rare rationale for plague-time (mis)behaviors:

Myself hath been perplexed now and then
With the wind Colic, years above thrice ten.
Within the country, I durst not repeat [this],
Although my pangs and gripes and pains were great,
For, to be sick of any kind of grief,
Would make a man worse welcome than a thief.
To be drunk sick, which erst did credit win,
Was fear'd infectious and held worse than sin.
This made me, and many more beside,
Their griefs to smother and their pains to hide,
To tell a merry tale with visage glad,
Whenas the Colic almost made me mad.
Thus mere dissembling, many practis'd then,
And mid'st of pain, seem'd pleasant amongst men,
For why, the smallest sigh or groan, or shriek
Would make a man his meat and lodging seek. (151)

In what is an ironic digression on how one "dares not be sick" in plague-time,
Taylor comments on his own pains, caused by thirty years of the "wind colic" (the

---

[57]   Among those to prescribe this rope-based nosegay was seventeenth century
housewife, Gervase Markham. See her "A preservative against the plague" in *The English
Housewife: Containing the Inward and Outward Virtues Which Out to Be in a Complete
Woman,* edited by Michael R. Best (Toronto: McGill-Queen's University Press, 1998),
12.   On scents and miasma theory, see Totaro, "Chicken Soup (and Orange Juice) for the
Plague-Time Soul?" 25–33.

wind colic being "paroxysmal griping pains in the belly" caused by gas, no less).[58] This condition was a common one, but it was undoubtedly uncomfortable and exacerbated by the need to keep the wind within one's body when it so desperately sought release. In plague-time, such efforts at relief were more complicated, as were expressions of discomfort resulting from their suppression. Routine troubles like this might be said to pose ethical challenges if indeed "many" were led to "mere dissembling," forced "to tell a merry tale with visage glad" when in "mid'st of pain." If one could suffer but still seem "pleasant amongst men," the implication is that those "many more beside" Taylor who stifled the symptoms of lesser diseases may also have stifled some of the symptoms of plague. In addition, Taylor's digression gives us insight into what many then cited as a fact about diseases: as with odors in the air, one could only have one major condition at a time, the strongest one dominating. If one had syphilis, for example, one could not also have gout, and if one had plague one could not also have the stone or the wind colic.[59] It appears from Taylor's confession that we can account for this seeming fact in at least one way: people did not report other diseases in plague-time for fear that reporting any ailment might lead to quarantine or at least to being avoided by others. And certainly, those suffering from buboes and headed for a swift death would be unlikely themselves to report (or even to notice) if their gout or hemorrhoids were aggravating them as well.

Offering a view of himself quite different than the one Taylor provides, Abraham Holland nevertheless similarly calls attention to his subjective condition. As he walks London's streets, he is a man full of emotion. Referring to the city as "A Theatre of Tragedies," Holland seems unable to resist attendance, in spite of the fact that he lives outside of London's walls:

---

[58]   OED *s.v.* wind (Compounds)

[59]   On the idea that it was only possible to have one major disease at a time, see for example Holland, who says that the plague "may affright the rest [of the diseases], we nam'd before" (163), and see Thomas Sprat's Pindaric ode, *The Plague of Athens* (1659): "Whatever lesser Maladies men had, / They all gave place and vanished; / Those petty Tyrants fled, / And at this mighty Conqueror shrunk their head" (10). Sprat's plague poem was reprinted at least 11 times between 1659 and 1743; please compare it with Pitt's in the volume. With respect to syphilis, itself an horrific, plague-like disease in many ways, see the only known epic on syphilis, *Syphilis, or, A poetical history of the French disease written in Latin by Fracastorius ; and now attempted in English by N. Tate* (1686), a work that served equally as a didactic poem of instruction on how to manage the disease. On this poem, in relationship to other poems on illness in the period, see Anselment 46–7, 150–51; on the poem as a precursor to Fracastoro's prose treatise *De Contagione*, see Geoffrey Eatough, *Fracastoro's Syphilis: Introduction, text, translation and notes with a computer-generated word index*, ARCA: Classical and Medieval Texts, Papers and Monographs, 12, (Liverpool: Francis Cairns, 1984); Stephen Jay Gould, *I Have Landed: The End of a Beginning in Natural History* (New York: Turbo, Inc., 2003), 194–205; and Douglas Biow, *Doctors, Ambassadors, Secretaries: Humanism and Professions in Renaissance Italy* (Chicago: University of Chicago, 2002), 71–100.

> I live not in it but in Chelsea air,
> Where Death but in his Outroads doth repair,
> And thence do only hear the murmuring Bells
> Disclose the slaughter by the frequent Knells.
> Yet, as a tender Mother, though she have
> A Child interr'd and sleeping in the grave,
> Yet will she oft go see the tomb and dew
> His dust with pious tears and oft renew
> His Posthume exequies, so sometimes I
> Go to behold the City and espy
> As I do walk along the widow'd streets
> Nothing but sorrow in each face that meets,
> In the Large ruin nothing but a grief
> That speaks itself in silence, true and brief. (158)

Holland is drawn to the city of London proper, within the walls—drawn there, he says, like a mother to the tomb of her dead child. By simile, then, he changes out his own experience for another's, even to the point of changing his gender to heighten the description of his passionate reaction to London's pain: "Yet, as a tender Mother ... so sometimes I."[60] Unlike Taylor, Holland expresses no wish to relieve London's "grief / That speaks itself in silence, true and brief." Rather, he implies that by witnessing her silence, he gets as close as possible to what is "true" about London in plague-time. The once bustling city is a graveyard, and his poem becomes *her* "Posthume exequies"—ironically so, because, as we know, between the two of them, he will be the one who in that year will not rise again. In this light, these words from earlier in his poem are heartbreaking: "we wretches try / What other Ages shall hold Poetry" (157).

An examination of the "I" inserted into *The Plague of Athens* (1659), by Royal Society historian and poet Thomas Sprat (bap. 1635, d. 1713), is instructive in this regard. Sprat fashioned the poem as a Pindaric ode based on the content of Lucretius' account of the plague in *De Rerum Natura*. Among the many changes he made to the Lucretian content is his inclusion of a first person witness to plague's destruction.[61] Sprat makes room in his translation for the voice of a solitary Athenian soldier struck with plague and who "in open streets did roar":

---

[60]   On early modern male authors appropriating the female voice for expressions of lament, see Phillippy, *Women, Death, and Literature,* 121-35.

[61]   Sprat followed the work of Abraham Cowley, champion of the Pindaric ode and of the biblical epic in England. By the time Sprat wrote *The Plague of Athens*, he was contributing to a trend in the Protestant appropriation of the Pindaric ode for serious matters of national and Christian import, as evident from the full title: *The plague of Athens, which happened in the second year of the Peloponnesian War. First described in Greek by Thucydides, then in Latin by Lucretius; now attempted in English, after incomparable Dr. Cowley's Pindaric way* (1659). In the excerpt cited, I have modernized the text, especially to highly the soldier's words by the addition of quotations marks. Known for his Christianized epic, *Davideis* (1656), Cowley also contributed a Pindaric ode in praise of Francis Bacon as

"How have I, Death, so ill deserv'd of thee,
That now thyself thou shouldst revenge on me?
Have I so many lives on thee bestow'd?
Have I the earth so often dy'd in blood?
Have I, to flatter thee, so many slain?
And must I now myself thy prey remain?
   Let me at least, if I must die,
Meet in the field some gallant enemy.

. . . . . . . . . . . . . . . . . . . . . . . . . . . . .

 Give me, great Heavns, some manful foes.
Let me my death amidst some valiant Grecians choose.
 Let me survive to die at Syracuse,
 Where my dear Country shall her Glory lose
For you, Great Gods! …

. . . . . . . . . . . . . . . . . .

Oh! might I die upon that glorious stage.
Oh, that …!" but then he grasp'd his sword, and death concludes his rage. (16)

This is the individual who rages against the plague, aware that his death is coming to him on terms unexpected and unacceptable, robbing him of a frame of reference for processing it and a community to offer him consolation. This is a rage also against creation, and the poem ends *sans* hope. This soldier is also entirely Sprat's creation, an individual voice that cries out against the cruel joke that is life, when one's sense of purpose becomes the source of one's greatest torment: "Oh! Might I …/ Oh that!" Sprat gives us an "I" that he does not claim for his own, but it is nevertheless a powerful, plague-time expression of exasperation in isolation, all the more poignant for its originality.

This exasperation of the isolated plague-time subject takes a less dramatic but arguably more intimate form in the plague epics transliterated here, each of which calls attention to the poet as witness. In the title to his poem, Richard Milton alerts the reader to just this role that he will play: *London's Misery, The Country's Cruelty, with God's Mercy: Explained by remarkable observations of each of them during this last Visitation.* Among the "remarkable observations" Milton makes are those of his own journey of faith. After describing the horrifying conditions

part of the prefatory material for Sprat's *History of the Royal Society* –both pieces turning Bacon into what John Steadman calls the "scientific hero," a new form of non-martial hero that would eventually replace the Protestant, suffering hero of the biblical epic (*Milton and the Paradoxes of Renaissance Heroism* [Louisiana: Louisiana State University Press, 1987], chapter 3, "Bacon and the Scientist as Hero"). On the Pindaric ode and Milton's epic poetry, see Phillip Edward Phillips, *John Milton's Epic Invocations: Converting the Muse,* Renaissance and Baroque Studies and Texts 26 (New York: Peter Lang, 2000), 55; Stella P. Revard, *Pindar and the Renaissance Hymn-Ode: 1450–1700* (Tempe: Arizona Center for Medieval and Renaissance Studies, 2001); and Lewalski, *The Life of John Milton: A Critical Biography,* Blackwell Critical Biographies (Malden, MA; Oxford: Blackwell, 2000), 46–7.

in London, Milton, chastises the plague for taking the lives of the innocent and upright: "Know you what you have done? Y'ave slain a woman, / That for her virtuous carriage, I think no man / Will find the like again" (121). Later, he scolds more generally: "Leave off, for shame. Away, now get you gone. / Go take the worst sort. Leave the best alone!" (122). In these angry outbursts against the plague, Milton speaks as many in the time might have wanted to do, crying out for a halt to the injustices perpetrated against London's citizens. As if overhearing the problem with his logic as he speaks it, however, Milton then performs a narrative maneuver of didactic simultaneity in which he turns his scrutiny upon himself and changes the direction of the narrative:

> Lord if 'twere so, what would become of me
> That know myself to be as bad may be?
> For there's not only one but thousands more
> That I go far behind that went before:
> Many a brave Scholar, many a worthy Teacher,
> Many a good liver, many a zealous Preacher,
> That liv'd as lights, and were to thee right dear.
> So carefully they walked in thy fear,
> But I, alas, have much abused thy will,
> Had not a care, thy hests for to fulfill,
> Have sin'd extremely and assuredly
> Had long before this time deserved to die.
>     But yet, O Lord, I see 'tis not thy will;
> Thou spar'st my life, wilt have me tarry still.
> And now I pray thee, whilst I have my being,
> Sith that thou hast vouchsaft to me the seeing,
> (Wretch that I am) of this thy mighty power,
> Grant that hereafter, daily and each hour,
> For that same small time, and the little space
> Of life that thou shalt grant me by thy grace,
> I may redeem time, which I lewdly spent,
> Bewail my sins and heartily repent. (122)

Determining by outward shows those whom the plague should and should not spare, Milton then turns his scrutiny upon himself, realizing he merits no special dispensation. Placing himself "far behind" the many others—"brave Scholar," "worthy Teacher," "good liver," and "zealous Preacher"—who deserved to live but did not, Milton gives voice to the very kind of inward doubt afflicting many plague-time survivors: Why me? Why him? Why not her? How can I make meaning from these extraordinary circumstances? This is a version of the spiritual reckoning that had in the same century gained public recognition and sanction in the form of the spiritual autobiography.[62] Unable to identify the fleas that, as

---

[62]    On the spiritual biography, particularly as one of the few permissible forms of privileging in sustained fashion the "I" of the author in seventeenth-century writing, see George A. Starr, *Defoe and Spiritual Autobiography* (1965; Princeton: Princeton

we now know, were spreading the *Y. pestis* bacteria among the rat and human populations, people like Milton looked to God, and Protestants in particular looked inward for answers, desperate in their self-reckonings to account for what they were witnessing.[63] Milton does not explain why he is spared when others die, but he does justify the act of uttering what he has witnessed: "Sith that thou hast vouchsaft to me the seeing." He has been trusted with witnessing to the power of God, who spares those whom He wishes to spare—even the most sinful. Milton's "remarkable observations" warrant if not compel him to share his account: I, a "wretch," still live—a line anticipating the last in Daniel Defoe's 1722 *A Journal of the Plague Year*: "*A dreadful Plague in* London *was* / *In the Year Sixty Five,* / *Which swept an Hundred Thousand Souls* / *Away; yet I alive!*"[64]

In *Britain's Remembrancer*, George Wither spends much more time assessing his own spiritual growth as it results from what he witnesses. In the process of self-reckoning, he offers details regarding the lived experience of those more afflicted than he:

> Upon an Evening (when the waning light
> Was that which could be call'd nor day nor night)
> I met with one of these, who on me cast
> A ruthful eye, and as he by me pass'd,
> Methought I heard him, softly, somewhat say,
> As if that he for some relief did pray,
> Whereat (he seeming in good clothes to be)
> I stayed and askt him if he spake to me.
> He bashfully replied that indeed,
> He was asham'd to speak aloud what *Need*
> Did make him softly mutter. Somewhat more
> He would have spoken, but his tongue forbore
> To tell the rest, because his eyes did see
> Their tears had (almost) drawn forth tears from me,
> And that my hand was ready to bestow
> That help which my poor fortunes could allow. (196–7)

In a reporterly style that also in some ways anticipates Defoe's in *A Journal of the Plague Year*, Wither takes us with him onto the streets of London. This effort primarily serves as a representation of Wither's own spiritual challenges in plague-

---

University Press, 1971); on the spiritual autobiography in relation to biblical models and organized around crisis points, such as illness, see Adam Smythe, *Autobiography in Early Modern England* (Cambridge and New York: Cambridge University Press, 2010), especially 145–48; and on the appearance of just this tension between standard form and resistance to standardization in the elegy, see Howard, "'Mine Own Breaking'" and Andrea Brady, *English Funerary Elegy in the Seventeenth Century: Laws in Mourning*. (Basingstoke: Palgrave Macmillan, 2006), 10.

63   On self-reckoning in plague-time, see Erin Sullivan, "Physical and Spiritual Illness: Narrative Appropriations of the Bills of Mortality," in Totaro and Gilman, 76–94.

64   Daniel Defoe, *A Journal of the Plague Year,* in Backscheider, 248.

time—how frequently he is tormented by fear and pity. The scene also opens a window in time, offering the reader a glimpse into a regularly occurring plague-time phenomenon: the citizen (in "good clothes") who has lost his livelihood during London's economic stagnation and who must resort to begging on the street.

The next step Wither takes in his representation of the scene reinforces its seventeenth-century literary context and genre, which is not able to admit something closer to a real dialogue between Wither and the man. Instead, Wither leads with his imagination in the place of this man's words, explaining,

> Nor his, nor all men's tongues, could more relate,
> Than I myself conceiv'd of his estate.
> Methought I saw, as if I had been there,
> What wants in his, and such men's houses were;
> How empty, and how naked it became;
> How nasty *Poverty* had made the same.
> Methought I saw, how sick his wife might lie;
> Methought I heard his half starv'd children cry;
> Methought I felt, with what a broken heart
> He lookt upon them, e're he could depart
> To try, if (by God's favor) he could meet
> With any means of comfort in the street. (197)

Careful to manage the scene of pathos, Wither places upon it the strict literary markers of an inexpressibility topos, anaphora, and a parenthetical insertion. Moreover, the description of the man is kept to a minimum, with Wither's many "methought"s in its place. So too is mention of God's place in the account both highlighted, as an insertion into an otherwise mundane scene, and reduced, by its location in a parenthetical. Wither performs a fine balancing act, reinforcing his own authority as key witness and credible interpreter of events, while admitting two additional perspectives—the unnamed man's clearly the most compelling.

Part of Wither's spiritual self-reckoning is evident in his frequent meditation on the roles he plays in life and in the poem, where he is citizen, Christian, prophet, and poet. In one of his many demonstrations of didactic simultaneity, Wither troubles at some length in the poem over the degree to which he has suitably represented what he has seen and done right by those whom he has described, as here:

> It may be that to some it will appear
> My Muse hath only poetized here,
> And that I fain'd expressions do rehearse,
> As most of those that use[d] to write in verse.
> But in this Poem I pursue the story
> Of real Truth, without an Allegory,
> And many yet surviving witness may,
> That I come short of what I more might say.
> But what I can, I utter...
> . . . . . . . . . . . . . . . . . .

> Methinks I cannot speak enough of that
> Which I have seen, nor full enough relate
> What I declare, but still it seems to me
> I leave out somewhat that should utt'red be. (211)

Here Wither's "I" is prominent as well, all but replacing the muse as the best judge for what counts as the "real Truth" in a plague visitation. At the same time, however, Wither carefully articulates a self-consciousness regarding whether he has related "enough" without leaving out what "should utt'red be."[65] His "should" implies that he measures his work by a higher standard, but at the same time this standard will be applied by a court of "the many yet surviving witness[es]." Wither has at least two very different audiences and agendas to satisfy; it is not enough, then, for this self-appointed, prophetic voice of Britain (who has dedicated his poem to King Charles I, no less) to tell the tale entirely on his own. It is not enough, alternatively, to rely entirely on a muse and risk losing a readership that already knew the plague and its local and epic terrors first hand.

Thomas Clark knew better than most what it was to be that London man whom Wither only partially describes. Clark knew the plague intimately, felt the pains of helplessness and rejection, and survived. Perhaps for this reason Clark is bold enough to state his purpose plainly:

> *No* elegancy *here is interlac'd,*
> *Which might the Reader* Court *to be embrac'd.*
> Courtship *with me was then quite out of* fashion,
> *When whole months pass'd and scarce a salutation.*
> Sighs *here* are Accents, Periods *end with* tears,
> *And for the* Burden, *'tis a Mass of* fears.
> *I have no argument that may incline*
> *You for to read this* Tract, *but that,* 'tis mine. (258)

One of the poets about whom we know the least here presents himself, his body and emotions, as intimately connected to his writing—an expression of authorship rare for its time. He breathes out his own "Sighs" into "Accents," his own "tears" into "Periods," as if they could only belong where his passions land them. Writing in heroic measures, Clark could not have allowed his emotions quite as much range as he suggests; yet his expression of authentic representation, of emotionally pouring out his verse, even to the sighing out of each accent, is in many ways an ideal preface to his unique account of plague. His proximity to the plague gives his voice as much authority as Wither's, if not more; there are no "methought"s in Clark's verse, no removes separating him from his subject. He is hero and victim, as if Hector had lived to write a first-hand account of the fall of Troy.

---

65   On the didactic narrator as distinctly a self-conscious one who practices poetic simultaneity, related here to Wither's self-questioning within the narrative, see Volk, *The Poetics of Latin Didactic,* especially pages 6–24.

The combination of content derived from epic suffering and of a form intended to serve the highest of literary aims with respect to artfulness has never been so poignantly rendered as in plague epics like Clark's. In the tension exhibited between the I and the we, the individual and the nation, between doubt and faith, and, again, between epic conventions and personal, passionate content, these poems articulate a peculiar seventeenth-century response to the plague, the severity and endurance of which called out for heroic measures and at the same time found them lacking. As if the epic container could no more hold the contents of a plague visitation than a proper muse could give it voice, the next century of poets all but uniformly denied the capacity of long-standing literary forms to serve such turns.[66] The proliferation of the mock epic, starting as early as 1684 with the publication of Samuel Butler's *Hudibras*, and of the proto-novel, with an early debut in Daniel Defoe's *A Journal of the Plague Year*, would follow—the latter an early embodiment of the genre that would come both to serve and define the needs of the next century of readers.[67] But before this, the works of poets from Muggins to Pitt testify that even during some of England's deadliest years, when authority and convention had failed them time and again, people were not entirely ready to relinquish the belief that the plague was part of a larger plan for the world, that England would again reassert her exceptionalism, that a patient Job could triumph over Satan, and that individuals taking their solitary ways out of a golden age and into a world of increased war and disease could learn by experience how to do better.

---

[66]  Christopher Pitt emerges as the eighteenth-century outlier by choosing heroic measures rather than prose for his plague account.

[67]  On the mock epic, see Richard Terry, *Mock-Heroic from Butler to Cowper: An English Genre and Discourse* (Aldershot and Burlington: Ashgate 2005). See also Samuel Garth's 1699 mock epic *The Dispensary* with its battle between Royal College physicians and the London apothecaries over who should be in charge of dispensing medicine.

# Part 2
# The Poems

## Editorial Policy

My goal has been to make these early modern texts accessible without compromising their character. In each case, I have based my transcription on the earliest available and complete edition of the poem listed in the English Short Title Catalog, noting for easy identification their Short Title Catalog (STC) number, always from the second edition of the STC. For accuracy, I have compared available copies from research libraries, including the Folger, Huntington, Bodleian, Cambridge, and British libraries. Spelling has been modernized, except in the cases of archaic verb endings, obsolete words, and when modernization would alter the meter, rhyme, or play on words.

Unusual, archaic, and field-specific terms appear defined in the General Glossary, to which I direct readers as a first stop, prior to turning to online queries. Definition of terms in the glossary is based on cross referencing the texts collected here with *Oxford English Dictionary* entries and occasionally with the notes and glossaries provided by Totaro, *The Plague in Print,* and by Taylor and Lavagnino, *Thomas Middleton: The Collected Works.* Identification of proper and place names listed in the Index of Names derives primarily from cross-referencing entries in the *Oxford Dictionary of National Biography* with those in other sources, including dictionaries of London printers and booksellers edited by McKerrow and by Plomer.

I have altered punctuation when necessary for clarity; this includes the addition of apostrophes for possessives and a modern management of comma, colon, and semi-colon usage as well as the addition of quotation and question marks where appropriate. I have retained the original capitalization and italics in all texts, except when a change of punctuation necessitated capitalization or its removal for clarity or when consistency within a text or across later editions of the same text recommended it.

The original marginal notes have been moved to the footnotes and are always preceded by [marginal note]. All other footnotes, not marked by [marginal note] are my additions to the original text. In the few cases where I offer such additional information, as in offering the full biblical quotation to which an original marginal note citation refers, the added information itself appears in separate brackets. In the rare case where I offer clarification for context-specific meaning, such as a rephrasing or other explanation, the words from the text in question are first noted in italics, followed by my findings in plain text.

Whenever I have adopted an editorial change, the effort has been to apply it consistently throughout the text in question and across texts as useful. This does not mean that I have provided a flawless execution of transliteration, the task being cumbersome and complicated, but every effort has been taken to provide clarity while maintaining the integrity of the original in meaning and in prosody. As a rule when conducting the transliterations, I have limited my own speculations on the texts and on the terms within them, leaving this level of analysis to the reader.

The necessity of setting limits extends to the selection of poems that appear in this volume. A single volume cannot hold them all; for additional titles, I direct the reader to the Works Cited section and, specifically, to Thomas Brewer's *The Weeping Lady: Or London Like Nineveh in Sack-Cloth* (1625) and *A dialogue betwixt a citizen, and a poor country-man and his wife, in the country, where the citizen remaineth now in this time of sickness* (1636); Thomas Sprat's *The Plague of Athens* (1659); John Quarles' *The Citizen's Flight* (1665); the syphilis epic of Girolamo Fracastoro, translated into English by Nahum Tate in 1686; Samuel Garth's 1699 *The Dispensary*; and other plague-time epics by Du Bartas, Dryden, and Tabor.

\*

# William Muggins,
## *London's Mourning Garment*

One copy of the only edition of this poem from 1603 (STC 2nd ed., 18248) resides in each of the following library archives: the British Library; the Bodleian Library; University of Oxford; and the Henry E. Huntington Library and Art Gallery. A short piece of dedicatory prose addressed to "Sir John Swynnerton, Knight, one of the worshipful Alderman of the honorable City of London" precedes the poem, and following it are "A godly and zealous Prayer unto God, for the surceasing of his ireful Plague and grievous Pestilence," in prose, as well as collated data from London's plague bills from 14 July to 17 November 1603.

## LONDON'S MOURNING GARMENT,

or Funeral Tears, worn and shed for the death of her wealthy Citizens and other
her inhabitants. To which is added a zealous and fervent Prayer, with a true
relation how many have died of all diseases in every particular parish within
London, the Liberties, and outparishes near adjoining, from the 14 of July 1603
to the 17 of November following.

At London printed by Ralph Blower 1603

With heavy heart and sighs of inward Cares,
With wringing hands, explaining sorrow's woe,
With blubbered cheeks, bedewed with trickling tears,
With mind opprest, lamenting griefs that flow—
London, lament, and all thy losses show.
What all? Nay, some. All were too much to tell;
The learned Homer could not pen it well.
    Ay me poor London, which of late did flourish,
With springing MARCH, the tidings of a King,
And APRIL showers, my blossoms so did nourish,        (10)
That I in MAY was called a famous thing.
Yea, Towns and Cities did my glory ring.
Nay, through the world my golden fame so grew
That Princes high crost Seas, my seat to view.
    And like to AGAMEMNON'S gallant train,
Throughout my streets, with stately steps did go,
Where them with welcomes, I did entertain,
Pleasing their liking, with each several show,
Where they in me, much treasure did bestow,
Honoring the Church with Prayers, the Change[1] with gold,        (20)
Where Princes bought, and beauteous Virgins sold.
    To add more glory to my prosperous state,
My Sovereign Lord, most high and mighty King,
Made oft repair both Morning, Ev'en, and late
To me, both gainful and a pleasant thing:
My heart was glad; my voice "SOL, FA," did sing.
My head did muse, not struck with sorrows sad,
But how to make my crowned Sovereign glad.
    And as a Bride, against her Nuptial day,
Doth deck herself with fair and rich attire,        (30)
Accompanied with Damsels fresh and gay,
To plight her faith to him she did desire,
Even so did I with zeal as hot as fire.
Prepare myself against this day of joy,

---

[1]  *the Change*. The Royal Exchange.

To give him welcome, with "VIVE LE ROYE."
 My Magistrates were all so ready prest
In scarlet rich, this potent Prince to greet.
My wealthy Free-men also wrought their best,
Preparing Pageants in each famous street.
My Merchant-strangers labored hands and feet, (40)
And scattered coin, like JUPITER'S showers of Gold,
Hoping with joy this CAESAR to behold.
 And as those men the wealthiest in my Bower,
Was never sparing in this good intent,
So did my Artisans with all their power,
For love or gain, to work were ready bent.
PYGMALION forth his skillful Carvers sent
Cunning APPELLES with his pencil drew
Prospectious strange for King and Peers to view.
 But oh, a sudden qualm doth cross my heart. (50)
Twixt cup and lip are dangers oft we see.
Unwelcome death approacheth with his dart,
Yelping, "Oh, LONDON, thou must yield to me.
I must have roots and branches for my fee.
The fruits full ripe and blossoms that might grow
Are mine, not thine; the Fates decreed it so."
 Drown'd in deep seas (poor Lady) thus I lie,
Unless some speedy help a comfort yield.
Is there no wife nor widow that will hie,
And reach a hand that hath some sorrows felt? (60)
My griefs are more than I myself can wield.
Help, some good woman with your soul's-sigh deep,
For you are tender-hearted and can weep.
 What none? Nay, then I see the Proverb old is true:
The widow's care is studious where to love.
Sith women are so fickle, men, to you,
LONDON laments. Will ye her plaints remove?
I hear no Echo. Men like women prove:
Widowers for wives, widows for husbands seek,
Before the tears are dried from their cheeks. (70)
 To children then I will my sorrows show,
Whose Parents lately in the grave were laid,
Their hearts with sighs will cause fresh tears to flow,
And reach a hand for sorrowing LONDON'S aid.
Come children mourn. I cry but am denied:
Their Parents' riches so inflames their breast,
That they long since did wish them at their rest.
 Where or to whom may I my voice set forth?

Men mourn for men, where friendship long hath bred.
Fie no (good Lady) there is found small troth.                           (80)
The living Friend deceives the friend that's dead,
Robbing his children with a subtle head.
By reason, he executor, made them drown.
By wresting Law, the riches are his own.
    Oh (helpless Lady) whither shall I fly
To find true mourners in this sad lament?
To aged people? No, their heads are dry;[2]
They cannot weep; long since, their tears were spent.
To middle age? (Alas) Their wits are bent
To purchase lands and livings for their heirs,                           (90)
Or by long life to gain which other spares.
    The loving servant may yet help at need,
That now hath lost his Master and his stay,
Sending forth sighings till the heart doth bleed.
Oh, LONDON, thou in vain to him dost pray.
His power and wits he bends another way:
His Master's custom, shop, and trade to get,
Is all the tears, the blithe young man can let.
    Is there none, then, that will take London's part
And help to sing a welcome unto woe?                                     (100)
Is there none found that feels a present smart?
Nor none alive that can cause Tears to flow?
If any be, then freely them bestow.
Two mourn together, 'suage each other's grief.
Weep on a while, and I will be the chief.
    I hear no answer yet in these estates.
Let me but study where and whom to seek,
Oh, now I have bethought me: come on mates,
For you and I must mourn it by the week,
And never will new tears be long to seek,                               (110)
For Parents' love, unto their Children dear,
In judgment sound, nothing can come more near.
    The love of Parents are like Grafts that grow,
Ever increasing, till it prove a tree.
The love of Children, like the melting Snow,
Ever decreasing, till an end there be.
Daily experience proves this true we see:
Love to the Children, evermore depends,
But to the Parents, seldom re-descends.

---

   [2]   *their heads are dry.* According to humoral theory, as one aged, the body grew increasingly colder and drier.

And now I have, with travail, grief, and pain, (120)
Found forth two mourners that will Agents be.
Choose which of us shall settle to complain.
Or, if you will, leave all the charge to me—
Only I with you, to abandon glee.
And, to my voice, prepare your glowing Ears,
With sighs and groans and sometimes scalding Tears.
    And if too high my warbling note ascends,
Judge me not bold but zealous in my love;
If that too low, think that with sighs for friends,
My voice is hoarse, yet I again will prove, (130)
The utmost power I can for to remove
Your too forgetful sorrows which are dry,
And place them now, afresh in memory.
    Art thou a Father or a Mother dear?
Hadst thou a Son or Daughter of thy side?
Were not their voice sweet music in thy Ear,
Or from their smiles, could'st thou thy countnance hide?
Nay, were they not the glories of thy pride?
I doubt too much, thy love on them were set,
That whilst thou livest, thou canst not them forget. (140)
    Remember well, you Dames of London City.
As for you men, I'll leave you for a while,
Because small pains deserves the lesser pity,
And you are stronger, sorrows to beguile.
A space we will your company exile,
And bid you farewell till another day,
When time and place will give you cause of stay.
    And now my hearts, old Widows and young wives,
You that in silence sit so sad and mute,
You that wring hands, as weary of your lives, (150)
Hear London speak; she will express your suit.
I know your sighs is for your tender fruit—
Fruit in the bud, in blossom ripe and grown,
All dear to you, now death hath made his own.
    And as the greedy Wolf from harmless Ewes,
Robs them of Lambs, sucking their tender Tett,
And in his Rigor, no compassion shews,
But gormandizing, kills them for his meat,
Even so death's fury now is grown so great,
The tender Lamb will not his fury stay. (160)
Both Lambs and Ewes, he swallows for his prey.
    Witness I can, poor LONDON for my part,
What palefac't Death within five Months hath wrought:

Seven hundred Widows, wounded to the Heart,
With their sweet Babes, which they full dearly bought,
Some dead new born, some never forth were brought.
You Mothers weep, if ever you bore any,
To think how sore Death did perplex so many.

    Not yet content, he Rageth up and down,
And, secretly, his heavy visage shows,                    (170)
In every street and corner of the Town,
Emptying whole houses, soon, whereas he goes,
Taking away both old and young, God knows:
The weeping Mother, and the Infant clear,[3]
The loving Brother, and the Sister dear.

    Oh mothers sigh, sit, and shed tears a while.
Expel your idle pleasures, think on woes.
Make not so much as countenance of a smile,
But with down looks, which inward sorrow shows,
And now afresh, remember all your throws,                 (180)
Your gripes, your pangs, your bodies pincht with pain,
As if this instant you did them sustain.

    Let not so much forgotten be of you,
As the least qualm that then your hearts opprest,
No nor the smallest dolor did ensue,
As heavy winks and too too little rest.
Remember all the sorrows of thy breast,
Which in the breeding, bearing and delivery,
You did endure with pain yet willing.

    Again bethink you, at that instant hour,          (190)
The little difference was twixt life and death,
When as the infant, with his naked power,
Labored for life to have his rightful birth,
And with the sickly Mother gaspt for breath,
The one near dead, as nigh to death the other,
Sore to the babe, worse Travail for the Mother.

    If any Mother can forget this smart,
Her for a woman, I will never take,
And out of London's favor may she part,
And all such brutish strumpets for her sake,              (200)
For such light huswives, I a wish will make,
That never any may approach my City,
Ever to want, and no heart them to pity.

    And now return I to you honest wives—

---

    [3]   *clear.* Fair, bright.

Who grieving fits and sighing send forth Tears—Which to your Husbands
live chaste and true lives
And with your Children, passeth forth your years.
To you that London's Lamentations hears,
And are true partners in my plaints and moans,
Experience shows it by your inward groans.                        (210)
　　　The Child new born, the Mother some deal well—
Are all the griefs and sorrows at an end?
No. Cares and troubles yet I have to tell.
Though Child be swath'd, and sickly Mother mend,
The feeble Infant, many a fret doth send,
Which grieves the Mother, till she weep again,
To hear and see the Infant in such pain.
　　　And with her feeble hand and weakly strength,
She plays and dallies for the baby's good,
And to her milk-white breasts doth lay at length             (220)
The pretty fool, who learns to take his food,
His only means to nourish life and blood.
He fed, she pained, he draws, poor Mother yields,
Whose loving breasts both shoots and prickings feels,
　　　And when the Babe doth gather strength amain,
Most strongly laboring at his mother's dug.
She patiently endureth all the pain,
Suffering his lips her nipple still to lug,
And with her arms most closely doth it hug,
As she should say, "draw child and spare not me;             (230)
My breasts are thine, I feel no pain with thee."
　　　Though that poor heart, her breast doth ache full sore,
And inwardly fell prickings she endures,
Till eyes gush tears, and lips reach kisses store,
Which in true mother's gladsome joys procures,
And to more ardent love them still allures,
That tears and kisses greet the Babe together,
Like to sunshine when it is dropping weather.
　　　Imagine here, the pretty Lamb doth cry,
The Mother strong, and times of Custom[4] pass'd,            (240)
Will she then leave it to the world's broad Eye?
No. Whilst her life and vital powers last,
The Mother's love to Child is fixt so fast,
She stills it straight and lays it to her breast,
With kisses more than VENUS could disgest

---

　　[4]　*times of Custom.* Formal rituals associated with childbirth, such as lying in or
churching.

And with her Arms, she heaves it high and low,
As if a cradle, it, sweet fool, lay in.
Doubt you not too, she kisses did bestow,
And if it smile, afresh she doth begin.
One pretty look, a hundred kisses win.                              (250)
"My more than sweet," unto her Child she saith,
"I would not for a Kingdom wish thy Death."
    Now is her mind full straight with inward joy,
As if all things she thought should come to pass.
Uttering forth Sighs, unto her pretty boy,
"Shall Death have thee, and lay thee in the grass,
I'll rather go to Earth from whence I was.
Fell Death go seek for crooked age and old;
My Child is fair, unfitting for the mould.
    I hope to see more comfort and more joy,                 (260)
Of this sweet Babe, which cost my life almost.
I pray thee, grim Death, do not him annoy.
Go get thee further, to some other Coast.
To kill an Infant gives small cause of boast.
There's many living that would gladly die,
Take them away, but spare my Child and I."
    Chaste LONDON wives, methinks I see you all,
Each several Mother, having griefs to show,
And with your griefs, I see the Tears do fall—
The only Physic women can bestow.                                  (270)
Oh, that I could, but ease your heartsick woe,
LONDON would spare no labor, cost, nor time,
To wipe the water from your blubbered Eyen.
    But I a skillful Surgeon's part will play:
First search the sore, then minister things meet
Unto your memories; I your plaints will lay,[5]
Causing afresh your heavy eyes to greet,
Then gentler salves, I mean persuasions sweet.
This is the surgery wounded LONDON lays
To all her Patients that her [be]hests obeys.                       (280)
    One tender mother cryeth loud and shrill,
Wringing her hands, "My children both are dead:
Sweet loving Henry, and my eldest girl.
Ah Bess, my wench, thou hadst thy mother sped
With sorrows that will never from my head.
Thy forward wit to learning and to awe,
A sweeter daughter never woman saw.

---

   [5]  *Lay.* Allay.

"Thy flaxen hair, thy color red and white,
Thy years full ten, thy body straight and tall,
Thy count'nance smiling, neither sad nor light,    (290)
Thy pleasant eyes, thy hands with fingers small,
Thy manners mild, thy reading best of all,
With needle pregnant, as thy Sampler shows,
Patient in death like sucking Lamb she goes.
 "My hopes were that I might have kept thy life
To see more years and be a beauteous Maid,
To see thee match't and be a LONDON wife,
To see thy child-bed and be safely laid,
To see thy children in the street have playd,
To cheer my age, as should a loving daughter,    (300)
But thou art gone, and I must follow after.
 "My little HENRY, oh, that pretty fool
That oft hath made my sorrowing heart full glad.
His words were 'Mamma, sit. Here is a stool,
Some bread and butter I have nothing had.
I'll busse you well (good Mamma) be not sad,
Up on cock-high, I will sit in your lap,'
Where oft (poor sweeting) he hath caught a nap.
 And if sometimes, he heard his Father chide,
As household word may pass twixt man and wife,    (310)
Unto my Husband, presently he hied
As he should say, 'I will appease the strife,'
And with his Childish mirth and pleasures rife,
Abates the heat and makes us both to joy,
To see such nature in the little Boy.
 "But Death, oh Death, that hater of my wealth
Hath slain my Daughter and my little Son:
Both of them props unto my wished health
Both to have kept I would barefoot have run.
Fell ATROPOS, her fatal stroke hath done.    (320)
With the eternal, I believe they rest,
Oh, happy Babes, forever they are blest."
 Step after Step, I see another come,
Casting her hands abroad, as she were would,
Seeming to tell a heavy tale to some,
But silly Dame, thou art not understood.
Speak mildly, lowly, not with chafing blood,
For hasty speech hath seldom reason shown,
When soft deliverance makes the matter known.
 "I am a Widow poor; Christ show me pity,    (330)
Feeble and weak of years, three score and ten.

I had two Daughters, married in the City,
Both of them well, and unto honest men;
They had my loves, and I had theirs again.
With them I hop't to spend my aged years,
And to be buried with their funeral tears.
 "To them I gave, that little I possest,
With them to dwell, as long as life ensured:
Three Months with one, my Custom was to rest;
Then, with the other, I like space endured.    (340)
With us, the Devil, no jars nor brawls procured,
But lived and lov'd, as quiet as might be.
I bore with them, they daily honoring me.
 "But now alas, a heavy Tale to tell,
As with my Chickens, I at pleasure slept,
Comes the great Puttock, with his Talons fell,
And from me quite, my youngest Chicken swept.
Then to the other, he full nimbly leapt,
Seizing on her, as he had done the other.
Oh greedy Death, could'st thou not take their Mother?  (350)
 "My age is fitter for the yawning Grave;
Their years more tender in the world to stay.
My bones are dry and would their portions have;
Their Limbs were nimble and a while might play.
My blood is cold; theirs hot; mine wears away.
They both were matched and fruit might bring forth store;
I old and withered, and can yield no more.
 "Thou cruel, lean, and ill-deformed Death,
Thou great intruder and unwelcomed guest,
Thou palefac't hog, thou shortner of long breath,   (360)
Thou mighty murdrer of both man and beast,
Why dost thou not invite me to thy feast
And on my body show thy fury great
That lacks house, lodging, sight, and what to eat?!"
 With lamentations and with Tears good store,
Imagine now you hear a Mother's grief.
She most of all her sorrows doth deplore,
Uttering forth words as helpless of relief,
She is depriv'd of all, both less and chief,
As well her Children as her Husband good,    (370)
With laboring servants that did earn their food.
 "Ah my sweet Babes, what would not I have done
To yield you comfort, and maintain you here?
Early and late, no labor would I shun,
To feed your mouths, though hunger pincht me near.

All three at once, I would your bodies cheer.
Twain in my lap, should suck their tender Mother,
And with my foot, I would have rockt the other. [6]
　　"Methinks I see them still and hear their cries,
Chiefly a nights, when I on bed am laid, (380)
Which make fresh tears go from my watry eyes,
When I awake and find I am deceived.
Sweet pretty Babes, Christ hath your souls received.
Fair Babes to me, you nere shall come again,
But where you are, I trust aye to remain.
　　"Your loving father took a great delight,
Often in Arms to have those children small,
And now he hath them ever in his sight:
Not one or two, the heavens possess them all.
Father and Babes obeyed when Christ did call. (390)
They all are gone; I only left with breath,
To bide more sorrows in this wretched earth.
　　"Poor and in want, young widow left am I,
Kindless and friendless, lacking means to live;
Had but my servants stayed, their work to ply,
Their labor would some comfort to me give.
My hopes are like to water poured in sieve.
Only, I trust God will increase my health,
That I may work and hate dishonest wealth."
　　Many more sorrows might I here repeat, (400)
Of grieved Mothers for their children dear,
But times are precious and work too great
For my hoarse voice to show and utter here.
Only, I pray you, listen and give ear
To LONDON'S sorrows, which so many are,
My clacking tongue cannot them half declare.
　　And as with pain I did endure to tell
Your too too heavy and unwelcom'd woes,
Wherein poor LONDON labor'd to do well,
But wanting gifts, the best she can she shows. (410)
The willing mind—that all she hath bestows—
Must needs be reckoned for a friendly part,
Deserving thanks with as cheerful a heart.
　　Excuse me then, and hear me too, a while,
For many sorrows compass me throughout.
Never since BRUTE set footing in this Isle,

---

　　[6] *All three at once.* A reference to the image of Charity as a mother with at least two
and often three children of or near nursing age attempting to nurse.

Nor nere since it was walled round about,
More blessed news nor happy spring could sprout,
Than did to LONDON in this present year,
When England's CAESAR came this City near.　　　　　　(420)
　　　All went askant. Happy that Merchant was
Which had rich wares to please his Chapman's eyes:
The finest shags, wrought stuffs, and purest glass,
Rare cloth of gold, and silks of every dye.
Who, for his money could know where to buy,
Both went and sent to fetch in wares good store,
Not doubting sale for that and three times more.
　　　And as they thought a while it did continue,
Doings waxt quick, and wares apace did sell.
Great men of honors with their retinue　　　　　　(430)
Approach't my City minding here to dwell.
Houses and Chambers were let dear and well.
There was no corner in me did remain,
But the true Owner might employ to gain,
　　　With ICARUS, I soaring then aloft,
Bathing my limbs in heat of highest sun,
Till waxen wings with melting heat were soft,
And had no power me from the waves to shun.
Down must I fall, my glory quite undone.
He sits above that looketh down below,　　　　　　(440)
Commanding powers, his justice here to show.
　　　And with King DAVID'S chance[7] doth me correct,
Spreading his Plague, where pleaseth him to strike,
Because in health his laws I did reject,
Trusting in means, in man, in horse, and pike,
Boasting of riches, beauty, and such like,
Never redeeming of swift passing times,
But still committing new and ugly crimes.
　　　And, to the end, none dwelling in my City
Should think themselves more safer than the rest,　　　　　　(450)
Judging their slights, and not God's lasting pity,
To be the cause why they with health are blest.
God's judgment upon all degrees are prest,
From poorest beggar to the wealthiest Squire,
From youngest infant to the oldest Sire.
　　　For if the aged people he should spare,

---

[7]　*King David's chance.* Likely a reference the biblical King David's choice that resulted in punishment by plague instead of war or famine (1 Chronicles 7–14 and 2 Samuel 24.13–15).

They would attribute to themselves too much,
And say their bloods are dry, their bones so bare,
The Pestilence their bodies cannot touch.
If middle age should scape, their wits are such,                    (460)
That through their diet or by letting blood,
They won the victory and the Plague withstood.
    The frolic youths would judge the strengths the mean,
Boasting of joints, arms, legs and sinews strong.
The little infant being weak and lean,
Wants substance for the Plague to work upon.
These are excuses, but effects have none.
God's Messenger (the Plague) doth fear no States,
But strikes both lowest and the highest Mates.
    Now, for the rich which have of gold such store,                    (470)
Feeding their bodies with delicious fare,
Keeping great fires, stir not out of door,
Using perfumes, shunning infected air.
Shall they escape? No, the Plague will them not spare,
Because they shall not think their heaped treasure
Can keep them longer than it is God's pleasure.
    If rich men die, and poorer people stay,
They will exclaim with hate and deadly ire,
Saying with surfeits they consume the day,
Wallowing in ease like dirty Swine in mire,                    (480)
Judging their scarcity and their thin attire
The only Physic, poisons to withstand,
But they like others have given death their hand.
    If any then should scape death's heavy sight,
And claim a pardon for a longer day,
The zealous Preacher and the godly wight,
Which for themselves, and for their hearts pray,
Might have some favor in this world to stay.
But God saith, "No, they shall yield to their kind,
Lest they prove haughty which remain behind."                    (490)
    There are a people that do lewdly live,
Swaggering and swearing, prone to every sin.
Shall those men scape? No, they account shall give
Of all the vices they have wallowed in.
Such wretched Caitiffs made the Lord begin,
To strike poor LONDON with thy heavy rod,
For pleasing Satan and offending God.
    What should I say? My sorrows are so many,
One for a thousand, I cannot repeat.
Within my liberties, scarce any,                    (500)

Which have not felt God's wrath and mighty threat,
Either by death or sickness fell and great.
If Parents scap'd, the children had their part.
If both remain, their servants felt some smart.
    The sick bequeather of his wealth by Will,
Not only dead, but his executors too,
And eke the Scrivener that did make the Bill,
All in one fortnight have paid death their due.
The like unto the Landlord doth ensue:
Both wealthy father and succeeding heir,           (510)
With their poor tenants, ended have their care.
    The joyful Bridegroom married as today,
Sick, weak, and feeble before table laid,
And the next morrow dead and wrap't in clay,
Leaving his Bride, a widow, wife, and maid.
Which sudden change doth make her so dismayed,
That griefs and sorrows doth perplex her heart.
Within three days she takes her husband's part.
    Much might I speak of other sad laments,
And fill your ears with new and several woes,       (520)
Spending a week, repeating discontents,
Which needless is, where all both sees and knows
How many thousands death and graves enclose,
Making me (LONDON) which long time hath flourish't
Scorned of those which I both fed and nourish't.
    And those that have my glory most set forth,
Boasting that I for beauty did excel,
Now to approach unto me are so loath,
As if my presence were a swallowing hell.
Within their houses they refuse to dwell,         (530)
And to the Country fly like swarms of Bees,
Where wealth and credit many of them lease.
    But most of all my sorrowing heart doth grieve,
For such as work and take exceeding care,
And by their labor know not how to live,
Going poor souls in garments thin and bare,
The belly hungry, of flesh lean and spare,
Pawning and selling clothes, and what they have,
To feed their children which for food do crave.
    And when poor hearts their hunger once is stayed,    (540)
The day ensuing brings the like distress:
The painful Parents working all their trade
For new supply, fell famine to suppress,
But all in vain their woes are nere the less.

Their work being made, abroad poor souls they trot,
From Morn to Noon, from Noon to Night, God wot[8],
 Offering their wares, and what they have to sell,
Unto such Tradesmen as have small pity,
But they like NABAL'S, will not with them mell,
Unless for half the worth they may it buy.      (550)
The rich man laughs; the poor in heart doth cry,
Shedding forth tears in sorrow to his wife,
"This world doth make me weary of my life."
 The Wife doth weep; the needy servants play;[9]
The Children cry for food where none is bought.
The Father saith, "I cannot sell today,
One jot of work that all of us have wrought.
In every shop, I have for money sought,
And can take none, your hunger to sustain."
Tears part from him; the Children cry amain.     (560)
 "What shall we do?" A counsel straight they take.
"Meat must be had; our people must not starve.
Wife, take such things and go without a loate.[10]
In HOUNDSDITCH, pawn them, our great need to serve.
They will make sure, if that a day we swerve,
All will be lost: our garments are their own,
Though for a pound we give a shilling loan.
 Besides the Bill, a polling groat will cost,
And every Month our pawn must be renew'd,
So was my Lease to griping usury lost,      (570)
The first beginner of my sorrows brew'd,
And ever since want upon want ensued.
My bedding forfeit for a thing of naught,
My brass and Pewter, want of conscience bought.
 If now our clothes which clad our naked skin,
Should thus be lost, as was our other good,
Alas, poor Wife, what case are we then in?
Such shamefast Beggars never asked food,
If honest labor could this grief withstood;
We would have reckoned day and night as one,    (580)
To work for meat, rather than make such moan."
 O you of LONDON, now hear LONDON speak,
Especially you Magistrates of might,
And wealthy Citizens, whose store is great.

---

8 *God wot.* God knows.
9 *Play.* Occupy oneself, in this case with work.
10 *Loate.* Unidentified term.

I gently woo you to have good foresight,
And cast your eyes upon the needy wight,
Though fear of sickness drive you hence as men,
Yet leave your purse and feeling heart with them.
　　　Remember all your riches are but lent,
Though in this world, you bear such power and sway.          (590)
Remember too how soon your years are spent.
Remember eke your bodies are but clay.
Remember death that rangeth at this day.
Remember when poor Lazar's woes did end:
The full fed glutton, to hell, did descend.
　　　Remember rulers, of each public charge,
The several branches of your private oath.[11]
Remember, them that use a conscience large
And on themselves the needy's stock bestow'th,
He robs his God and his poor neighbors both.          (600)
He that grants blessings to the poor, that lends,
Gives treble cursings to those it misspends.
　　　Remember likewise, God hath plac't you here
To be as nursing fathers to the poor.
Let then your kindness, now to them appear.
Give much and be no niggards of your store.
God in his wisdom gave it you therefore.
Put forth your talents, and gain ten for five,
so shall you in the heavenly City thrive.
　　　One other boon doth mournful LONDON crave,          (610)
Of you on whom her weal and woes depend.
When in the senate house with counsel grave,
You sit debating causes how to end,
Make some decree, poor working trades to mend.
At least set down some order for their good,
That each man may with labor earn his food.
　　　Restrain the number of devouring drones,
That sucks the honey, from the laboring bees,
Catching by piece-meal, in their bribes and loans,
Men's whole estates, which are of poor degrees,          (620)
And brings them quickly, on their naked knees.
Four groats a month for twenty shillings lent,
Is like winds, tempest, till the house be rent.[12]
　　　The number, numberless, of houses vain,
Which beer and ale, forsooth make show to sell,

---

[11]　*oath.* Civic leaders took oaths upon assumption of duties.
[12]　*Rent* Torn to pieces.

Under which color[13] doth such vices rain,
My cheek doth glow, my tongue refrains to tell,
Offending God, and pleasing Satan well.
Like wicked SODOM doth my Suburbs lie,
A mighty blemish to fair LONDON'S eye.                    (630)
    Reform these things, you heads of LONDON City.
Punish lewd vice; let virtue spring and grow.
Then God's just wrath, now hot, will turn to pity,
And for his children, you again do know,
Your former health on you he will bestow.
The Plague and Pestilence, wherewith he visits still,
To end or send are in his holy will.
    You see the runner in his race is tript:
Well when he went, dead ere his journey's done.
You see how sudden beauty's blaze is nipt,                (640)
Which sought all means, death's danger for to shun.
You hear what success follow them that run:
Most true report doth tell us where and how
The Country's plague exceeds the City's now.
    Sith then it resteth in God's mighty power,
Who, when he please, can bid his Angel stay,
Or, if he will, destroy you in an hour,
A thousand years being with him as one day,
Why should you not to him for mercy pray,
Desiring pardon, with a contrite heart,                  (650)
And from your former wickedness depart?
    If this you will incontinently do,
The Lord in pity will his judgments cease,
And many blessings will he pour on you:
Health and long life, honor and happy peace;
Your Foes shall quail; your friends shall still increase;
Your Wives shall flourish like a fruitful Vine;
Your Children prosper, and your griefs decline;
    Your Terms shall hold; your men of Worth shall stay;
Your Merchants, traffic and great riches, gain;          (660)
Your Tradesmen's sorrows shall be done away;
True loyal servants shall with them remain;
Your Artisans shall never more complain;
Their honest labor so shall thrive and speed,
That they shall give to others that have need.
    And I, that long have been a loathed Dame,
Shall frolic then with mirth and inward glee.

---

[13]   *Under which color.* Under pretext or pretence of.

"Renownd Lady" now must be my name.
O famous LONDON, who is like to thee?
Thy God is serv'd by men of each degree,                    (670)
Thy Churches filled, thy Preachers burn with zeal,
Thy glory shines, O blessed Common-weal.
    My crowned CAESAR and his Peerless Queen,
Comes now triumphing with their princely son,
Deckt with rich robes the like was never seen,
Nor never none more welcome to LONDON.
Methinks I see the people how they run,
To get them room this happy sight to see.
That this may come, say all, "Amen," with me.
FINIS

\*

# Thomas Dekker and Thomas Middleton, *News from Graves-end*

The following libraries house the only edition of this poem from 1604 (STC 2nd ed., 12199): the Bodleian Library; University of Oxford; Harvard University Library; and the Henry E. Huntington Library and Art Gallery. Preceding the poem is a prose epistle to "Sir Nicolas Nemo, alias Nobody," the same Nobody mentioned in the poem's full title below.

NEWS
from Graves-end,
Sent to *Nobody*.
Nec Quidquam nec Cuiquam.[1]


LONDON
Printed by T[homas] C[reed] for Thomas Archer,
and are to be sold at the long Shop
under S. Mildred's Church in the Poultry
1604


    To Sickness and to Queasy Times,
We drink a health in wholesome Rhymes.
Physic, we invoke thy aid,
Thou (that born in heaven) art made
A lackey to the meanest creature,
Mother of health, thou nurse of nature,
Equal friend to rich and poor,
At whose hands, Kings can get no more
Than empty Beggars—O thou, wise
In nothing but in Mysteries!                                    (10)
Thou that hast of earth the rule,
Where (like an *Academy* or School);
Thou readst deep Lectures to thy sons,
(Men's *Demi-gods*) Physicians,
Who thereby learn the abstruse powers
Of Herbs, of Roots, of Plants, of Flowers,
And suck from poisonous stinking weed
Preservatives, man's life to feed;
Thou nearest to a God (for none
Can work it but a God alone),                                   (20)
O grave *Enchantress*, deign to breath
Thy Spells into us and bequeath
Thy sacred fires, that they may shine
In quick and virtual medicine.
Arm us to convince this Foe,
This King of dead men, conquering so,
This hungry Plague, Cater to death,
Who eats up all, yet famisheth.
Teach us how we may repair
These Ruins of the rotten Air,                                  (30)
Or if the Air's pollution can

---

[1]    *Nec Quidquam nec Cuiquam.* Nothing dedicated to nobody.

So mortal strike through beast and man,
Or if in blood, corrupt Death lie,
Or if one dead, cause others die,
Howere thy sovereign cures disperse,
And with that glory crown our verse,
That we may yet save many a soul
(Perchance now merry at his Bowl)
That ere our Tragic Song be done,
Must drink this thick Contagion.                              (40)
        But (oh grief) why do we accite
The charms of Physic, whose numb'd sprite
Now quakes, and nothing dare or can,
Checked by a more dread Magician?
Sick is Physic's self to see
Her *Aphorisms* prov'd a mockery,
For whilst she's turning o're her books,
And on her drugs and simples looks,
She's run through her own armed heart
(Th'infection flying above Art).                              (50)
        Come, therefore, thou the best of Nine,
(Because the Saddest)² every line
That drops from *Sorrow's* pen is due
Only to thee, to thee we sue.
Thou Tragic Maid, whose Fury's spent
In dismal and most black Ostent,
In Uproars, and in Fall of Kings,
Thou of Empire's change that sings,
Of Dearths, of Wars, of Plagues—and laughs
At Funerals and Epitaphs—                                     (60)
Carouse thou to our thirsty soul
A full draught from the *Thespian* bowl,
That we may pour it out again,
And drink, in numbers, Juice to men,
Striking such horrors through their ears
Their hair may upright stand with fears,
Till rich Heirs meeting our strong verse
May not shrink back before it pierce
Their marble eyeballs and there shed
One drop (at least) for him that's dead,                      (70)
To work which wonder, we will write
With Pens pulled from that bird of night

---

² *thou ... Saddest.* The nine muses of Greek mythology, the "best" here being Melpomene, the muse of Tragedy.

(The shrieking Owl); our Ink we'll mix
With tears of widows (black as Styx);
The paper where our lines shall meet,
Shall be a folded winding sheet;
And that the Scene may show more full,
The Standish is a dead man's skull.
Inspire us therefore how to tell
The *Horror* of a *Plague*, the *Hell*.                    (80)

## The Cause of the Plague

Nor drops this venom from that fair
And crystal bosom of the Air,
Whose ceaseless motion clarifies
All vaporous stench that upward flies
And with her universal wings,
Thick poisonous fumes abroad she flings,
Till (like to Thunder) rudely tosst,
Their malice is (by spreading) lost.
Yet must we grant that from the veins
Of Rottenness and Filth that reigns,                    (90)
O're heaps of bodies, slain in war,
From Carrion (that endangers far),
From standing Pools or from the wombs
Of Vaults, of Muckhills, Graves, and Tombs,
From Bogs, from rank and dampish Fens,
From Moorish breaths and nasty Dens,
The Sun draws up contagious Fumes,
Which falling down burst into Rheums,
And thousand maladies beside,
By which our blood grows putrefied.                    (100)
Or, being by winds not swept from thence,
They hover there in clouds condense,
Which suckt in by our spirits, there flies
Swift poison through our Arteries,
And (not resisted) straight it chokes
The heart with those pestiferous smokes.
Thus, Physic and Philosophy
Do preach, and (with this) Salves apply,
Which search and use with speed. But, now,
This monster breeds not thus, for how                    (110)
(If this be prov'd) can any doubt
But that the Air does (round about)
In flakes of poison drop on all,

The Sore being spread so general?
Nor dare we so conclude, for then
Fruits, Fishes, Fowl, nor Beasts, nor Men
Should scape untainted; Grazing flocks
Would feed upon their graves; the Ox
Drop at the plough; the traveling Horse
Would for a Rider bear a Coarse;                         (120)
Th'ambitious Lark (the Bird of state)[3]
Whose wings do sweep heaven's pearled gate,
As she descended (*Then*) would bring,
Pestilent News under each wing.
Then Rivers would drink poison'd air,
Trees shed their green and curled hair,
Fish swim to shore, full of disease,
(For Pestilence would Fin the seas),
And we should think their scaly barks,
Having small speckles, had the marks.                   (130)
No soul could move. But, sure there lies
Some vengeance more than in the skies,
Nor (as a Taper at whose beams
Ten thousands lights fetch golden streams,
And yet itself is burnt to death)
Can we believe that one man's breath,
Infected and being blown from him,
His poison should to others swim,
For then who breath'd upon the first?
Where did th'embulked venom burst?                      (140)
Or how scapte those that did divide
The selfsame bits with those that died,
Drunk of the selfsame cups, and lay
In Ulcerous beds, as close as they?
Or those, who every hour (like Crows)
Prey on dead carcasses, their nose
Still smelling to a grave, their feet
Still wrapt within a dead man's sheet!
Yet (the sad execution done)
Careless among their Cans they run,                     (150)
And there (in scorn of Death or Fate)
Of the deceast they widely prate,
Yet snore untoucht and next day rise
To act in more new Tragedies,

---

[3]  *Th'ambitious ... of state.* The lark sings as is rises aloft, attributed with dignity, of high estate.

Or (like so many bullets flying)
A thousand here and there being dying,
Death's Text-bill clapt on every door,
Crosses on sides, behind, before,
Yet he (i'th midst) stands fast. From whence
Comes this? You'll say, "From *Providence*."        (160)
'Tis so, and that's the common Spell
That leads our Ignorance (blind as hell)
And serves but as excuse to keep
The soul from search of things more deep.
No, no, this black and burning star
(Whose sulfured drops do scald so far)
Does neither hover o're our heads,
Nor lies it in our bloods nor beds,
Nor is it stitcht to our attires,
Nor like wild balls of running fires,        (170)
Or thunderbolts, which where they light
Do either bruise or kill outright,
Yet by the violence of that Bound,
Leap off and gives a second wound.
    But this fierce dragon (huge and foul)
Sucks virid poison from our soul,
Which being spit forth again, there reigns
Showers of Blisters and of Blains,
For every man within him feeds
A worm which this contagion breeds.        (180)
Our heavenly parts are plaguey sick,
And, there, such leprous spots do stick,
That God in anger fills his hand
With Vengeance, throwing it on the land.
Sure 'tis some capital offence,
Some high, high Treason doth incense
Th'Eternal King that thus we are
Arraign'd at Death's most dreadful bar,
Th'Inditement writ on England's breast,
When other Countries (better blest)        (190)
Feel not the Judge's heavy doom,
Whose breath (like Lightning doth consume)
And (with a whip of Planets) scourges
The Veins of mortals, in whom, Surges
Of sinful blood, Billows of Lust,
Stir up the powers to acts unjust.
Whether they be Princes' Errors
Or faults of Peers, pull down these Terrors,

Or (because we may not err)
Let's sift it in particular,                                    (200)
The Courtier's pride, lust, and excess;
The Churchman's painted holiness;
The Lawyer's grinding of the poor;
The Soldier's starving at the door,
Ragged, lean, and pale through want of blood,
Sold cheap by him for Country's good;
The Scholar's envy; Farmer's curse,
When heav'ns rich Treasurer doth disburse
In bounteous heaps (to thankless men)
His universal Blessings—then,                                  (210)
This delving Mole for madness eats
Even his own lungs and strange oaths sweats,
Because he cannot sell for pence
Dear years, in spite of *Providence.*
Add unto these the City['s] sin
(Brought by seven deadly monsters in)
Which doth all bounds and blushing scorn,
Because 'tis in the Freedom born.
What Trains of Vice (which even Hell hates)
But have bold passage through her gates?                       (220)
Pride in Diet, Pride in Clothing,
Pride in Building, pure in nothing,
And, that she may not want[4] disease,
She sails for it beyond the Seas:
With *Antwerp,* will she drink up *Rhine*;
With *Paris,* act the bloodiest Scene;
Or in pied fashions pass her folly,
Mocking at heaven, yet look most holy.
Of Usury she'll rob the Jews;
Of Luxury, *Venetian* Stews;                                   (230)
With Spaniards, she's an Indianist;
With barbarous Turks, a Sodomist.
So low her Antique walls do stand,
These sins leap o're even with one hand,
And He, that all in modest black,
Whose Eyeball strings shall sooner crack,
Than seem to note a tempting face,
Measuring streets with a Dove-like pace,
Under that oily vizard wears,
The poor man's sweat and Orphan's tears.                       (240)

---

[4]   *Want.* Lack.

Now, whether these particular Fates
Or general Moles (disfiguring States),
Whether one sin alone, or whether
This Main Battalion joined together,
Do dare these plagues, we cannot tell,
But down they beat all human Spell.[5]
Or, it may be, *Jehovah* looks
But now upon those Audit Books
Of forty-five years' husht account,[6]
For hours misspent (whose sums surmount          (250)
The price of ransomed Kings), and there
Finding our grievous debts, doth clear
And cross them under his own hand,
Being paid with *Lives* through all the land.
For since his Maiden Servant's gone,
And his new Viceroy fills the Throne,[7]
Heaven means to give him (as his bride)
A Nation new and purified.

    Take breath a while our panting Muse,
And to the world tell gladder news,          (260)
Than these of Burials; strive a while
To make thy sullen numbers smile.
Forget the names of Graves and Ghosts,
The sound of bells, the unknown coasts
Of Death's vast Kingdom, and sail o're
With fresher wind to happier Shore.
For now the maiden Isle hath got
A Royal Husband (heavenly *Lot*)
Fair *Scotland* does fair *England* wed,
And gives her for her maidenhead,          (270)
A crown of gold, wrought in a Ring,
With which *She's* married to a King.
Thou Beldame (whisperer of false Rumors)
Fame, cast aside those Antique humors.
Lift up thy golden Trump, and sound
Even from *Tweed's* utmost crystal bound,
And from the banks of Silver Thames
To the green Ocean, that King *James*
Had made an Island that did stand
(Half sinking) now the firmest land.          (280)

---

5   *Spell*. Discourse; tale.
6   *45 years*. Since 1558, when Queen Elizabeth I came to the throne.
7   *Maiden Servant's ... Viceroy*. Queen Elizabeth I followed by King James VI and I.

Carry thou this to *Neptune's* ear,
That his shrill Tritons it may bear
So far, until the Danish sound
With repercussive voice rebound,
That *Echoes* (doubling more and more)
May reach the parched Indian shore,
For 'tis heav'ns care so great a wonder,
Should fly upon the wings of Thunder.

## The Horror of the Plague

O Thou, my Country, here mine eyes
Are almost sunk in waves that rise                       (290)
From the rough wind of Sighs to see
A spring that lately courted thee
In pompous bravery, all thy Bowers,
Gilt by the Sun, perfumed with flowers,
Now like a loathsome Leper lying,
Her arbors withering, green Trees dying,
Her Revels and May-merriments,
Turned all to Tragic drearyments,
And thou (the mother of my breath)[8]
Whose soft breast thousands nourisheth,                  (300)
Altar of *Jove*, thou throne of Kings,
Thou Font, where milk and honey springs,
Europe's Jewel, England's Gem,
Sister to great *Jerusalem,*
*Neptune's* minion, 'bout whose waist
The Thames is like a girdle cast,
Thou that (but health) canst nothing want,
Empress of Cities, *Troynovant*—
When I thy lofty Towers behold,
(Whose Pinnacles were tipt with gold                     (310)
Both when the Sun did set and rise
So lovely wert thou in his eyes)
Now like old Monuments forsaken,
Or (like tall Pines) by winter shaken,
Or seeing thee gorgeous as a bride,
Even in the height of all thy pride,
Disrob'd, disgraced, and when all Nations
Made love to thee in amorous passions,

---

8     [marginal note] *Apostrophe ad Civitatem.* [An apostrophe on citizenship, on being a member of a community.]

Now scorned of all the world alone,
None seek thee, nor must thou seek none,                    (320)
But like a prisoner must be kept
In thine own walls, till thou hast wept
Thine eyes out to behold thy sweet,
Dead children heapt about thy feet.
    O Dearest! say, how can we choose
But have a sad and drooping Muse,
When Corpses do so choke thy way
That now thou lookst like *Golgotha*,
But, thus, the altring of a State
Alters our Bodies and our Fate,                             (330)
For Princes' deaths do even bespeak
Millions of lives; when Kingdoms break,
People dissolve, and (as with Thunder)
Cities' proud glories rent asunder.
Witness thy walls, whose stony arms
But yesterday receiv'd whole swarms
Of freighted English: Lord and Lowne,
Lawyer and Client, Courtier, Clown—
All sorts did to thy buildings fly,
As to the safest Sanctuary.                                 (340)
And he that through thy gates might pass,
His fears were lockt in Towers of brass.
Happy that man, now happier they,
That from thy reach get first away,
As from a shipwreck, to some shore;
As from a lost field, drowned in gore;
As from high Turrets, whose Joints fail;
Or rather from some loathsome Jail.
But note heav'ns Justice: they by flying,
That would cozen Death and save a dying,                    (350)
How like to chaff abroad th'are blown,
And (but for scorn) might walk unknown.
Like to plumed Ostriches they ride,
Or like Sea-pageants all in pride
Of Tacklings, Flags, and swelling Sails,
Borne on the loftiest wave, that vails
His purple bonnet and, in dread,
Bows down his snowy curled head—
So from th'infected city fly
These Swallows in their Gallantry,                          (360)
Looking that wheresoe're they light,
Gay Summer (like a Parasite)

Should wait on them, and build'em bowers,
And crown their nests with wreathed flowers,
And Swains to welcome them should sing
And dance, as for their Whitsun King.
Feather of Pride, how art thou tost?
How soon are all thy beauties lost?
How easily golden hopes un-wind?
The russet boar, and leathern hind,                (370)
That two days since did sink his knee,
And (all uncovered) worshipt thee,
Or being but poor and meanly clothed,
Was either laught to scorn or loathed;
Now thee he loathes and laughs to scorn,
And though upon thy back be worn
More Satin than a kingdom's worth,
He bars his door and thrusts thee forth.
And they whose palate Land nor Seas,
Whom fashions of no shape could please,                (380)
Whom Princes have (in ages past)
For rich attires and sumptuous wast[e],
Never come near—now sit they round
And feed (like beggars) on the ground,
A field their bed, whose dankish Sheets
Is the green grass, and he that meets
The flattringest Fortune does but lie
In some rude barn or loathsome sty,
Forsook of all, flouted, forlorn.
Own brother does own brother scorn;                (390)
The trembling Father is undone,
Being once but breath'd on by his son.
Or if in this sad pilgrimage
The hand of vengeance fall in rage,
So heavy upon any's head
Striking the sinful body dead,
O shame to ages yet to come!
Dishonor to all Christendom!
In hallowed ground, no heaped gold
Can buy a grave; nor, linen sold                (400)
To make (so far is pity fled)
The last apparel for the dead,
But, as the fashion is, for those
Whose desperate hands the knot unloose
Of their own lives. In some highway
Or barren field, their bones they lay,

Even such his burial is, and there
Without the balm of any tear,
Or pomp of Soldiers, but (oh grief!)
Dragged like a Traitor or some thief                          (410)
At horses' tails, he's rudely thrown,
The corpse being stuck with flowers by none,
No bells (the dead man's Comfort) playing,
Nor any holy Churchman saying
A Funeral Dirge, but swift th'are gone,
As from some noisome carrion.
      O desolate City! now thy wings
(Whose shadow hath been lov'd by Kings)
Should feel sick feathers on each side,
Seeing thus thy sons (got in their pride)                     (420)
And heat of plenty, in peace born,
To their own Nation, left a scorn.
Each cowherd fears a Ghost him haunts,
Seeing one of thine inhabitants,
And does a Jew or Turk prefer,
Before that name of Londoner.
Would this were all, but this black Curse,
Doing ill abroad, at home does worse,
For in thy (now dispeopled) streets,
The dead with dead so thickly meets,                          (430)
As if some Prophet's voice should say
"None shall be Citizens, but they."
Whole households and whole streets are stricken.
The sick do die; the sound do sicken,
And "Lord have mercy upon us," crying.
Ere Mercy can come forth, th'are dying.
No music now is heard but bells,
And all their tunes are sick men's knells,
And every stroke the bell does toll,
Up to heaven it winds a soul.                                 (440)
Oh, if for every corpse that's laid
In his cold bed of earth were made
A chime of bells; if peals should ring
For everyone whom death doth sting,
Men should be deaf, as those that dwell
By *Nylus'* fall, but now one Knell,
Gives with his Iron voice this doom,
That twenty shall but have one room.
There, friend and foe, the young and old,
The freezing coward and the bold,                             (450)

Servant and master, Foul and fair—
One Livery wear and fellows are,
Sailing along in this black fleet
And at the New *Graves-end* do meet;
Where Churchyards banquet with cold cheer,
Holding a feast once in ten year,
To which comes many a Pilgrim worm,
Hungry and faint, beat with the storm
Of galping *Famine*, which before
Only pickt bones and had no more.                              (460)
But now their messes come so fast,
They know not where or which to taste,
For before "Dust to Dust" be spoken,
And thrown on One, more Graves be broken.
    Thou, Jealous man, I pity thee,
Thou that liv'st in hell to see
A wanton's eye cheapening the sleek
Soft Jewels of thy fair wife's cheek.
My verse must run through thy cold heart:
Thy wife has played the woman's part,                          (470)
And lyen with Death, but (spite on spite)
Thou must endure this very night
Close by her side the poorest Groom,
In selfsame bed and selfsame room.
But ease thy vext soul; thus, behold:
There's one, who in the morn with gold
Could have built Castles; now he's made
A pillow to a wretch that prayed
For half-penny Alms (with broken limb);
The Beggar now is above him.                                   (480)
So he that yesterday was clad
In purple robes and hourly had
Even at his fingers' beck, the fees
Of bared heads and bending knees,
Rich men's fawnings, poor men's prayers
(Though they were but hollow airs)
Troops of servants at his calling,
Children (like to subjects) falling
At his proud feet—lo (now he's taken
By death) he lies of all forsaken.                             (490)
  These are the Tragedies, whose sight
With tears blot all the lines we write.
The Stage whereon the Scenes are played
Is a whole Kingdom, who was made

By some (most provident and wise)
To hide from sad Spectators' eyes
Acts full of Ruth, a private Room
To drown the horror of death's doom.
That building, now, no higher rear;
The *Pest-House* standeth everywhere,[9]          (500)
For those that on their Biers are born,
Are numbered more than those that mourn.
    But you grave *Patriots*, whom *Fate*
Makes Rulers of this walled State,
We must not lose you in our verse,
Whose Acts we one day may rehearse
In marble numbers that shall stand
Above *Time's* all-destroying hand.
Only (methinks), you do err
In flying from your charge so far.          (510)
So coward Captains shrink away,
So Shepherds do their flocks betray,
So Soldiers and so Lambs do perish,
So you kill those, y'are bound to cherish.
Be therefore valiant, as y'are wise.
Come back again; the man that dies
Within your walls is even as near
To heav'n as dying anywhere.
But if (oh pardon our bold thought)
You fear your breath is sooner caught          (520)
Here than aloof and, therefore, keep
Out of Death's reach, whilst thousands weep
And wring their hands for thousands dying,
No comfort near the sick man lying,
—'Tis to be fear'd (you petty-kings),
When back you spread your golden wings,
A deadlier siege (which heaven avert)
Will your replenisht walls engirt.
'Tis now the Beggar's plague, for none
Are in this Battle overthrown          (530)
But Babes and poor; the lesser Fly
Now in this Spider's web doth lie.
But if that great and goodly swarm
(That has broke through, and felt no harm)
In his envenom'd snares should fall,
O pity! 'twere most tragical,

---

[9]   [marginal note] Pest-house.

For then the Usurer must behold
His pestilent flesh, whilst all his gold
Turns into Tokens, and the chest
(They lie in), his infection's breast.                                    (540)
How well he'll play the Miser's part
When all his coin sticks at his heart?
He's worth so many farthings then,
That was a golden God mongst men.
And 'tis the aptest death (so please
Him that breath[ed] heaven, earth, and Seas)
For every covetous, rooting Mole
That heaves his dross above his soul,
And doth in coin all hopes repose
To die with corpse stampt full of those.                                    (550)
        Then the rich Glutton, whose swollen eyne
Look fiery red (being boiled in wine)
And in his meals adores the cup,
(For when he falls down, that stands up;
Therefore a goblet is his Saint,
To whom he kneels with small constraint.
When his own goblet Skull flows o're,
He worships *Bacchus* on all four,
For none's his God but *Bacchus* then,
Who rules and guides all drunken men)                                    (560)
When He shall wake from wine and view
More than Tavern-tokens new
Stampt upon his breast and arms,
In horrid throngs and purple swarms,
Then will he loathe his former shapes,
When he shall see blue marks mock grapes,
And hang on clusters on each vein,
Like to wine-bubbles, or the grain
Of staggering sin, which now appears
In the December of his years,                                    (570)
His last of hours, when he'll scarce have
Time to go sober to his Grave,
And then to die! (dreadful to think!)
When all his blood is turned to drink,
And who knows not this Sentence given,
Mongst all sins, none can reel to Heaven?
But woe to him that sinks in wine,
And dies so (without heav'd up eyne)[10]

---

[10]   *Without ... eyne.* Without looking up to heaven.

And buried so! O loathsome trench!
His grave is like a Tavern bench.                                    (580)
'Tis fearful and most hard to say,
How he shall stand at latter day.
      The adulterous and luxurious spirit,
Pawned to hell and sins hot merit,
That bathes in lust his leprous soul,
Acting a deed without control
Or thought of Deity, through whose blood,
Runs part of the Infernal flood—
How will he freeze with horror lying
In dreadful trance before his dying,                                 (590)
The heat of all his damned desires
Cold with the thought of gnashing fires?
His Riots ravisht all his pleasures,
His marrow wasted with his treasures,
His painted harlots (whose embraces
Cost him many silver faces,
Whose only care and thought was then
To keep them sure from other men)—
Now they dance in Ruffian's hands,
Lazy Lieutenants (without bands)                                     (600)
With muffled half-fac'd Panders, laughing;
Whilst he lies gasping, they sit quaffing,
Smile at this plague and black mischance,
Knowing their death's come o're from *France*.
'Tis not their season now to die,
Two gnawing poisons cannot lie,
In one corrupted flesh together;
Nor can this poison then fly thither.
There's not a Strumpet 'mongst them all,
That lives and rises by the fall,                                    (610)
Dreads this contagion or her threats,
Being guarded with French Amulets.[11]
Yet all this while, thyself liest panting,
Thy Luxurious hours recanting,
Whilst before thy face appears
Th'adulterous fruit of all thy years
In their true form and horrid shapes,
So many Incests, violent Rapes,
Chambered adulteries, unclean passions,

---

[11]   *Strumpet ... Amulets.* No prostitute fears contracting plague, because they all already have syphilis.

Wanton habits, riotous fashions,                                  (620)
And all these Antics drest in hell,
To dance about the passing bell,
And clip thee round about the bed,
Whilst thousand Horrors grasp thy head.

## The Cure of the Plague

And therefore this infectious season
That now arrests the Flesh for Treason
Against heaven's everlasting King,
Anointed with th'eternal spring
(Of life and power) this stroke of Force,
That turns the world into a Coarse,                               (630)
Feeding the Dust with what it craves,
Emptying whole houses to fill graves,
These speckled Plagues (which our sins levy)
Are as needful as th'are heavy,
Whose cures to cite, our Muse forbears,
Though he, the *Daphnean* wreath that wears
(Being both Poesy's Sovereign King,
And God of medicine)[12] bids us sing
As boldly of those policies,
Those Onsets, and those Batteries,                                (640)
By Physic cunningly applied,
To beat down Plagues (so fortified)
And of those Arms defensive,
To keep th'assaulted Heart alive,
And of those wards and of those slights,
Used in these mortal single fights,
As of the causes that commence
This civil war of Pestilence.
For Poets' souls should be confined
Within no bounds; their towering minds                            (650)
Must (like the Sun) a progress make
Through Art's immensive Zodiac,
And suck (like Bees) the virtuous power,
That flows in learning's seven-fold flower,[13]
Distilling forth the same again
In sweet and wholesome Juice to men.
But for we see the Army great
Of those whose charge it is to beat

---

[12]  *he ... medicine.* Apollo, god of music, poetry, war, medicine, and plague.
[13]  *learning's seven-fold flower.* The seven liberal arts.

This proud Invader and have skill
In all those weapons that do kill (660)
Such pestilent foes, we yield to them
The glory of that stratagem,
To whose Oraculous voice repair,
For they those Delphic Prophets are,
That teach dead bodies to respire
By sacred Aesculapian fire.
We mean not those pied Lunatics,
Those bold fantastic Empirics,
Quack-salvers, mishrump Mountebanks,
That in one night grow up in ranks (670)
And live by pecking Physic's crumbs.
O, hate these venomous broods; there comes
Worse sores from them, and more strange births,
Than from ten plagues or twenty deaths.
   Only this Antidote apply,
Cease vexing heaven, and cease to die.[14]
Seek therefore (after you have found
Salve natural for the natural wound
Of this Contagion) Cure from thence
Where first the evil did commence, (680)
And that's the Soul: each one purge one,
And *England's* free, the Plague is gone.

## The Necessity of a Plague

Yet to mix comfortable words—
Though this be horrid, it affords
Sober gladness, and wise joys,
Since desperate mixtures it destroys,
For if our thoughts sit truly trying,
The just necessity of dying
How needful (though how dreadful) are
Purple Plagues or Crimson war. (690)
We would conclude (still urging pity)
A Plague's the Purge to cleanse a City.
Who amongst millions can deny
(In roughprose or smooth Poesy)
Of Evils, 'tis the lighter brood—
A dearth of people, than of food!
And who knows not, our Land ran o're
With people and was only poor

---

[14] [marginal note] *The cure.*

In having too too many, living—
And, wanting living, rather—giving                                    (700)
Themselves to waste, deface, and spoil,
Than to increase (by virtuous toil)
The bankrupt bosom of our Realm,
Which naked births did overwhelm!
This begets famine and bleak dearth,
When fruits of wombs pass fruits of earth.
Then Famine's only Physic, and
The medicine for a riotous Land
Is such a plague; so it may please
Mercy's Distributer to appease                                    (710)
His speckled anger and now hide
Th'old rod of Plagues, no more to chide
And lash our shoulders and sick veins
With Carbuncles and shooting Blains.
Make us the happiest amongst men,
Immortal by our prophesying pen,
That this last line may truly reign:
The Plague's ceast; heaven is friends again.
FINIS

*

# John Davies,
## *The Triumph of Death*

The following libraries house copies of the only edition of this poem, published in 1609 (STC 2nd ed., 6332): the British; the Bodleian at the University of Oxford; the University of Edinburgh (two copies); California State University; the Henry E. Huntington Library and Art Gallery; and the University of Texas. Davies' plague epic appears as part of a larger collection of lengthy poems, *Humours heau'n on earth, with the civil wars of death and fortune. As also the triumph of death, or the picture of the plague, according to the life, as it was in anno Domini. 1603. By John Davies of Hereford.* These works are preceded by short verses of praise by others, including Edward Sharphell, Robert Cox, and Anthony Greys. In addition, the poems are preceded and followed by shorter dedicatory verses written by Davies and addressed separately to Algernon, *Lord* Percy; Ladies Dorothy and Lucy Percy; Sir Philip Cary; Sir Humphrey Baskerville of Eardisley; Mistresses *Elizabeth Dutton,* and *Mary* and *Vere Egerton; and Thomas Bodenham*, Esquire.

## THE TRIUMPH OF DEATH
### Or The Picture of the *Plague*,
According to the Life, as it was in *Anno Domini*
*1603*

So, so, just Heav'ns, so, and none otherwise,
Deal you with those that your forbearance wrong.
Dumb Sin (not to be nam'd) against us cries,
Yea, cries against us with a tempting tongue,
And it is heard, for Patience oft provokt
Converts to Fury's all-consuming flame,
And foulest sin (though ne'r so cleanly cloakt)
Breaks out to public plagues and open shame!
Ne'r did the Heav'ns' bright Eye such sins behold
As our long Peace and Plenty have begot.                        (10)
Nor ere did Earth's declining props uphold
An heavier plague than this outrageous Rot!
Witness our Cities, Towns, and Villages,
Which Desolation, day and night, invades[1]
With Coffins (Cannon-like) on Carriages,
With trenches ram'd with Carcasses, with Spades!
    A shiv'ring cold (I sensibly do feel)
Glides through my veins and shakes my heart and hand
When they do prove their virtue to reveal
This plague of plagues that overlays this Land!                 (20)
Horror stands gaping to devour my Sense
When it but offers but to mention it.[2]
And Will, abandon'd by Intelligence,
Is drown'd in Doubt, without her Pilot Wit!
But thou, O thou great giver of all grace,
Inspire my Wit so to direct my Will,
That notwithstanding either's wretched case,
They may paint out thy Plagues with grace, with skill,
That so these Lines may reach to future times,[3]
To strike a terror through the heart of Flesh,                  (30)
And keep it under, that by Nature climbs.
For Plagues do Sin suppress when they are fresh,

---

[1]     [marginal note] Therefore hath the curse devoured the Land, and the inhabitants thereof are desolate. Isaiah 24.6.

[2]     [marginal note] Who among you shall harken to this, and take heed and hear for afterwards. Isaiah 42.23.

[3]     [marginal note] Now go and write it before them in a Table, and note it in a book, that it may be for the last day forever and ever. Isaiah 30.8.

And fresh they be, when they are so exprest
As though they were, in being, seen of Sense,
Which divine Poesy performeth best,
For all our speaking Pictures come from thence!
The object of mine outward Sense affords[4]
But too much Matter for my Muse to form.
Her want (though she had words at will) is words,
T'express this Plague's unutterable Storm!          (40)
Fancy, thou needst not forge false Images
To furnish Wit t'express a truth so true.
Pictures of Death stop up all Passages,
That Sense must needs those obvious objects view.
If Wit had power t'express what Sense doth see,
It would astonish Sense that hears the same,[5]
For never came there like Mortality,
Since Death from *Adam* to his Children came!
    Scarce three times had the Moon replenished
Her empty Horns with light but th'empty Grave       (50)
(Most ravenous) devoured so the Dead,
As scarce the dead might Christian burial have!
Th'Almighty's hand that long had, to his pain,
Offer'd to let his Plagues fall by degrees,
And with the offer pull'd it back again,
Now breaks his Vial, and a Plague out-flees
That gluts the Air with Vapors venomous
That putrefy, infect, and flesh confound,[6]
And makes the Earth's breath most contagious,
That in the Earth and Air but Death is found!       (60)
A deadly Murrain, with resistless force,
Runs through the Land and levels All with it!
The Coast it scoured in uncleanly Course,
And thousands fled before it to the Pit![7]
For ere the breath of this Contagion,
Could fully touch the flesh of Man, or Beast,
They, on the sudden sink, and straight are gone,

---

4   [marginal note] I am the man that hath seen affliction in the rod of his indignation. Lamentations 3.1.

5   [marginal note] Hear, ye deaf, and ye blind, regard that ye may see. Isaiah 42.18.

6   [marginal note] Thou hast forsaken me, saith the Lord, and gone backward: therefore will I stretch out mine hand against thee, and destroy thee, for I am weary with repenting. Jeremiah 15.6.

7   [marginal note] The fear, and the pit, and the snare are upon thee, O inhabitant of the earth. Isaiah 24.17.

So, instantly, by thousands, are decreast!
    No Physic could be found to be a mean[s]
But to allay their Pain, delay their Death                                    (70)
In this Physician's Harvest, they could glean[8]
But corrupt Air and Danger by that Breath.
All Arts and Sciences were at a stand,
And All that liv'd by them, by them did die,
For death did hold their heads and stayed their hand,
Sith they nowhere could use their Faculty.
The nursing Mothers of the Sciences
Withdrew their Foster-milk while wit did fast,
For both our forlorn Universities
Forsaken were and Colleges made fast!                                        (80)
    The Magistrates did fly, or if they stayed,
They stayed to pray, for if they did command,
Hardly, or never, should they be obeyed,
For Death dares all Authority withstand.
And where's no Magistrate, no Order is;
Where Order wants, by order doth ensue
Confusion straight, and in the neck of this
Must silent Desolation all subdue!
For fear whereof, both king and kingdom shakes,
Sith Desolation threatens them so sore,                                       (90)
All hope of earthly help the Land forsakes,
And Heav'n pours plagues upon it more and more![9]
    Now, Death refreshed with a little rest
(As if inspired with the Spirit of Life)
With fury flies (like Air) through man and beast,
And makes eftsoons the murrain much more rife!
*London* now smokes with vapors that arise[10]
From his foul Sweat, himself he so bestirs.
"Cast out your Dead!" the Carcass-carrier cries,
Which he, by heaps, in groundless graves inters!                             (100)
Now scours he Streets, on either side, as clean
As smoking showers of rain the Streets do scour.
Now, in his Murdring, he observes no mean,
But tag and rag he strikes, and striketh sure.

---

[8]    [marginal note] Physicians; Universities.

[9]    [marginal note] Then said I, Lord, how long? and he answered, Until the Cities be wasted without inhabitant, and the houses without man, and the Land be utterly desolate. Isaiah 6.11

[10]    [marginal note] And the Cities that are inhabited shall be left void, the land shall be desolate, and ye shall know that I am the Lord. Ezekiel 12.20.

He lays it on the skins of Young and Old,
The mortal marks whereof therein appear.
Here swells a Botch as high as hide can hold,
And Spots (his surer Signs) do muster there!
The South wind blowing from his swelling cheeks,
Sultry hot Gales did make Death rage the more,                    (110)
That on all Flesh to wreak his Wrath he seeks,
Which flies, like chaff in wind, his breath before![11]
He raiseth Mountains of dead carcasses,
As if on them he would to Heav'n ascend,
T'assuage his rage on divine Essences,
When he of Men, on Earth, had made an end.
Nothing but Death alone could *Death* suffice,
Who made each Mouse to carry in her Coat[12]
His heavy vengeance to whole Families,
Whilst with blunt Botches he cuts other's throat!                (120)
And if such Vermin were thus all employed,
He would constrain domestic fowls to bring[13]
Destruction to their haunts, so, men destroy'd,
As swiftly as they could bestir their wing!
So, Death might well be said to fly the field,
And in the House foil with resistless force,
When he abroad all kind of Creatures kill'd
That he found living in his lifeless Corse!

    Now like to Bees in Summer's heat from Hives,
Out fly the Citizens, some here, some there,[14]                 (130)
Some all alone, and others with their wives,
With wives and children some fly, All for fear!
Here stands a Watch with guard of Partisans
To stop their Passages, or to, or fro,
As if they were nor Men, nor Christians,
But Fiends, or Monsters, murdring as they go!

    Like as an Hart, death-wounded, held at Bay,
Doth fly, if so he can, from Hunter's chase,
That so he may recover (if he may)

---

[11]   [marginal note] Zephaniah 2.2 ["Before the decree bring forth, before the day pass as the chaff, before the fierce anger of the LORD come upon you, before the day of the LORD's anger come upon you."]

[12]   [marginal note] Even the mouse shall be consumed together, saith the Lord. Isaiah 66.17.

[13]   [marginal note] Tame Pigeons, Cocks, Hens, Capons, etc.

[14]   [marginal note] Arise and depart, for this is not your rest, because it is polluted, it shall destroy you even with a sore destruction. Micah 2.10.

Or else to die in some more easy place,    (140)
So might ye see (dear Heart) some lusty Lad
Struck with the Plague, to hie him to the field,
Where, in some Brake or Ditch (of either, glad),
With pleasure, in great pain, the ghost doth yield![15]
Each Village free now stands upon her guard;
None must have harbor in them but their own,
And as for life and death, all watch and ward,
And fly for life (as Death) the man unknown!
For now men are become so monsterous
And mighty in their power, that with their breath    (150)
They leave no ills, save goods, from house to house,
But blow away each other from the Earth!
The sickest Suckling's breath was of that force,[16]
That it the strongest Giant overthrew,
And made his healthy corpse a carrion Corse,
If it (perhaps) but came within his view!
  "Alarm, alarm," cries *Death*, "Down, down with All;
I have and give Commission All to kill.
Let not one stand to piss against a wall,
Sith they are all so good in works so ill.    (160)
Unjoint the body of their Commonweal.
Hew it in pieces; bring it all to naught.
With Rigor's boist'rous hand all Bands cancel,
Wherein the heav'ns stand bound to Earth in aught.
Wound me the scalp of human Policy,
Sith it would stand without the help of heav'n
On rotten props of all impiety.
Away with it; let it be life-bereav'n.
With plagues, strike through Extortion's loathed loins,
And rivet in them glowing pestilence.    (170)
Give, give Injustice many mortal foins,
And with a plague, send, send the same from hence.
Wind me a Botch (huge Botch) about the Neck
Of damn'd, disguis'd, man-pleasing Sanctity,
And Simony with selfsame Choler deck:
Plague these two Plagues with all extremity,
For these are Pearls that quite put out the eyes
Of Piety in Christian Commonwealths.

---

[15] [marginal note] And he that flyeth from the noise of the fear shall fall into the pit, etc. Isaiah. 24.18.

[16] [marginal note] Ye shall conceive chaff, and bring forth stubble, the fire of your breath shall devour you. Isaiah 33.11.

These, these are they, from whom all plagues do rise;
Then plagues on plagues, by right, must reave their healths.          (180)
Dash Veng'ance['s] vial on the cursed brow
Of *Sodomy*, that ever-crying sin,
And that it be no more, whole Pelions throw
Through black *Avernus* (Hell's mouth); send the same
Into the deepest pit of lowest hell.[17]
Let never more the nature nor the name
Be known within the Zones where men may dwell.
Oppress Oppression, this Land's burning-fever,
With burning sores of fevers-pestilent,
And now or never, quell it now and ever,          (190)
For it doth quell the Poor and Innocent.
Bring down damn'd Pride with a pure pestilence
Derived from all plagues that are unpure,
Extracted to th'extremest quintessence,
For Pride, all Sins and plagues for sin, procures.[18]
In Atheism's breast (instead of her curst heart)
Set an huge Botch, or worse plague, more compact,
That it may never convert or pervert,
Nor have power to persuade, much less coact.
Beblaine the bosom of each Mistress[19]          (200)
That bares her Breasts (lust's signs) guests to allure;
With a plague, kiss her (that plagues with a kiss),
And make her (with a murrain) more demure.
Our puling puppets, coy, and hard to please,
My too strait-laced, all-beguarded Girls
(The scum of Niceness, *London* Mistresses),
Their skins embroider with plague's orient Pearls,
For these, for First-fruits, have Fifteens to spare[20]
But to a Beggar say, '*We have not for ye.*'
    Then, do away this too-fine, wasteful Ware          (210)
To second death, for they do most abhor me.
Then, scour the Brothel-houses; make them pure
That flow with filth that wholesomest flesh infects.

---

[17] [marginal note] Ask now among the Heathen, who hath heard such things? The virgin of Israel hath done very filthily Jeremiah 18.13.

[18] [marginal note] Pride, the cause of Adam's fall, and so of all sin.

[19] [marginal note] They are waxen fat, and shining, they do overpass the deeds of the wicked, etc. Jeremiah 5.2.

[20] [marginal note, for *First-fruits*] Strawberries, Cherries, etc. when they first come in; [marginal note, for *Fifteens*] Shillings, Crowns, or Pounds.

Fire out the Pox from thence with plagues unpure,[21]
For they do cause but most unpure effects.
Plague carnal Colleges, wherein are taught
Lust's beastly lessons, which no beast will brook,
Where *Aratine* is read, and nearly sought,
And so Lust's Precepts practis'd by the Book.
Who knows not *Aratine*, let him not ask                    (220)
What thing it is; let it suffice, he was,
But what? No Mouth can tell without a Mask,
For Shame itself will say, 'O let that pass!'
He was a Monster, Tush, O nothing less,
For Nature monsters makes (how ere unright),
But Nature ne'r made such a Fiend as this,
Who, like a Fiend, was made in Nature's spite!
Therefore, away with all that like his Rules,
Which Nature doth dislike as she doth Hell.
Break up those free (yet dear and damned) Schools,          (230)
That teach but gainst kind Nature to rebel.
Rough-cast the skin of smooth-fac'd, glozing Guile
With burning blisters to consume the same,
That swears to sell crackt wares, yet lies the while,
And of gain, by deceiving, makes her game.[22]
Who, but to utter, but a thing of naught,
Utters all oaths, more precious than her Soul,
And thinks them well bestowed, so it be bought:
So, utters wares with oaths, by falsehood foul.
This foul offence to Church and Commonwealth,               (240)
Sweep clean away with Wormwood of annoy,
For it consisteth but by lawful stealth.[23]
Then, let the truest Plagues, it quite destroy.
    "Of Taverns, reeking still with vomitings,
Draw, with the Owners, all the Drawers out.
Let none draw Air that draw on Surfeitings,
But Excess and her Slaves, botch all about.
Sith such, by drawing out and drawing on,

---

[21] [marginal note] Then will I turn mine hand upon thee, and burn out thy dross, till it be pure, and take away thy Tin. Isaiah 1.25.

[22] [marginal note] And every one will deceive his friend and will not speak the truth, for they have taught their tongues to speak lies, and take great pains to do wickedly. Jeremiah. 9.5.

[23] [marginal note] As a Cage is full of Birds, so are their houses full of deceit, thereby they are become great and waxen rich. Jeremiah. 5.27; For all their Tables are full of filthy vomitings: no place is clean. Isaiah 28.8.

Do live, let such be drawn out on a Bier,
For they with wine have many men undone,                          (250)
And famisht them, in fine,[24] through belly-cheer.
Brown-paper Merchants (that do vent such trash
To heedless heirs, to more wealth born than wit,
That gainst such Paper-rocks their houses dash,
While such sly Merchants make much use of it),
Use them as they do use such heirs to use,
That is, to plague them without all remorse.
These with their Brokers, plague, for they abuse
God, King, and Law, by Law's abused force.
Then, petty-botching-Brokers, all bebotch                         (260)
That in a month catch eighteen pence in pound:
Six with a Bill, and twelve for use they catch,[25]
So, use they all they catch, to make unsound,
That they may catch them and still patches make,
Which in the pound do yield them eighteen pence,
Forc'd, like sheep trespassing, the Pound to take,
Leaving their Fleece, at last, for recompense.
Hang in their hangman's wardrobe plagues to air
That all may fly or die that with it mell,
And so, when none will to their rags repair,                      (270)
They must forsake their lives, or labor well.
    "Briefly, kill cursed Sin in general,
And let Flesh Be no more to harbor it.
Away with filthy Flesh; away with all
Wherein still-breeding Sin on brood doth sit."
    This was *Death's* charge, and this charge did he give,
Which was perform'd (forthwith) accordingly,
For now the dead had wasted so the live,
(Or wearied so) that some unburied lie,
For All observ'd the Pestilence was such                          (280)
As laught to scorn the help of Physic's art,
So that to death All yielded with a touch,
And sought no help but help with ease to part.[26]
    An hell of heat doth scorch their seething veins,
The blood doth boil, and all the Body burns,
Which raging Heat ascending to the Brains
The powers of Reason there quite overturns!

---

[24]  *in fine.* In the end, at last.

[25]  [marginal note] Their Bill of Sale.

[26]  [marginal note] And death shall be desired rather than life of all the residue that remain of this wicked family. Jeremiah 8.3.

Then, 'tis no sin to say a Plague it is
From whence immortal miseries do flow;
That makes men, reason, with their rest, to miss,                    (290)
And Souls and Bodies do endanger so.
    Here cry the parents for their Children's death;
There howl the children for their parents' loss,
And often die as they are drawing breath
To cry for their but now inflicted cross.
Here goes an husband heavily to seek
A Grave for his dead wife (now hard to have)
A wife there meets him that had done the like,
All which (perhaps) are buried in one Grave.
The last survivor of a Family,                                      (300)
Which yesterday (perhaps) were all in health,
Now dies to bear his fellow's company,
And for a Grave for all, gives all their wealth.
There wends the fainting Son with his dead Sire[27]
On his sole shoulders borne, him to inter;
Here goes a father with the like desire,
And to the Grave alone, his Son doth bear.
The needy, greedy of a wealthy Prey,
Run into houses cleans'd of Families,
From whence they bring, with goods, their bane away,                (310)
So end in wealth their lives and miseries.
No Cat, Dog, Rat, Hog, Mouse, or Vermin vile,
But usher'd Death, where ere themselves did go,
For they the purest Air did so defile,
That whoso breath'd it, did his breath forgo.
    At *London* (sink of Sin) as at the Fount,
This all-confounding Pestilence began,
According to that Plague's most woeful wont,
From whence it (flowing) all the realm o'reran,
Which to prevent, at first, they pestered                          (320)
Pest-houses with their murrain-tainted Sick,
But though from them, and thence the healthy fled,
They, ere suspected, mortified the Quick.
Those so infected, being ignorant
That so they are, converse with whomsoere,
Whose open Shops and Houses all do haunt,
And find most danger where they least do fear.
And so not knowing sick-folk from the sound

---

[27] [marginal note] Thy Sons have fainted, and lie at head of all the streets, as a wild Bull in a net, and are full of the wrath of the Lord, and rebuke of thy God. Isaiah 51.20.

(For such ill Air's not subject to the sense)
They One with Other do themselves confound,[28]                    (330)
And so confound all with a pestilence.
Out flies one from the Plague and bears with him
An heavy Purse and Plague more ponderous,
Which in the highway parteth life from limb,
So, plagues the next of his coin, covetous.
In this ditch lies one breathing out his last,
Making the same his Grave before his death!
On that Bank lies another, breathing fast,
And passers by he baneth with his breath.
Now runs the Rot along each bank and ditch,[29]                   (340)
And with a murrain strikes Swine, Sheep, and all
(Or man, or beast) that chance the same to touch,
So all in fields as in the Cities fall.
The *London* Lanes (themselves thereby to save)
Did vomit out their undigested dead,
Who by cartloads are carried to the Grave,
For all those Lanes with folk were overfed.
    There might ye see Death (as with toil opprest
Panting for breath, all in a mortal sweat)
Upon each bulk or bench, himself to rest,                         (350)
(At point to faint) his Harvest was so great!
The Bells had talkt so much, as now they had
Tir'd all their tongues and could not speak a word,
And Grief so toiled herself with being sad,
That now at Death's faint threats, she would but bourd.
Yea, Death was so familiar (ah) become
With now-resolved *London* Families,
That, wheresoere he came, he was welcome
And entertain'd with joys and jollities.
Goods were neglected, as things good for naught;                 (360)
If good for aught, good but to breed more ill.
The Sick despis'd them; if the Sound them sought,
They sought their death which cleaved to them still!
So, Sick and Sound, at last neglected them,

---

[28]  [marginal note] I will dash them one against another even the fathers and the sons together, saith the lord; I will not spare I will not pity, not have compassion upon them, but destroy them. Jeremiah 13.14.

[29]  [marginal note] Therefore will I be unto Ephraim as a moth, and to the house of Judah as a rottenness. Hosea 5.12.

As if the Sound and Sick were near their last,[30]
And all, almost, so fared through the Realm
As if their Souls the Judgment day were pass'd.
    This World was quite forgot; the World to come
Was still in mind, which, for it was forgot,
Brought on our World this little day of Doom,                    (370)
That choked the Grave with this contagious Rot!
No place was free for Free-men, ne for those
That were in Prisons, wanting Liberty.
Yet Prisoners freest were from Plagues and Woes
That visit Free-men but too lib'rally.
For all their food came from the healthy house,
Which, then, would give God's plagues from thence, to keep
The rest shut up, could not like bounty use—
So, woeful Pris'ners had least cause to weep.
    The king himself (O wretched Times the while!)               (380)
From place to place, to save himself did fly,
Which from himself, himself did seek t'exile,
Who (as amaz'd) not safe, knew where to lie.
It's hard with Subjects when the Sovereign
Hath no place free from plagues his head to hide,
And hardly can we say the King doth reign,
That nowhere, for just fear, can well abide,
For nowhere comes He but Death follows him
Hard at the Heels, and reacheth at his head.
So sinks all Sports that would like triumphs swim,[31]          (390)
For what life have we, when we all are dead,
Dead in our Spirits, to see our Neighbors die,
To see our King so shift his life to save,
And with his Council all Conclusions try
To keep themselves from th'insatiate Grave.
    For hardly could one man another meet,
That in his bosom brought not odious Death.
It was confusion but a friend to greet,
For like a Fiend, he baned with his breath.
The wildest wastes and places most remote                       (400)
From Man's repair are now the most secure.

---

[30] [marginal note] Neither their silver nor their gold shall be able to deliver them in the day of the Lord's wrath, etc. Zephaniah 1.18; Her filthiness is in her skins; she remembered not her last end, therefore she came down wonderfully; she had no comforter, etc. Lamentations 1.9.

[31] [marginal note] The mirth of tabrets ceaseth: the noise of them that rejoice endeth; the joy of the harp ceaseth. Isaiah 24.8.

Happy is he that there doth find a Coat
To shroud his Head from this Plague's smoking shower.
A Beggar's home (though dwelling in a Ditch)
If far from *London* it were situate[d]
He might rent out, if pleas'd him, to the Rich,
That now as Hell their *London* homes do hate.
    Now had the Sun the Balance entered,[32]
To give his heat by weight, or in a mean,
When yet this Plague more heat recovered,                              (410)
And scour'd the towns that erst were cleansed clean.
Now, sad Despair (clad in a sable weed)
Did All attend, and All resolv'd to die,
For Heat and cold, they thought, the Plague would feed
Which, like a Jerffe, still sinned in gluttony.[33]
The heav'nly Cope was now ore-canopied,
(Near each one's Zenith, as his sense suppos'd)
With ominous impressions, strangely dyed,
And like a Canopy at top it clos'd,
As if it had presag'd the Judge was nigh,                             (420)
To sit in Judgment his last doom to give,
And caus'd his cloth of State t'adorn the Sky
That All his near approach might so perceive.
Now fall the people unto public Fast,
And all assemble in the Church to pray.
Early, and late, their souls, there take repast,
As if preparing for the later day!
Where (fasting) meeting with the sound and sick,
The sick the sound do plague while they do pray,
To haste before the Judge the dead and quick,                         (430)
And pull each other so, in post, away.
    Now Angels laugh to see how contrite hearts
Encounter *Death* and scorn his Tyranny.
Their Judge doth joy to see them play their parts,
That erst so liv'd as if they ne'r should die.
Up go their hearts and hands, and down their knees,
While Death went up and down, to bring them down,
That up they might at once (not by degrees)

---

[32]   [marginal note] Libra September.
[33]   [marginal note] A Beast never but feeding, and when he hath eaten as much as his paunch can hold, goes to a forked tree, and there strains out his food undigested between the twist of the tree, and so again presently falls to feed, and being full, again to the tree, and so eftsoons to feed.

Unto the High'st that doth the humble crown!³⁴
O how the thresholds of each double door                                    (440)
Of Heav'n, and Hell, were worn with throngs of ghosts.
Ne'r since the Deluge did they so before,
Nor ever since so polisht the side-posts.
The Angels, good and bad, are now all toil'd
With entertaining of these ceaseless throngs:
With howling some (in heat and horror broiled)
And othersome in bliss, with joyful Songs.
Th'infernal Legions, in Battalions,
Seek to enlarge their kingdom, lest it should
Be cloyed with Colonies of wicked ones,                                     (450)
For now it held more than it well could hold!
The Angels, on the Crystal walls of Heav'n,
Holp thousands ore the Gates (so glutted were),
To whom authority by Grace was giv'n
(The press was such) to help them over there.
The Cherubin, eye-blinding Majesty
Upon his Throne (that ever blest hath been)
Is compast with unwonted Company,³⁵
And smiles to see how Angels help them in.
The heav'nly streets do glitter (like the Sun)                              (460)
With throngs of Sons but newly glorified,
Who still to praise their Glorifier run
Along those streets, full fraught on either side.
        Now was the earthly Mammon, which had held
Their Hearts to Earth, held most contagious:
A Beggar scorned to touch it (so defiled).
So, none but castaways were covetous.
Now Avarice was turned Cherubin,
Who naught desir'd but the extremest Good,
For now she saw she could no longer sin.                                     (470)
So, to the Time she sought to suit her mood.
The loathsome Lecher loath'd his wonted sport,
For now he thought all flesh was most corrupt.
The brainsick brawler waxed all-amort,
For such blood-suckers Bane did interrupt.

---

³⁴   [marginal note] Isaiah 37.15 ["And Hezekiah received the letter from the hand of
the messengers, and read it: and Hezekiah went up unto the house of the LORD, and spread
it before the LORD / And Hezekiah prayed unto the LORD" (verses 14–15)]

³⁵   [marginal note] The world is divided into twelve parts, and ten parts of it are gone
already, and half of the tenth part: and there remaineth that which is after the half of the
tenth part. 2. Esdras 14.10, 11.

The Pastors now steep all their words in Brine,
With "woe, woe, woe," and naught is heard but "woe."
"Woe and alas," they say, "the powers divine
Are bent Mankind, for sin, to overthrow.
Repent, repent" (like *Jonas*)[36] now they cry, (480)
"Ye men of *England*, O repent, repent,
To see if so ye may move Pity's Eye
To look upon you, ere you quite be spent."[37]
And oft whilst he breathes out these bitter Words,
He, drawing breath, draws in more bitter Bane,
For now the Air, no Air but death affords,
And lights of Art (for help) were in the wane.
Nor people praying, nor the Pastor preaching,
Death spared ought but murd'red one and other.
He was a walm; he could not stay impeaching, (490)
Who smokt with heat and chokt all with the smother.[38]
    The babe new born nipt straight in the head
With air that through his yet unclosed Mould
Did pierce his brains, and through them poison spread,
So left his life, that scarce had life in hold.
The Mother after hies; the Father posts
After the Mother; thus, at Base they run
Unto the Goal of that great Lord of Hosts,
That for those keeps it, that run for his Son.
The rest, Death trips and takes them prisoners; (500)
Such lose the Goal without gainsaying-strife.
But all, and some, are as Death's Messengers
To fetch both one and other out of life.
The Sire doth fetch the Son, the Son the Sire.
Death, being impartial, makes his Subjects so.
The Private's not respected, but entire
(Death pointing out the way) away they go.
    The ceremony at their Burials
Is Ashes but to Ashes, Dust to Dust—
Nay not so much, for straight the Pitman falls (510)
(If he can stand) to hide them as he must.
A Mount thus made, upon his Spade he leans

---

[36]  *Jonas.* Jonah.

[37]  [marginal note] Nevertheless saith the lord, at those days I will not make a full end of you. Jeremiah 4.18.

[38]  *He was a walm . . . smother* Metaphorically, he (Death) was a flood and suffocated all; [marginal note] For it is the day of the Lord's vengeance, and the day of recompense for the judgment of Sion. Isaiah 34.8.

(Tired with toil) yet (tired) prest to toil
Till Death, an heap in his inned Harvest, gleans,
That so he may, by heaps, eft seed the Soil.
Not long he stays, but (ah) a mightier heap
Than erst he hid is made straight to be hild.
The Land is scarce, but yet the Seed is cheap,
For all is full, or rather overfill'd.
The Bier is laid away, and Cribs they get[39]                          (520)
To fetch more dung for Fields and Garden-plots.
Workmen are scarce, the labor is so great,
That (ah) the Seed, unburied, often rots.
It rots and makes the Land thereby the worse,
For, being rotten, it ill vapors breeds,
Which many mortal miseries do nurse,
And the Plague (overfed) so, overfeeds.
　　Here lies an human Carcass half consum'd,
And there some sow or beast, in selfsame plight,
Dead with the Pestilence, for so it fum'd,                             (530)
That all it touched, it consumed quite.
Quite through the host of Nature's Animals,
Death like a Conqueror in Triumph rides,
And ere he came too near, each Creature falls;
His dreadful presence then no flesh abides.
Now man to man (if ever) fiends became,
Fear of infection chokt Humanity.
The empty Maw (abandon'd) got but blame
If it had once but sought for Charity.
The Poor must not about to seek for food,                             (540)
And no man sought them, that they might be fed.
Two Plagues, in one, invaded so their blood;
Both Famine and Infection strikes them dead.
Some stayed, in hope that Death would be appeas'd,
And kept the towns, which them and theirs had kept,
Till their next neighbors were (perhaps) diseas'd,
Or with Death's fatal Fan away were swept;
Then, fain would fly but could not (though they would)
For will they, nill they, they must keep their house,
Till through some chink, on them Death taketh hold,                   (550)
And us'd them, as he did their neighbors use.
If any at some Postern could get out,

---

[39]    [marginal note] Dung-cribs; They shall die of deaths and diseases, they shall not
be lamented, neither shall they be buried, but they shall be as dung upon the earth, etc.
Jeremiah 16.4.

As good they stayed, sith sure they stayed should be,
For all the Countries watcht were round about,
That from the town, none might a furlong flee.[40]
    Then, who from Death did fly, the fear of Death
Made Free-men keep the fliers in his Jaws,
Where (poison'd with his foul infectious breath)
Their flesh and bones he (ne'r sufficed) gnaws.
Now might ye see the Plague devour with speed        (560)
As it near famisht were, lest in a while
It might be so and want whereon to feed.
So fed, the future hunger to beguile.
Now doth it swell (hold hide) nay,[41]
Till skin doth crack, to make more room for meat,
Yet meat, more meat it (never cloyed) doth cry,
And all about doth run the same to get.
The Graves do often vomit out their dead;
They are so over-gorg'd with great and small,
Who hardly with the earth are covered—        (570)
So, oft discover'd when the Earth did fall.
    Those which in highways died (as many did),[42]
Some worthless wretch, hir'd for no worthless fee,
Makes a rude hole, some distance him beside,
And rakes him in far off, so there lies he.
But if the Pitman have not so much sense
To see nor feel which way the wind doth sit
To take the same, he hardly comes from thence,
But for himself (perhaps) he makes the pit,
For the contagion was so violent,        (580)
(The will of Heav'n ordaining so the same)
As often struck stone-dead incontinent,
And Nature's strongest forces straight orecame.
Here lieth one upon his burning breast,
Upon the Earth's cold breast, and dies outright,
Who wanting burial, doth the Air infest,
That like a Basilisk he banes with sight!
There reels another like one deadly drunk,
But newly struck (perhaps) then down he falls,

---

[40]  [marginal note] They have compassed her about, as the watchmen of the field, because she hath provoked me to wrath, saith the Lord. Jeremiah 4.17.

[41]  [marginal note] If the botch break not, the Patient liveth not; It kills others with breaking.

[42]  [marginal note] They that feed delicately perish in the streets; they that were brought up in scarlet, embrace the dung. Lamentations 4.5.

Who in the Streets or ways no sooner sunk,[43]                    (590)
But forthwith dies and so lies by the walls.
The Haycocks in the Meads were oft opprest
With plaguey Bodies both alive and dead,
Which being us'd, confounded Man and Beast,
And us'd they might be ere discovered.
For some (like Ghosts) would walk out in the night,
The City glowing (furnace-like) with heat
Of this contagion, to seek, if they might,
Fresh air, where oft they died for want of meat.
The Traveler that spied (perhaps his Sire)                    (600)
Another far off coming towards him,
Would fly, as from a flying flame of fire
That would, if it he met, waste life and limb.
So, towns fear'd towns, and men each other fear'd.
All were (at least) attainted with suspect,
And sooth to say, so was their envy stirr'd,
That one would seek another to infect,[44]
For whether the disease to envy mov'd,
Or human nature's malice was the cause,
Th'infected often all Conclusions prov'd                    (610)
To plague him that from them himself withdraws!
Here do they Gloves and there they Garters fall;
Ruffs, Cuffs, and handkerchers, and such like things
They strew about, so to endanger all,
For Envy now most pestilently stings!
    So, heav'n and earth, against Man did conspire,
And Man against Man, to extirp his Race,
Who Bellows were t'augment Infection's fire,
And blow abroad the same from place to place.
Sedition thus marcht (with a pestilence)                    (620)
From town to town, to make them desolate.[45]
The Brownbill was too short to keep it thence,
For further off it raught the Bill-man's pate,
Nor walls could keep it out, for it is said
(And truly too) that Hunger breaks stone-walls.
    The plague of Hunger with the Plague array'd

---

[43]  [marginal note] And their corpses shall lie in the streets of the great city, etc.
Revelation 11.8.

[44]  [marginal note] Because of their pride the Cities shall be troubled the houses shall
be afraid; men shall fear. 2. Esdras 15.18.

[45]  [marginal note] Destruction upon destruction is cried, for the whole Land is wasted
etc. Jeremiah 4.20.

Itself to make way where ere Succor calls,
For hungry Armies fight as Fiends they were:
No human power can well their force withstand.
They laugh to scorn the shaking of the Spear,[46]                    (630)
And gainst the gods themselves, themselves dare band.
Some ran as mad (or with wine over-shot)
From house to house, when botches on them ran,
Who, though they menac'd were with Sword and Shot,
Yet forward ran, and fear nor God nor man!
As when a Ship at Sea is set on fire,[47]
And (all on flame's) wind-driven on a Fleet,
The Fleet doth fly, sith that Ship doth desire
(Maugre all force oppos'd) with it to meet,
So flies the Bill-man and the Musketeer                              (640)
From the approaching desperate plaguey wight,[48]
As from a flying flame of quenchless fire.
For, who hath any life with Death to fight?
"At all," cries *Death*, then down by heaps they fall.
He draws in, By and Main; amain[49] he draws
Huge heaps together, and still cries, "At all."
His hand is in, and none his hand withdraws.
For look how Leaves in Autumn from the tree[50]
With wind do fall, whose heaps fill holes in ground,
So might ye (with the Plague's breath) people see,                   (650)
Fall by great heaps and fill up holes profound.
       No holy Turf was left to hide the head
Of holiest men, but most unhall'wed grounds
(Ditches and Highways) must receive the dead,
The dead (ah, woe the while) so oreabounds![51]
Here might ye see as t'were a Mountainet
Founded on Bodies, grounded very deep,
Which like a Trophy of Death's Triumphs set
The world on wonder that did wondring weep.
For to the middle Region of the Air,                                 (660)

---

[46]   [marginal note] Job 41.20. ["Out of his nostrils goeth smoke, as out of a seething pot or caldron."]

[47]   [marginal note] Similitude.

[48]    [marginal note] Plagues are sent unto you, and who can drive them away. 2 Esdras 16.4.

[49]   *By and Main; amain.* With all his might.

[50]   [marginal note] Similitude.

[51]   [marginal note] Many dead Bodies shall be in every place, they shall cast them forth with silence. Amos 8.3.

Our earthly Region was infected so,
That Fowls therein had cause of just despair,
As those which over *Sodom* dying go!
Some common Carriers for their own behoof,
And for their good, whose Souls for gains do groan
Fetching from *London* packs of Plagues and stuff,
Are forc'd to inn it in some Barn alone,
Where, lest it should the Country sacrifice,
Barn, Corn, and Stuff, a Sacrifice is sent
(In Air-refining Flames) to th'angry Skies.                              (670)
While th'owners do their Faults and Loss lament,
The Carriers, to some Pest-house or their own,
Carried, clapt up, and watcht for coming out,
Must there with Time or Death converse alone,
Till Time or Death doth free the world of doubt,
Who though they Carriers were, yet being too weak,
Such heavy double Plagues as these to bear.
Out of their houses some by force do break,
And drown themselves, themselves from plagues to clear.[52]
    These are revenges fit for such a God,                              (680)
Fit for his Justice, Power, and Majesty.
These are right jerks of divine Fury's Rod,
That draw from Flesh the life-blood mortally.
If these are but his temp'ral Punishments,
Then what are they, surmounting Time and Fate?
Melt Flesh to think but on such Languishments,
That Soul and Body burn in endless date.
His utmost Plagues extend beyond the reach
Of comprehension of the deepest Thought,
For he, his wisdom infinite doth stretch                                (690)
To make them absolutely good for naught.
Then, O what heart of sensible Discourse,
Quakes not, as if it would in sunder fall
But once to think upon such Fury's force,
As doth so far surmount the thoughts of all?
If human Wisdom in the highest strain
Should yet stretch, further Torments to devise,
They would be such that none could them sustain
Through weight of woes and raging agonies.

---

[52]  [marginal note] This no fiction, nor inserted by poetical license. But this verily
was performed in the borough of Leominster in the county of Hereford: the one at the
commandment of Sir Herbert Croft knight, one of the Council of the Marches of Wales; the
other by the instigation of Satan, and provocation of the disease.

Then (Oh) what be they that devised are                              (700)
By Wisdom, that of Naught made all this All,[53]
That stretch as far past speech as past compare,
Surmounting Wonder, supernatural!?
They be the Judgments of that Trinity,
Which (like themselves) are most inscrutable;
Then can man's heart but either swoon or die,
To think on anguish so unthinkable.
And can our Sense, our Sense so much besot,
To think such worlds of woe nowhere exist,
Sith in this sensual World it feels them not,                        (710)
And so in sin (till they be felt) insist?
    Then happy That, that is insensible,
Since we employ our happiness of Sense
To feel and taste but pleasures sensible,
And see no Pain that at their end commence
To break the Belly of our damn'd Desires
With honeyed Sweets that soon to poison turn,
And in our Souls enkindle quenchless fires,
Which all the frame thereof quite overturn,
To please itself a Moment and displease                             (720)
Itself forever, with ne'r-ending pains;[54]
To ease the Body with the Soul's disease;
To glad the Guts; to grieve the Heart and Brains;
To make the Throat a Throughfare for Excess,
The Belly a *Charybdis* for the same;
To use Wit still but only to transgress,
And make our Sense the Sponge of Sin and Shame.
    Then happy are sweet Flowers that live and die[55]
(Without offence) most pleasing unto all,
And hapless Man that lives unpleasingly                              (730)
To Heav'n and Earth, so lives and dies to fall.
The Rose doth live a sweet life but to please,
And when it dies, it leaves sweet fruit behind,
But Man in Life and Death doth none of these,
If Grace by Miracle ne'r mend his mind.[56]
Blush Man, that Flowers should so thyself excel
That wast created to excel—what not—
That on the Earth created was to dwell;

---

[53]   [marginal note] Torments, devised by infinite wisdom, are infinite in pain.
[54]   [marginal note] Mortal life is no more (at the most) compared to Eternity.
[55]   [marginal note] So fares it with sensual Epicures and Libertines.
[56]   [marginal note] The conversion of a sinner is most miraculous.

Then blush for shame to grace thy Beauty's blot.
Art thou Horizon made (unholy one)                                    (740)
Betwixt immortal Angels and brute beasts,
Yet wilt twixt beasts and fiends be Horizon,
By that which Angels grieve and God detests?
Then Plagues must follow thy misguided Will,
So to correct thine ill-directing Wit,
Such as these are, or others much more ill,
The worst of which Sin (ill of Ills) befit.

    And lo, for Sin, how yet the Plague doth rage
(With unappeased fury) more and more,
Making our Troynovant a tragic Stage                                   (750)
Whereon to show Death's power, with slaughters sore.
Great Monarch of Earth's ample world he is,
And of our little Worlds (that world's content)[57]
He gives ill Subjects Bale, good Subjects Bliss,
So, though he reigns, just is his Regiment.
Our sins (foul blots) corrupt the Earth and Air;
Our sins (soul's botches) all this All defile,
And make our Souls most foul that were most fair,
For naught but sin we all, all naught the while!
When sharpest wits are whetted to the point,                          (760)
To pierce into all secrets, but to sin!
And all the corpse of Luxury unjoint,
To see what sensual joy might be therein;
Whenas such tricks, as no Sun ever saw,
Devis'd are daily by the Serpent-wise,
To cram all Flesh into the Devil's maw
By drifts, as scarce the Devil can devise!

    Can God (most just) be good to men so ill?
And can the Earth, and Air, wherein such live,
Keep such alive? O no, all Plagues must fill                          (770)
That Air, and Earth, that do such plagues relive.
What are those men but plagues, that plague but men?
All men are such that teach sin in effect,
And all do so that sin but now and then,
If now and then they sin in overt act.

    What can contain us if these plagues cannot?
If neither these we feel, nor those we shall,
Be not of force to keep our lives from blot,
What then remains but plagues to scour us all?
Till we wax less, and they so multiplied,                             (780)

---

[57]  [marginal note] Man is Microcosmos.

That we be nothing less, than what we are,
Converted or confounded we abide
In or without God, with or without care!
If when his iron Rod draws blood from us,
And is upon our backs, yea breaks our bones,
We cease not yet to be rebellious,
What can convert us but plagues for the nones![58]
For Nature's heart doth yearn with extreme grief,
When well she weighs her children's strange estate,
Subject to sin and so to sorrow's chief,                        (790)
For both in counterchange renew their date,
For now we sin (yea with a witness sin;
Witness, our conscience) then we plagued are,
Plagu'd with a witness (witness plagues that race
With fury on us); then, when so we fare
Fall we to pray and creep to Grace for grace,
Which being got, and ease, and weal at will,
We fall to sin, and so our soul's disgrace.

    Thus sin and plagues run round about us still.
This ever-circling Plague of plagues and sin,                   (800)
Surroundeth Mankind in an hell of woe.
Man is the *Axis* standing still therein,
And goes with it wherever it doth go,
For since he fell, who at this Center stays
By Nature (most unnatural the while)
Here moves man moveless as the *Axis* plays,
And Time's turns (turning with him) doth beguile.
And yet this Plague (if Grief's tears quench it not)
Is like a spark of fire in flax too dry,
And may, if our Lusts cool not, burn more hot                   (810)
Than erst it did, so waste us utterly.
We see it will not out, but still it lies
In our best City's Bowels like a Coal
That threats to flame and still doth fall and rise,[59]
Wasting a part, thereby to warn the whole.
None otherwise than when (with grief) we see
Some house on fire, we straight to save the town,
Watch, fast, and pray, and most industrious be,
With hook and line to pull the Building down,
So doth this fire of heav'n's still-kindling ire               (820)
Blister our City's public Body so,

---

[58]   *for the nones*. For the nonce; for the occasion.
[59]   [marginal note] As appeareth by the Plague bills every week. Similitude.

As we are blister'd, but with so much fire,
As we may quench with tears if they do flow.
But if it should break forth in flames afresh,
(As [ah] what stays it but unstinted Grace?)
What thing should quench it but a world of Flesh,
Or desolation, it away to chase?
    Time never knew since he began his hours,
(For aught we read) a Plague so long remain
In any City as this Plague of ours,                    (830)
For now six years in *London* it hath lain.
Where none goes out but at his coming in,
If he but feels the tendrest touch of smart,
He fears he is Plague-smitten for his sin,
So, ere he's plagu'd, he takes it to the heart,
For Fear doth (Loadstone-like) it oft attract,
That else would not come near, or steal away,
And yet this plaguey-fear will scarce coact
Our Souls to sin no more, this Plague to slay.
    But thou, in whose high hand all hearts are held,    (840)
Convert us, and from us this Plague avert,
So sin shall yield to Grace, and Grace shall yield
The Giver glory for so dear desert:
Too dear for such too worthless, wicked Things,
At best but clods of base Infirmity;
Too dear for sin that all this murrain brings;
Too dear for those that live, but twice to die.
In few, what should I say? The best are naught
That breathe, since man first breathing did rebel.
The best that breathe are worse than may be thought,    (850)
If Thought can think the best can do but well,
For none doth well on Earth, but such as will
Confess (with grief) they do exceeding ill!
    The best is but a Briar, and none doth good,
But He that makes Us blameless in his Blood.[60]
FINIS

---

[60]  [marginal note] Micah 7.4; Psalm 14.1; Ephesians 5.12 [Respectively, "The best of
them is as a brier: the most upright is sharper than a thorn hedge: the day of thy watchmen
and thy visitation cometh; now shall be their perplexity"; "The fool hath said in his heart,
There is no God. They are corrupt, they have done abominable works, there is none that
doeth good"; For it is a shame even to speak of those things which are done of them in
secret."]

\*

# Richard Milton,
## *London's Misery*

The British Library holds the only copy of this poem from 1625 (STC 2nd ed., 17939). A short prose epistle to "Uncle, Master *Richard Gough,* of the City of Hereford Gentleman" precedes the poem that otherwise stands alone. Within the poem itself is a plague bill and prose explanation for the bill's inclusion.

LONDON'S MISERY,
The Country's Cruelty
with
God's Mercy
Explained by remarkable observations
of each of them during this last Visitation

*Written by* Richard Milton
London
Printed by Nicholas Okes
1625

No far fetcht Story brought from Foreign land
Or such like matters do I take in hand;
No lovesick Sonnet or sweet roundelays
No Epigrams or such like pleasing toys;
Nor do I write the deeds of Martial men
That have been done: the place, time, where, and when.
This I refer unto some other men,
To paint and set forth with their fluent pen,
Whilst I with sighing do most sadly sing,
The fearful judgments of the Heavenly King,                    (10)
That in his wrath by his most heavy hand,
Puts to amazement this most sinful Land—
A task too hard for me, whose slender skill,
Is far unfit, although God knows my will
Be very good; for matter, it befits
The industrious penning of more curious wits.
My wit is mean, God knows, I understand
But little, and for me to take in hand
This worthy work, I might presume too much
To meddle with, for answer unto such                    (20)
Shall so oppose me; this poor simple skill
I here have shown is meant by me no ill
In any kind, but only for to show,
The good affection I to duty owe
Unto this City (where I have my being)
Whose great calamities I daily seeing,
Makes me break forth and with grieved soul
Her miserable state for to condole.
Amongst the rest, should I not be unkind
As not to show grief where such cause I find                    (30)
In th'ighest manner to a place I love so,
As none in the earth more dearer? Surely no,

But in this Action will be so far bold,
Not fearing what I write shall be controlled.
    And first to thee Lord, do I humbly bow,
For pardon for our sins, whose angry brow
Still Frowns as if no mercy thou wilt have
Upon this City but will send to Grave
All the inhabitants within a little space.
Oh be not angry still, afford us grace                    (40)
For to repent, and stay thine angry hand,
For who thy powerful judgments can withstand?
Lord, we have sinned and have done amiss;
Wherefore thine anger fiercely kindled is.
Upon this city, vengeance thou hast pour'd,
And we like sheep to slaughter are devour'd.
Our sins forgive; behold our watery eyes,
Our grievous groans, our lamentable cries.
Long have we sighed, but thou hast not heard;
Oft have we prayed, but thou hast not spar'd,        (50)
As if even with our prayers thou wer't offended,
As if thy judgments never would be ended.
    Faintness possesseth all our vital parts,
Our courage fails us; daunted are our hearts.
In this extremity, whither shall we fly,
But unto thee oh God; prostrate we lie
Before thy Throne of grace and with bleeding wound
And sobbing sighs, our miseries we sound.
Do we not know, Lord, thou didst send thy Son
To pay a ransom for our deeds misdone,          (60)
Even from the Heavens where thou sits above?
So dear the life of sinners thou didst love,
And when, by our transgression, mankind all,
Were subject to thy wrath, fast bound and thrall,
And we believe, Lord help our unbelief,
For of the same thou are our stay and chief,
Prop and upholder; we believe, I say,
For on so sure a ground, safe build we may:
What thou has promised in thy sacred Word,
What thou hast vowed, oh most gracious Lord,    (70)
That thou the death of sinners not desirest,
But rather life to them, for thou requirest,
That of their sinful lives, they would amend,
And so gain mercy where they did offend.
With patience therefore we attend thy will,
Not doubting but thy words thou wilt fulfill.

Tis not unknown to many a Foreign Nation,
The beauty of *London* and the situation:
The strength, the wealth, and multitude of men
It did contain at such good time, as when                    (80)
God was at peace with us, the Famous Sparks
Of sweet invention and the learned Clarks,
Worthy Divines and Physicians store,
Attorneys, Counselors and penmen more
I think than need is; there the reverend Judges
Gave many a sentence at which ill men grudges,
For there the Courts of justice have been kept,
Where many a Client hath full sorely wept.
The cause is known to God; what shall I say
That, to this City, in some sort, I may                       (90)
Express good will? There 'twas the liberal Arts
Did chiefly flourish, men of excellent parts
Did there abide, as being the very spring,
That to their Studies sweet refresh did bring.
There liv'd our King, also his noble Peers,
To whom the Lord grant life and many years
Of happiness on earth, fame and renown,
And in the end an everlasting Crown
Of glory; there his Subjects at command
In multitude were like unto the sand,                         (100)
That on the Seashore, Seamen used to see,
When waves are pass'd, and waters calmed be.
The several sorts of Tradesmen and of Arts,
The several merchandise from Foreign parts,
The multitude of rich and wealthy men,
I am not able to express with pen,
And though for four years pass'd, it so fell out
That many Tradesmen here were in great doubt
They should have been undone (for trading fail'd
And so long time their hearts were cold and quaild).         (110)
    Yet the late marriage of our Royal King
We thought a settling to this Realm would bring,
In such a wise that now our fear was pass'd,
And well was he that did hold out till last,
That all men so with doings should abound,
That work-men for our work would nere be found.
Oh God, how of our hopes we are deceived,
And of our long expected joys bereaved.
How thou our foolish wisdom sets at naught,
And even ourselves unto destruction brought.                 (120)

Vain is the help of man, also are vain
The imagination of a mortal brain.
    OH *London, London*, thou didst feel the Rod,
But never rightly lookt up to thy God
That struck thee with it, when thou feltst the smart,
Even at the first, then with a grieved heart.
Thou of thy grievous sins shouldst have repented,
And so God's angry Judgments have prevented.
This was neglected, and, O most unkind,
God's former benefits, imprint in mind              (130)
Thou didst not do; for, assuredly,
Before thy wickedness to him did cry
For heavy vengeance, he was wondrous kind
To thee, and thou didst many favors find
From him; we are apt to forget God wot,
Or if we do remember, we bear not
The thankful minds we should, and therefore we
Even for our sins most justly plagued be.
Should we persuade ourselves Almighty Jove,
This Famous City did more dearly love            (140)
Than others that his power could not withstand,
But in the former ages felt his hand?
Or shall we think that shortned is his Arm
Or that he will not suffer so much harm
To come upon us as he did to those
That sinn'd as well as we? O, no repose,
Nor harbor in your hearts so vain a thought,
For even as they were to destruction brought,
Even so shall we if we do still offend
And do not of our sinful lives amend.             (150)
For as the Lord is by his mercy known
To be a gracious God, and he hath shown
That in his mercy he doth far surpass,
Which plainly doth appear, but yet whereas
Almighty God in mercy doth abound,
Take this for certain and a constant ground,
As on his mercies we may boldly trust,
So in his Judgments is he always just.
    Aye me! I need not long to treat of this,
How many demonstrations daily is,             (160)
How many several bells do sadly ring
The doleful tune of this most certain thing,
In this our present sad disastrous plight,
Whilst many souls have bid the world goodnight.

My flesh do tremble; I amazed stand,
To see the force of God's Almighty hand;
My hand do quake and eke my joints do shiver
To see what deadly Arrows from his Quiver
Are now sent forth to this forsaken City,
Whose very miseries my soul doth pity.                    (170)
 Go on my muse now, and right sadly tell,
The doleful sound that every Parish bell
Within this poor afflicted City make
That we may from our sinful lives awake.
Our daily sorrows and continual fears
Our loss of dear friends and our daily tears
That we for them do shed the sundry moans,
Deep hearted sighings and the grievous groans,
That many a husband for his tender wife
Sends forth for her that is bereav'd of life.             (180)
How many a wife mourns for her Turtle mate,
That now lies gasping, struck by cruel fate
Of conquering Death, and when thou hast so done,
Tell how the father grieves for his lost son;
The woeful screeches many a mother mild
Bitterly sends forth for their dying child;
How many a son weeps for his loving father
(Whose love so dear was that he would more rather
Have died himself even such as was his good will,
But we cannot our own desires fulfill);                   (190)
How many a daughter grieves for her dear mother,
And many a sister for her loving brother,
And many a brother for his loving sister,
That knew not what he lost before he misst her.
Here weeps the servant for this loving Master
And grieves that Death is grown so great a waster.
There sighs the Master for his loving man,
For that he is not able, neither can
Save his poor servant's life; with weeping eyes
The careful maiden for her Mistress cries.               (200)
The mistress likewise for her maid doth moan,
Because so good a servant's dead and gone.
Neighbor for neighbor, one friend for another,
Their loves were such, their griefs they cannot smother;
The Preacher for his flock, and they for him.
We wail and weep until our eyes are dim.
And then, O Lord, a sad thing for to see,
Yet daily such sad spectacles there be,

They that before so sadly mourned have
By other Friends are shortly brought to grave                    (210)
With much ado, for Friends are very few,
In this their last farewell, their loves to shew.
    Such is the force of Death's fell conquering hand,
That none in this world can his power withstand.
Tis not the power of a mighty King
Can serve to free him from Death's deadly sting,
Much less the title of a Lord or Knight
Can keep their persons from this pale-fac't wight.
Tis not the wisdom of a learned man,
No there is neither Art nor wisdom can                           (220)
Be forcible enough with Art or wile
Either to stay death's stroke or him beguile.
Mark it, I pray you, how he makes men reel:
His Bow is iron sure and his Arrows steel,
How many through his might do daily die,
How many likewise do there sprawling lie,
How many also dead in fields are found,
And suddenly in streets do fall to ground,
Even as they pass and then before were well
And felt but little pain until they fell.                        (230)
    Stay, gentle death, for I assure you can:
The party's held an upright honest man,
You are about to deal. I tell you more:
Of wealth he hath a great abundant store,
And liberally he giveth to the poor.
Of that he hath the like given at his door.
There's very few that doth, nay, hardly any,
Although there do in wealth surpass him many.
    Ay, that is well done, I commend you better,
And for your kindness will remain your debtor.                   (240)
That miserable, griping, rusty Chuff,
That always wanted, never had enough
And never car'd how many men were killed,
So he might have his Coffers stuft and filled—
Ah wretched Carle, I trust that there is none
True hearted wight will weep when thou art gone.
They in thy lifetime wept and were not heard;
Now at thy death they rightly may be spar'd.
    Know you what you have done? Y'ave slain a woman,
That for her virtuous carriage, I think no man                   (250)
Will find the like again; now, good Sir, tell,
To take the good away, do you do well?

Doth there not many an idle Gossip stay
Who long before we'd fain have had away?
Leave off, for shame. Away, now get you gone.
Go take the worst sort. Leave the best alone!
    Lord if 'twere so, what would become of me
That know myself to be as bad may be?
For there's not only one but thousands more
That I go far behind that went before:             (260)
Many a brave Scholar, many a worthy Teacher,
Many a good liver, many a zealous Preacher,
That liv'd as lights and were to thee right dear.
So carefully they walked in thy fear,
But I, alas, have much abused thy will,
Had not a care, thy hests for to fulfill,
Have sin'd extremely and assuredly,
Had long before this time deserved to die.
    But yet, O Lord, I see 'tis not thy will;
Thou spar'st my life, wilt have me tarry still.       (270)
And now I pray thee, whilst I have my being,
Sith that thou hast vouchsaft to me the seeing,
(Wretch that I am) of this thy mighty power,
Grant that hereafter, daily and each hour,
For that same small time and the little space
Of life that thou shalt grant me by thy grace,
I may redeem time, which I lewdly spent,
Bewail my sins and heartily repent.
    When hoary hymns now had chang'd his hue,
And for that year had bid the world adieu,      (280)
When trees gan sprout, the grass and everything
Lookt green and fair, lambs skipt, the birds did sing,
And with their warbling notes in woods did Ring,
Their maker's praise, according to their kind,
*April* the month was called, for so I find,
(for fore that time there died not any store,
That either had the tokens or plague sore),
Then did the Lord begin to lay his hand,
And plainly showed he'd give us understand,
That he was angry with us. At the first        (290)
Small quantity there dy'd—Death did not thirst
As now it doth—a dozen or a score,
We thought it much; soon after forty more,
Or such like number to the ground were sent,
But hardly any miss of those that went.
    Time slides away, our glass doth daily run,

And God will finish what he had begun,
For shortly after in the Bills are spied,
About a hundred of the sickness died.
    And, yet, at that at time, I remember well,                    (300)
There's very few of us could rightly tell,
Whether the sickness were the plague or no
So willingly we would have had it so.
The Searchers now brought into question be?
For that, poor aged folks, they could not see
God's handy-work; twas thought that they did wrong
To many people: thus did we prolong
Our miseries. Advice was taken then
Of Physic Doctors, all held worthy men
And such as for their skill did much surpass                    (310)
The meaner sort; they told us that whereas
Those that from us this sickness did divide,
Had caught a spotted fever, and so died.
    Thus the Almighty, though he hath and can,
Produce strange wonders by the Art of man,
Nevertheless, when he thinks good, he will
Confound the wisdom and the learned skill
Of mortal Creatures and us plainly show,
He can send judgments that they shall not know
How to prevent with all their art or skill                    (320)
If we rebel and not his will fulfill.
    The Former Searchers now are in hard case;
They are reprov'd, some forc't to lose their place,
And now with cheerful hearts we do agree
The former doubt but a mistake might be.
Yet still alas, the sickness doth increase,
And therefore of our fears we do not cease.
Those that they now appoint are bound with oath,
Upon their consciences to tell the troth,
That neither for reward or filthy fear,                    (330)
Or else for any favor that that they bear
Unto the person that are so infected,
Should stop their judgments, now to be expected.
    Their charge receiv'd, away now do they hie.
And to their business do they look more nigh.
Days quickly go, the nights likewise full fast,
And very suddenly a week is pass'd,
And now we lookt to be resolved well,
And who but searchers could us better tell?
The questions askt, and then they told their mind,                    (340)

That certainly the places which they find
So visited so far as they could see
No other sickness than the plague should be.
The reason now of this afore-said doubt
(As I have heard) by experience is found out,
That as the plague beginneth with the year,
So do the marks thereof at first appear
Much like the spotted Fever; as time goes on,
And year upon his back puts age upon,
The marks do alter to another hue,                              (350)
Leaving the red, and then is turn'd do blue.
     We study now and often cast about
And call to mind what heretofore fell out
Upon the Death of any Sovereign Prince,
Or in Successor's reign hath hapned since.
There's many of us do remember yet
It was so late, we can it not forget,
When first King *James*, came here this Crown to sway,
How many by the plague were caught away,
And now the most of us persuaded be,                            (360)
That such a sickness we again shall see.
     But being come unto the month of *June*
It sings to us a sad and mournful tune.
For now we think the sickness will not cease,
Because we find it weekly doth increase.
Orders are now prescribed and best invention
That we can use or find out for prevention.
The doors of sick are shut, and Dogs be killed;
'Tis better they should go than we be filled
With noisome smells, a reason some doth tell,                   (370)
That brings the sickness with us here to dwell.
It to avoid, houses and streets we wash,
And many a pail of water down we pash
Before our doors; the place of those infected,
We warily avoid. Though we respected
The visited before their sickness came,
Yet now to see them would redound much blame
Unto us; all the neighbors they would fear us,
And hearing it, few of them would come near us,
For so to do, can we tell what may chance                       (380)
To us or ours so far for to advance,
Or venture out ourselves, them to come near?
Pray, blame us not; we justly may forbear.
     Thus did we fear at first but time grows on

That which before we could not build upon:
*Trinity* Term was for that time put off.
Causes of suit in Law were driven off
Till longer time; they that came many a mile
With grief return, stay here but little while,
That hoped to have seen some happy end                    (390)
Of their long Suits, now vainly do they spend
Both time and money; *London* they forsake,
And many a long and weary step they make,
Before they come unto their wisht desire,
To see the smoke that issues from the fire
Of their own Chimneys. And to prevent
Danger of infection, the Parliament,
That ever commonly with us did sit,
Do now forbear, and think it far for more fit,
That kept it should be in some other place.                (400)
The City of *Oxford* 'twas that had the grace
Of that assembly; there they time did spend,
No doubt careful for to make an end
Of that they had in hand; statutes are acted,
And in a book together are compacted
For public good. There let them rest a while,
Whilst we go forwards in our homely style,
To tell you truly what did come to pass
        To month next following, which called *July* was.
Each week with longing we desire to see                    (410)
Whether the bills increase or lessened be,
But where the figures set for hundreds were
Now thousands, three and more, there do appear,
By hundreds three, fourscore, five in number.
        Due time it is for us to leave off slumber
And generally with one voice and accord,
We gin to weigh the judgments of the Lord,
And seek to him, our helper and our guide,
That we of mercy may not be denied.
In this affliction call to mind our sin,                   (420)
With humble prayers and fasting we begin,
That so we may appease God's angry hand,
(The only way his judgments to withstand),
Wherein assuredly we did do well.
We knew the gracious goodness which befell
To *Nineveh*, and other Cities moe,
Which else had been destroyed had't not been so
They had repented. This right godly thing,

First was commended by our noble King.
Thereby he show'd that he a Father was                                (430)
Unto this City, and what came to pass
He took to heart. Alas what better love,
Or friend for friendship can we further prove
Than at such times as we afflicted be,
That they are mov'd our miseries to see
And do their best endeavors, to be brief,
Use all the art they can for our relief?
    In this renowned King, great commendation
We much ascribe; welfare and preservation
Of us and ours was daily in thy mind,                                 (440)
As by thy provident care we did it find.
Should we unthankful be, it were most vild,
And we, hereafter, justly might be stild,
Ungrateful subjects; likewise know 'twas he
Gave special order that a book should be
Read in our Fasts of Prayers and Psalms selected
Fit for the times, so greatly he respected
The safety of our souls; another Book[1]
By him was set forth, wherein if you look,
Medicines for bodies' health did there insert,                        (450)
With wary visements, how we should divert
Or keep ourselves from causes of Infection,
What else to do he gave to us direction.
    But well-away, before the month is gone,
How many thousands, left us here alone,
And gave us leave to fast and eke to pray,
For neither wealth nor Counsel could them stay.
Both rich and poor away now do they hie.
Both old and young, they care not where they lie,
In barns or haycocks, fields, or under tree,                          (460)
Nor how they fare, so *London* they not see.
    *London* that heretofore had such Renown,
Is not respected as a common Town,
Her glories darkened and her strength decayed,
And those that trusted in her are afraid
For to come near her. *London* that heretofore,
Which for the bigness sure was people more

---

[1]   *a book ... another Book.* The first, a book of special common prayers for plague-time issued by successive kings, beginning with Elizabeth I; the second also initiated by Elizabeth I, the Orders for plague that included a medical regimen with inexpensive remedies.

Than any City in the world again,
Doth say when God is angry "'tis but vain
To trust in multitude," but I call to mind, (470)
When't did abound with men, then most unkind
Full many of us grudge to have it so,
Thinking the cause thereof procur'd us woe.
So many of a trade (thus did we grieve)
That one man by another could not live.
Sure, God was angry with us; now you see
The city of large multitudes are free.
Where is the doings that should now abound?
Sure, nothing else but wailing is there found,
For want of those that in the same did dwell, (480)
And when woe will be done, we cannot tell.
　　But shall I leave our fellow brethren so,
And not vouchsafe a little for to go
To bring them out of town? At least-wise know,
The favor jolly Countrymen did show
To strangers and to kin, but, first, alas,
You know 'tis fitting they should have a pass—
Whither he be a wiseman or an Ass,
Unless he mean to lie upon the grass—
The which unto the Countrymen they show, (490)
Contents whereof doth let all people know
That whereas Almightily God (more is the pity)
With sickness now had visited the City,
Yet notwithstanding (blest be his high hand)
Their dwelling house amongst the rest doth stand
Free from infection. Nay, some thought it meet,
To set down in their writing, "all the street"
Wherein they dwelled (praised be God) "was clear,"
And therefore, as for that, you need not fear
To give them entertainment; this safe kept, (500)
Made many that at first full sweetly slept
In wholesome beds and likewise to fare well.
But afterwards it otherwise befell:
*London* they thought all over was infected,
And therefore they no passes now respected.
　　Wandring in Fields, some here, some there do lie,
And by the way there's many of them die,
A grievous spectacle for to behold,
And causing tears may, for to hear it told,
To see that Christians should be so estrang'd, (510)
And from their mark Christianity so rang'd,

That from another they no love can have
So far as to vouchsafe them to their grave
But leave them merciless, ev'n where they die,
And so expose them to the ravenous eye
Of Fowls and other vermin, very unfit,
And surely shows small love, or little wit
In these our Countrymen. But I alas
Am gone too far with you; how shall I pass
From whence I came? You know I am expected,          (520)
And let not *London* be by me neglected.

    Fasts are continued, *Wensday* is the day,
And many of us I dare boldly say
Did carefully observe them; many moe,
(I do persuade me) did not keep them so
As fit they should. 'Tis goodly for to see
How yet our Churches filled with people be
And with attention do the Preacher hear,
Although so many durst not venture there,
For fear of further harm; I never heard          (530)
Such zealous Preaching that was still conferd
Unto the hearers, brave renowned men
That so encouraged us; I would my pen
Had all the art that might be to give praise
Unto your worthy actions; many ways
You did declare yourselves like Champions stout,
And were the only men that held us out
From fainting; Physicians they were fled,
Only a few amongst the rest, some dead,
And grief to speak, but true it is (God wot)          (540)
Of your own Coat too many tarried not.

    To those that stayed then, you gain double praise,
For taking pains when *Halcyon* were our days,
And stick not now your lives for us to spend,
Even your own bloods, so that you might but end
Twixt God and us the strife—this was your care,
Thus *Moses* humbly sought the Lord to spare
Hardhearted Jews; full often was he heard,
And I persuade myself God hath not bard
Sweet mercy's gate so fast, but one time he          (550)
Or other with our prayers will pleased be.
Go on therefore, surely of God y'blest,
And let not the Almighty yet take rest,
Until that by his mercies we do find
God's wrath appeasd and he of other mind.

And next on earth then you shall have the praise,
Men, wives, and children, shall with pleasing lays,
Have cause to sing your Victories about,
And say you were their Champions fell and stout,
That *Jacob*-like did wrestle with the Lord,                    (560)
And held him fast until he did afford
To hold his hand, and this great sickness stay;
This may be said of you another day.
    Although the Sun shined bright, the Heavens fair,
Yet still we thought corrupted was the air.
Great cause it was of sickness, so we thought,
And so by learned writers were we taught
It to avoid; the best advice we take,
To clear the *Air*, great *Bonfires* we make
Before our doors, as likewise pans of fire                      (570)
Ymixt with pitch, so greatly we desire
Cause of Infections cease, then thought it meet,
That everyone at home or else in street
(As they did pass) should to a Nosegay smell
Held in their hands, which would do very well:
Some made of Hemp and Pitch; others thought fit
To use some other Scents, which I omit.
And Frankincense in houses do we burn
And use all other means we can to turn
That into sweet, we thought corrupted was.                      (580)
    Let's leave off this and tell what came to pass.
And now imagine *July* we have pass'd.
*August* the Month is, wherein we so fast
Do leave this world, to seek another rest,
Wherein one week there died at the least
Five thousand souls, two hundreth and five.
They'd make a fair show to be seen alive.
So many thousands in the Country gone,
And we so few in number left alone,
And yet so many in one week should die,                         (590)
So many corpses that I think nere eye
Did ere behold daily and hourly pass
Within this City; infinite grief alas,
Must needs possess those that are left alive,
And for one safeguard, how do we now strive,
These lines ensuing will directly tell;
Please you peruse them and to mark them well.
    The eighteenth of the month that was the week,
Now not so much for human helps we seek,

But ready for Death's stroke we do prepare,                                    (600)
And for to gain heaven's Crown is all our care.
Daily we see our Friend and neighbors die
And who can say is next, ore he or I?
The shunning now of sick is not respected,
For who doth know whose house is not infected?
They are not now pent up; doors are open.
No coy there is with any to be spoken,
But one with other do consort together.
And as for danger few of us care whether,
The party we are with be sick or no,                                           (610)
Only we ask him whether it be so,
And where the pain proceeds, rising or spot,
And to their beds we go, for we are not
So timorous, but do approach them near,
And with our best advice we do them cheer.
And, being dead now, we such kindness have,
None will refuse to bring them to the grave,
But after Biers we throng without disdain,
And in our judgment hold it very vain,
If we should not our last performance lend                                     (620)
To such a neighbor or to such a Friend:
Discourteous, unfit and eke faint-hearted,
Thus did we meet and thus we kindly parted.
     Well may I say to many a Country lout
Of this our Kingdom, "Where's the valor stout
Possest your fearful hearts? What is the matter
That so for fear your very teeth do chatter
Within your heads? Why do your bones so shiver
As if you neither had nor heart nor liver?
To see a *London* man, oh y'are undone,                                        (630)
Venture not near, but as far from him run,
As Furlongs, two contain, at least. Oh fly!
His very breath will smell, as far as eye
Can ere behold him. Are you not asham'd
And in all good men's judgments to be blam'd?
I am not ignorant of your churlish dealing.
The wound that open is will need long healing,
Of your unkindness show'd to our poor City.
Hard-hearted men, you should have had more pity.
You think us Cowards; you the worthies are,                                    (640)
And who but you for sturdy men of war?
How is it now, do you not plainly see?
*London* doth yield as stout as any he

Lives on your clotted grounds as do appear.
We stand not in such dread, nor do we fear
The loss of our poor lives, for in a word,
Although we in a manner see the sword,
Of the Almighty's Justice ever waving
Over our heads, killing many, craving,
Yet from the venger do we never shrink.                    (650)
No, we persuaded be and surely think,
That he is everywhere and that he can
(And if please him) send to the Countryman,
As great a sickness as he hath to us;
Thus I persuade myself and even thus
Should you persuaded be and understand,
That the best means for to avoid God's hand,
Is not to fly but to approach him near
With hearty sorrow; take heed how we bear
Ourselves hereafter that we not offend,                    (660)
Else worser judgments God to us can send
Where're we be. With you I have now done."
    Lord with what longing do the people run,
To know what number this next week have died,
And now (blest be his name) we have espied
A happy ceasing of his anger past,
For in this week they died not so fast:
Four thousand, eight hundred, one and forty fell,
Though a great number, it rejoyct us well
To see a ceasing, and with thankful mind,                  (670)
We gave God thanks for that he was so kind.
    And by the way now this is to be noted,
And will be markt by those that are devoted:
When we are now even hurl'd into despair
And scarce car'd whether day was foul or fair,
Such a perplexity were we driven in,
That how the world went we weight'd not a pin.
When we were almost weare now with crying,
And almost past all hope for ought relying
At the Almighty's hands, lo even then,                      (680)
He gan to show unto us (sinful men)
Some tokens that his anger will not long
Continue if so be we sing the song
Of true repentance. I remember well
The Prohibition of our fast days fell
This very week; the ceasing was before.
We cannot, then, directly say therefore

That they were cause so many were infected.
I hope there's few that are so ill affected
As so to think did we not meet together,                    (690)
And as I said before, we car'd not whether
Daily and hourly 'bout our worldly ends,
Someone for one thing, others see their Friends
Lie visited; Sick with well we mingle.
Those that are well from sick we cannot single,
Yet many of us were both well and sound,
And I amongst the rest this favor found
(Blest be his holy name). No more of this.
     Now in my mind a homebred story is,
Of one I knew, a Countryman of mine,                        (700)
(Hardly deserving here to have a line)
Who did refrain the Churches (so wise was he)
So did his son, lest they infect might be.
What I insert I heard it to be true,
And I think God their judgment gave them due,
Neither in the Church or Churchyard did they die,
But in the open Fields there did they lie.
     And one thing more I thought good to observe.
Whether it observation do deserve
Or no, I pray you judge: this did I find                    (710)
When we unto each other were most kind
And feared not the visited to see,
Yet even at the time, I noted we
Did find a ceasing which did plainly show
That we unto the Almighty much did owe,
For his great love, beyond imagination
And far beyond all human expectation.
For, fore that time most were of judgment still,
The reason why so many there were ill,
Was cause they took not heed, nor much respected,          (720)
To keep themselves from those that were infected.
     The last great sickness it did fall out so,
(As I have heard). Well, let us forwards go,
Not that I think the sickness not infect,
For many then my judgment will reject,
For to the contrary it doth appear.
Therefore I'd wish no moral wight come near
Infected persons, to presume too much,
Unless occasions so great be such
As either them to help or help themselves,                 (730)
Else should I count them for presuming Elves.

Weary with toil and with sad cares opprest,
Let now my muse from this sad strain take rest,
Nevertheless but for a little while,
And give me leave but only for to smile
At worldings' folly, who with care they strive
To keep their earthly Carcasses alive,
Whilst others pining do desire to die,
Respectless of their lives: such misery
They do sustain, y'wrapt in cruel love,                                      (740)
Or else some higher crosses from above.
    For recreation I think best befits,
In time of sadness to revive our wits
With honest mirth, a story for to tell,
The best I have; mark then how it befell.
In *Gloucestershire* (a parcel of this Land)
There *Cheltenham,* my native Town, doth stand,
Many a brave lad hath there been bred and bore
As well in these our times as long before,
Who hand to hand in battle would men thrill,                                 (750)
Ere they from them would suffer any ill.
Howbeit now the sickness (as I hear)
Have brought these hardy men into great fear,
Yet to their kindred still their love is such,
To give them kind relief they will not grutch,
Provided always that they may be pent
In some remoted place, whereas the scent
May not annoy the dwellers of the Town,
Else one against another well might frown.
Some two miles off the same there stands a hill,                            (760)
That if you saw it, surely say you will,
It is a great one, likewise very high.
Not far upon, nor yet not very nigh
A wood doth stand—*Puckham* is called by name—
And thereabouts is of great note and fame
In nutting-time; then, famous let it be
A little more for that we now do see:
It proves a shelter to our *London* men,
Who there did lurk as Foxes in their den,
But if they chanc't abroad once for to stere[2]                            (770)
More dreadful far than wolves they did appear
To friend or foe: if once they do them spy
Their sight more fell than any *Basilisk's* eye.

---

[2]   *Stere.* Stir; so spelled to rhyme with appear.

There lodg'd that hard Squire, Sir *Henry* hight,
A valiant, doughty, and courageous sprite.
There lay that Lady bright, his partner dear,
That were most bravely brought on horseback there,
With diverse others, men of mickle worth,
That were resolv'd, none of them to come forth
But round about the wood to rove and range,　　　　　(780)
Until the Moon had pass'd her full and change.
This was the order then, but out, alas,
Whilst we on hills are, there's a *London* Ass
Or Carrier comes to Town within bowshot.
Whenas the sickness reign'd exceeding hot,
His pack he doth untie and *London* ware
Lies open to be catch't with *Cheltnam* air.
High time it is for safety to provide;
More harm, than ere aware, may them betide.
The matter known, some wise men of the Town,　　　　(790)
Bold affrappeth this foolhardy Clown,
With bitter threats and with a dire aspect;
This great presumptuous act they do detect,
And to him spake thus or to this effect,
"Thou *London* vagrant, bold presumptuous man,
All words too good for thee that name we can,
Is this a place for thee for to untie?
At such a time as this, now verily,
If straight thou do'st not truss and quickly run
From this same coast, we'll shoot thee with a Gun."　　(800)
At which hard words forthwith it did appear,
How much it deem'd him by the trembling fear
Of all his joints, for greatly he did quake,
And seem'd as if his very heart did ache,
Sighing, quoth he, "good sirs be not offended,
What's done amiss hereafter shall be mended."
　　　Courage, brave *London!* heart unto thee take,
For every week the sickness now doth slake.
What, shall we always faint, be drooping men
And think that nere good time will come again?　　　　(810)
Indeed 'tis true, many our Friends are gone,
And dear ones too; we cannot choose but moan
For them a while; God's hand we cannot stay
When he doth please to strike, well wish we may.
Time is for all, a time there is to die,
And as they are, so must be you and I.
A debt we owe, that is to God a Death;

Short is our life and soon gone is our breath.
Here is not resting place; Pilgrims we are
Within this world; unto a Country far (820)
We have to trace; it is to Heaven's high,
To which we cannot come before we die.
They are in rest no doubt, we still in care;
Sorrow we taste, but they do better fare.
 Like as in bloody field a battle fought,
By raging enemies that always sought
To work unto each other harm and scathe
And naught but death could swage their baneful wrath,
Where many thousands in one battle die,
And many groveling on the earth do lie, (830)
After a long and weary battle tried,
So many wounded eke so many died,
Upon retire, they do their losses count,
And find they do in number much surmount—
Of this poor City such now was the case,
When time had made so many run the race
Of this their mortal lives; the rest, behind,
To know the perfect number were inclin'd,
Of those that dy'd, the several Bills they view,
And cast them up to be informed true. (840)
The better to express, cease Verse a while,
And let us forwards in another style.

Gentle Reader, I am not ignorant what great mortality hath been reported and verily believed to be in *London,* in almost all places of this Kingdom, by reason of this sickness, and that they conceived a far greater number died than indeed there did, or at least-wise—not considering or once imagining such a multitude of people (men, women, and children) should be in one place or City—thought verily there were hardly any or very few of us left alive. Indeed the streets were empty in respect of the large multitudes that formerly before this great sickness pass'd to and fro in it, but there was no grass growing in any streets of note for want of trading, as thy conceived, for I persuade me as many people pass'd to and fro in the streets of the said City in the highest of the sickness upon their occasions as did at any time in the streets of any other City or great Town of this Kingdom where the sickness was not (setting Fairs and appointed assemblies aside); wherefore, we were not all dead. Indeed if God Almighty had gone on in wrath, as of long time you see he did continue, we should have all been ere long consumed. But he is a God of mercy and is graciously pleased to leave some behind—yea, very many— for a witness both of his Justice and Mercy.

 And as in my former similitude, after a battle fought as well the several armies as the several adverse Countries will hearken after and take notice of the loss received, although they may be much more moved for the same, so I persuade myself both City and Country in this Kingdom that have had no certainty of the number that have died in this present visitation, although they wish well to the City (it being the harbor of many of their kindred and friends and in a manner the beauty, wealth, and straight of this nation) will desire notwithstanding to be truly informed, and therefore as aiming altogether to make my poor subject profitable or pleasing or at leastwise not burdensome to all the whole hands it shall happen to come, I have taken this pains to set down the number, both in gross and as they died weekly, so may you perceive the increase and decrease.

*There died in London and the Liberties thereof*

|  | Total | Plague |
|---|---|---|
| From the 23 of *December* to the 30 of the same | 211 | 0 |
| From the 30 of *December* to the 6 of *January* | 220 | 1 |
| From the 6 of *January* to the 13 of the same | 196 | 1 |
| From the 13 of *January* to the 20 of the same | 240 | 0 |
| From the 20 of *January* to the 27 | 226 | 0 |
| From the 27 to the 3 of *February* | 174 | 3 |
| From the 3 to the 10 | 204 | 5 |
| From the 10 to the 17 | 211 | 3 |
| From the 17 to the 24 | 252 | 1 |
| From the 24 to the 3 of *March* | 207 | 0 |
| From the 3 to the 10 | 210 | 0 |
| From the 10 to the 17 | 261 | 4 |
| From the 17 to the 24 | 226 | 8 |
| From the 14 to the 31 | 243 | 11 |
| From the 31 to the 7 of *April* | 239 | 10 |
| From the 7 to the 14 | 256 | 24 |
| From the 14 to the 21 | 230 | 25 |
| From the 21 to the 28 | 305 | 26 |
| From the 29 to the 5 of *May* | 292 | 30 |
| From the 5 to the 12 | 332 | 45 |
| From the 12 to the 19 | 379 | 71 |
| From the 19 to the 26 | 401 | 78 |
| From the 26 to the 2 of *June* | 395 | 69 |
| From the 2 to the 9 | 434 | 97 |
| From the 9 to the 16 | 510 | 165 |
| From the 16 to the 23 | 640 | 239 |
| From the 23 to the 30 | 942 | 390 |
| From the 30 to the 7 of *July* | 1222 | 593 |
| From the 7 to the 14 | 1741 | 1004 |
| From the 14 to the 21 | 1850 | 1819 |
| From the 21 to the 28 | 3583 | 2471 |

| | | |
|---|---|---|
| From the 28 to the 4 of *August* | 4517 | 3659 |
| From the 4 of *August* to the 11 | 4855 | 4115 |
| From the 11 to the 18 | 5205 | 4463 |
| From the 18 to the 25 | 4841 | 4218 |
| From the 25 to the 1 of *September* | 3897 | 3344 |
| From the 1 of *September* to the 8 | 3157 | 2550 |
| From the 8 to the 15 | 2148 | 1672 |
| From the 15 to the 22 | 1994 | 1555 |
| From the 22 to the 29 | 1256 | 852 |
| From the 29 to this 6 of *October* | 838 | 538 |
| From the 6 of *October* to the 13 | 815 | 511 |
| From the 13 to the 20 | 651 | 331 |
| From the 20 to the 27 | 375 | 134 |
| From the 27 to the 3 of *November* | 357 | 89 |
| From the 3 of *November* to the 10 | 319 | 92 |
| From the 10 to the 17 | 274 | 48 |
| From the 17 to the 24 | 231 | 27 |
| From the 24 to the 1 of *December* | 190 | 15 |
| From the 1 of *December* to the 8 | 181 | 15 |
| From the 8 to the 15 of the same | 168 | 6 |

*Total from the 23 of December 1624 to the 15 of December 1625, 52914.*
*Whereof of the plague, 35417.*

The Total of the last great sickness happening in the beginning of the Reign of our late Sovereign Lord Kind *James* deceased, *viz.* from the 23 of *December* 1602 to the 22 of *December* 1603, there died of all diseases in *London* and the Liberties 38244, whereof of the plague 30578. Wherein the greatest number that died in one week was in *London* and the Liberties in all, 3385. Whereof the plague, 3035.

In Former times the Kingdom and City have been likewise visited, as soon after the Conquest of King *William* Duke of *Normandy* there happened a fearful plague; as likewise in the Reign of King Edward the third; and in the year of 1562 in which year there died of the Pestilence 20136. Also in *Anno* 1592, in which year there died in all 25886, where of the plague in and about *London*, 1503.

Other parts of the world have likewise felt God's hand, as you may read in Scripture of *Jerusalem,* etc. Further it is recorded of the City called the grand *Cair*o in *Turkey* once every seven years there hapneth a vehement Contagion, to the loss of most part of the people there. In *Rome* there have died 2000 a day, and 100,000 in a year. In *Constantinople* 5000 a day, and 700,000 within six months. In the City of *Paris* in *France,* 100,000 in a year, *viz.* in *Anno* 1348. In *Milan, Padua,* and *Venice* 100,000 in each City within two years. In *Bohemia* 300,000 in the like space, and so likewise in other Cities and Kingdoms, and at several times hath God shown his power.

As one asleep, of many pleasing toys
Oft times doth dream and thinks that he enjoys
That which indeed he doth not when he wakes,
Into his former dumps himself betakes,
So, after we such bitter storms had tasted,
For want of Trade whilst that the sickness lasted,
Luld with vain hope whenas we still did see
The sickness cease, that there a Term should be                    (850)
Without all questions kept, thus thought we then,
And for a while we were right joyful men.
Our shops begin to open, we prepare,
And set them out with sundry sorts of ware,
Although before this time windows stood bare,
Open or shut we did not greatly care.
When news doth come that sets us into passion:
The King proclaimeth by his Proclamation
That there no Term of *Michael*[3] *should be kept*
But where the Proclamation did direct,                             (860)
Which was to *Reading*, good for *Berkshire* men.
You may conjecture what a plunge we then
Were put unto; how shall our Rent be paid,
And other needments which we want defrayd?
Now many a poor soul in the streets we see
For want to beg and crave, which would not be,
But that the times so hard are; others sham'd
(Although their need is great) yet to be nam'd
A craving beggar; much they could endure
Ere they could btook to put the same in ure,                       (870)
And therefore far more harder was their case,
Than those that beg'd and car'd not to be base.
'Tis such a time that many a sigh is set
By those we "good-men" call, yet run in debt,
And further also, I think, like to run.
Good Lord, amend it, else we are undone.
     Albeit 'tis a comfort that we find
That King and great men were so well inclin'd,
Their charitable deeds for to express,
In these our great afflictions, to redress                         (880)
The want of poor men, which did so abound
Within this city, that no place was found
Without a multitude, and to prevent,

---

[3]    *Term of Michael.* One of four terms for the English Court of Common Law, held
2–25 November; also called Michaelmas Term and associated with St. Michael's day.

Means was collected; orders there were sent
By Proclamation how it should be used
That so their worthy deeds be not abused.
This was commended to the weighty care
Of *London's* Governor (the worthy Mayor),
Who in the same did show himself upright,
Got great applause in all the people's sight.                (890)
This worthy Act did many others move
To show their Charity and Christian love.
Yea, those that had not much themselves would give
Of that they had, poor people to relieve
In these sad times, abroad and at the door;
Thus were we mov'd, so far'd it with the poor.
    Examples surely are of wondrous force,
In such sad times as these to strike remorse
Into men's hearts, but more whenas we see
Before our eyes the woeful misery                            (900)
Of those that want; no doubt most that were here
And saw these things more liberal far they were
Than erst before, and to tell plain my mind,
What others write myself did daily find
Them very free, for wheresoere I was
At home or [a]broad, giving there always was
By one or other, unto those that cried,
Who hardly of an Alms-deed were deny'd
Of them they askt; foretimes, it was not so,
But many should be askt that would say no.                   (910)
Before that we would see one's wants relieved,
So hard our hearts were to poor souls y'grieved.
    And now to you that in the country be,
Hear not the cries of poor, nor yet do see
Their miserable wants, how they have far'd,
And how we to our powers have not spar'd
Our means for to relieve them—if we slack,
Let not our slackness you hard-hearted make
When you shall be required. I may say,
We have done well whilst you have been away.                 (920)
Still, need there is and like is so to be.
Twill be a pleasing thing for us to see
You home again in peace, if much you make
Of poor afflicted ones, for Christ his sake.
    Lastly, to all Residers of this Land
That at this time have felt the Almighty's hand
Or seen the heavy judgments that have been,

Sith that the cause thereof is only sin,
For which we have endured many a smart,
And oft times gone to bed with aching heart.                    (930)
Like dreaded children; let us now be wise,
And have a care that we do not despise,
Or set at light the anger of our God,
Lest he in fury with a greater rod
In vengeance come upon us; warning take,
By this most grievous chastment; now awake
And look about us; let us call to mind
What mighty City we in writings find,
That heretofore for glory bare the bell,[4]
And through the world did far and near excel                    (940)
The Famous *Nineveh, Jerusalem*,
*Troy, Carthage, Rome*, and many more with them,
Which for their sins were wholly overthrown,
Their standing places hardly to be known.
And, in this sad disaster, let us not
Forget the woeful state which now, God wot,
Renown'd *Judea* and the Eastern Lands,
That now lie groaning under Turkish bands,
The famous *Grecia*, many Countries more,
Who all one God and Savoir did adore,                          (950)
That we do now, but, going far astray,
Have wrought unto themselves such sad annoy,
That grief it is to tell. Oh, that my pen,
Or all the art I have could now move men
To leave their evil courses and to turn
Unto their maker, inwardly to mourn
For what hath been the cause of this sad woe,
And gain the love of him that now our foe
Appears to be; how have we wandred wide,
In vain excess of riot, sinful pride,                          (960)
Where the love that with us should be found,
And God's servants should to all abound?
Was it not turn'd to hatred and despite,
Or such a love as strayd far from the right?
Most filthy fraud, we lov'd, for to deceive,
And if we could our neighbors to bereave
Of that they had, be't but a good name,
(If we had none), we envi'd at the same.
Our swearing and blaspheming, hateful lies,

---

[4]    *bare the bell.* Have foremost rank or position.

Have pierc'st the very Heavens and there cries                    (970)
For flaming vengeance, and our great oppression
Have there been likewise and have made confession,
Before we'd do't ourselves; our beastly lust
And many other sins did stick as rust
Upon our sinful souls. Oh now, like men,
Let's rouse these dang'rous Adders from their den.
These have been they that have our sorrows sought,
And these were they that to destruction brought
The other woeful countries; these are they
That if we not forsake them will destroy                          (980)
Our woeful Land likewise; now, let us weep
And drench our eyes in floods of sorrows deep,
That we so great a God have not regarded,
Conclude that we most justly are rewarded
For our misdeeds, and let us from them cease.
This is the way to make a final peace
'Twixt God and us, so let all good men pray,
"Amen, Amen" with me, God grant we may.
FINIS

# John Taylor,
## *The Fearful Summer*

Copies of the edition of this poem transcribed here (STC 2nd ed., 23754) are housed in the archives of The British and Bodleian Libraries. Two additional editions exist: one from the same year, issued by the same printers (STC 2nd ed., 23755, with two copies at The British Library); and one printed by Elizabeth Purslowe for Henry Gosson, which appears ten years later, during the next large-scale plague visitation in 1636 (STC 2nd ed., 23756—one copy each in the British and Huntington Libraries). The remarkable cover image of *The Plague Epic in Early Modern England* is from the title page of this later, 1636, edition, reproduced with permission of The Henry E. Huntington Library. Preceding the poem in all three editions are a verse dedication in iambic pentameter to "Sir John Millicent, Sergeant Porter to the King's most Excellent Majesty"; a prose dedication "To the Printer"; and a full prose "Preface" explaining the occasion and purpose of the verse. In the first two editions from 1625, *Against Swearing*, a poem in iambic pentameter with rhyming couplets is appended following the poem. The first of these editions (23754), includes a prose preface to *Against Swearing* and a concluding prose work, "My farewell to the famous University of Oxford." The second edition of this poem in the same year as well as the third edition in 1636 offer "a conclusion in Prose" to *The Fearful Summer*, and both omit the farewell to Oxford. The 1636 edition also drops *Against Swearing*, which by this time had circulated separately as *A warning for swearers and blasphemers* (1626, STC 23812.7) and as *Christian admonitions against the two fearful sins of cursing and swearing* (1630, STC 23741.5).

THE FEARFUL SUMMER
OR
LONDON'S CALAMITY,
the country's courtesy, and both their misery

By JOHN TAYLOR
OXFORD
Printed by *John Litchfield* and *William Turner*,
Printers to the famous *University*.
*Anno Domini* 1625

The *Patience* and long-*suffering* of our *God*,
Keeps close his *Quiver* and restrains his *Rod*,
And though our crying Crimes to Heav'n do cry
For vengeance on accurst Mortality,
Yea, though we merit mischiefs manifold,
Blest *Mercy* doth the hand of *Justice* hold.
But when that *Eye* that sees all things most clear,
Expects our *fruits* of *Faith* from year to year,
Allows us painful[1] *Pastors* who bestow
Great care and toil to make us fruitful grow,                                    (10)
And daily doth in those weak *Vessels* send
The dew of *Heaven*, in hope we will amend,
Yet (at the last) he doth perceive and see
That we unfruitful and most barren be,
Which makes his dreadful Indignation frown,
And (as accursed *fig-trees*) cut us down.
Thus Mercy (mock'd) plucks Justice on our heads,
And grievous *Plagues*, our Kingdom overspreads.
Then let us to our *God* make quick returning,
With true contrition, fasting, and with mourning.                                (20)
*The Word is God*, and *God* hath spoke the Word;
If we repent, he will put up his sword.
*He's* griev'd in punishing, *He's* slow to Ire,
And *HE* a sinner's death doth not desire.
If our Compunction our Amendment show,
Our purple sins, *He'll* make as white as snow.
If we lament, our God is merciful;
Our scarlet crimes he'll make as white as wool.
Fair *London* that did late abound in bliss,
And wast our Kingdom's great *Metropolis*.                                       (30)
'Tis *thou* that art dejected, low in state,

---

[1]    *painful.* Painstaking.

Disconsolate, and almost desolate.
The *hand* of Heav'n that, only, did protect thee,
Thou hast provok'd most justly to correct thee,
And for thy pride of Heart and deeds unjust,
He lays thy Pomp and Glory in the dust.
Thou that wast late the Queen of Cities nam'd,
Throughout the world admir'd, renown'd, and fam'd;
Thou that hadst all things at command and will,
To whom all *England* was a Handmaid still.                (40)
For raiment, fuel, fish, fowl, beasts, for food,
For fruits,for all our Kingdom counted good.
Both near and far remote, all did agree
To bring their best of blessings unto *thee*.
Thus in conceit thou seem'dst to rule the *Fates*,
Whilst *peace* and *plenty* flourish'd in thy Gates.
      Could I relieve thy miseries as well
As part I can thy woes and sorrows tell,
Then should my Cares be eas'd with thy Relief,
And all my study, how to end thy grief.                   (50)
Thou that wer't late rich, both in friends and wealth,
Magnificent in state, strong in thy health,
As chiefest Mistress, of our country priz'd,
Now chiefly in the country are despis'd.
The name of *London* now both far and near,
Strikes all the Towns and Villages with fear,
And to be thought a *Londoner* is worse
Than one that breaks a house or takes a Purse.
He that will filch and steal—now is the Time—
No Justice dares examine him, his crime.                   (60)
Let him but say that he "from *London*" came,
So full of Fear and Terror is that name,
The Constable his charge will soon forsake,
And no man dares his *mittimus* to make.
      Thus Citizens, plagu'd for the City['s] sins,
Poor entertainment in the Country wins.
Some fear the City and fly thence amain,
And those are of the Country fear'd again,
Who 'gainst them bar their windows and their doors,
More than they would 'gainst *Turks*, or *Jews*, or *Moors*.    (70)
I think if very *Spaniards* had come there,
Their welcome had been better and their cheer,
Whilst Haycock lodging, with hard slender fare,
Welcome, like dogs unto a Church, they are.
Fear makes them with the Anabaptists join,

For if an Hostess do receive their coin,
She in a dish of water, or a pail,
Will new baptize it, lest it something ail.
Thus many a Citizen well stor'd with Gold,
Is glad to lie upon his mother *mould*,                    (80)
His bed the map of his mortality,
His curtains clouds, and Heav'n his Canopy.
The russet ploughswain and the Leathern Hind,
Through fear is grown unmannerly, unkind,
And in his house (to harbor) he'll prefer
An Infidel before a *Londoner*.
Milk-maids and Farmers' wives are grown so nice,
They think a Citizen a Cockatrice,
And country Dances are wax'd so coy and brisk,
They shun him as they'll shun a Basilisk,                  (90)
For every one, the sight of him would fly,
All fearing he would kill them with his eye.
Ah, woeful *London*, I thy grief bewail,
And if my sighs and prayers may but prevail,
I humbly beg of *God* that he'll be pleas'd,
In *Jesus Christ* his wrath may be appeas'd,
Withholding his dread Judgments from above,
And once more grasp thee in his arms of love,
In Mercy all our wickedness remit,
For who can give thee thanks within the pit?              (100)
    Strange was the change in less than three months' space,
In joy, in woe, in grace, and in disgrace.
A healthful *April*, a diseased *June*,
And dangerous *July*, brings all out of tune.
That city whose rare objects pleas'd the eyes
With much content and more varieties;
She that was late delightful to the ears
With melody Harmonious, like the *Spheres*;
She that had all things that might please her taste
That was by *Skies*, or *Earth*, or *Seas* embrac'd,      (110)
All odors and perfumes to please the *scent*,
And all she *felt* did give her *touch* content.
Her Cinque port *senses*, richly fed and cloy'd
With blessings bountiful, which she enjoy'd,
Now three months change hath fill'd it full with fear,
As if no Solace ever had been there.
    What do the eyes see there but grieved sights
Of sick, oppressed, and distressed wights?
Houses shut up, some dying, and some dead;

Some (all amazed) flying and some fled,                                    (120)
Streets thinly man'd with wretches every day
Which have no power to flee or means to stay;
Dead Corpses carried and recarried still,
Whil'st fifty Corpses scarce one grave doth fill;
With "LORD HAVE MERCY UPON US," on the door
Which (though the words be good) doth grieve men sore,
And o're the door-posts fix'd a *cross* of *red*
Betokening that there *Death* some blood hath shed.
Some with God's marks or tokens do espy
Those *Marks* or *Tokens* show them they must die.                          (130)
Some with their Carbuncles and sores new burst
Are fed with hope they have escap'd the worst.
Thus passeth all the week, till *Thursday's Bill*,
Shows us what thousands Death that week did kill.
That fatal *Bill* doth like a razor cut
The dead, the living in a maze doth put,
And he that hath a Christian heart, I know,
Is griev'd, and wounded with the deadly blow.
        These are the objects of the *Eye*; now hear
And mark the mournful music of the *Ear*.                                   (140)
There do the brazen Iron-tong'd loud bells
(Death's clamorous music) Ring continual knells.
Some lofty in their notes, some sadly tolling,
Whil'st fatal dogs make a most dismal howling;
Some frantic raving, some with anguish crying,
Some singing, praying, groaning, and some dying;
The healthful grieving and the sickly groaning—
All in a mournful diapason moaning.
Here, Parents for their Children's loss Lament;
There, Children's grief for parents' life that spent.                       (150)
Here, Sister mourns for sister, Kin for Kin.
As one grief ends, another doth begin.
There, one lies languishing with slender fare
Small comfort, less attendance, and least care,
With none but Death and he to tug together,
Until his corpse and soul part each from either.
In one house one, or two, or three doth fall,
And in another Death plays sweepstake all.
Thus, universal, sorrowful complaining
Is all the music now in London reigning.                                    (160)
Thus is her comfort sad Calamity,
And all her *Melody* is *Malady*.
These are the objects of the *eyes* and *ears*

Most woeful sights and sounds of griefs and fears.
    The curious *taste* that whilom did delight [2]
With cost and care to please the Appetite,
What she was wont to hate, she doth adore
And what's high priz'd, she held despis'd before.
The drugs, the drenches, and untoothsome drinks,
Fear gives a sweetness to all several stinks,                              (170)
And for supposed *Antidotes*, each Palate
Of most contagious weeds will make a Sallate.
And any of the simplest Mountebanks
May cheat them (as they will) of Coin and thanks,
With scraped powder of a shoeing-horn,
Which they'll believe is of an *Unicorn*.
*Angelica*'s distasteful root is gnaw'd
And *herb of Grace* most Ruefully is chaw'd.
*Garlic* offendeth neither *taste*, nor *smell*;
Fear and opinion makes it relish well,                                     (180)
Whilst *Bezoar* stone, and mighty *Mithridate*,
To all degrees are great in estimate,
And *Treacle's* power is wondrously exprest,
And Dragon Water in most high request—
These 'gainst the Plague are good preservatives.
    But the best cordial is t'amend our lives.
Sin's the main cause, and we must first begin
To cease our griefs by ceasing of our sin.
I do believe that *God* hath given in store
Good medicines to cure or ease each sore,                                  (190)
But first remove the cause of the disease,
And then (no doubt but) the effect will cease.
Our sin's the Cause; remove our sins from hence,
And *God* will soon remove the Pestilence.
Then every med'cine (to our consolation)
Shall have his power, his force, his operation,
And till that time, Experiments are not
But Paper walls against a Canon shot.
    On many a post I see *Quacksalvers'* Bills
Like *Fencers'* Challenges to show their skills,                           (200)
As if they were such *masters of defense*,
That they dare combat with the *Pestilence*,
Meet with the plague in any deadly fray,
And brag to bear the victory away.
But if their patients patiently believe them,

---

[2]    [marginal note] *Tasting.*

They'll cure them (without fail) of what they give them.
What though ten thousand by their drenches perish,
They made them purposely themselves to cherish.
Their Art is a mere Artless kind of lying
To pick their *living* out of other's *dying*.                              (210)
    This sharp invective no way seems to touch
The learn'd *Physician*, whom I honor much,
The Paracelsians and Galenists,
The Philosophical grave Herbalists—
These I admire and reverence, for in those,
God doth dame *Nature's* secrets fast enclose,
Which they distribute, as occasions serve
Health to reserve, and health decay'd conserve.
'Tis 'gainst such *Rat-catchers* I bend my pen,
Which do mechanically murder men,                                           (220)
Whose promises of cure (like lying knaves)
Doth beggar men or send them to their graves.
    Now *London* for the sense of *feeling* next,
Thou in thy *feeling* chiefly art perplext,[3]
Thy heart *feels* sorrow, and thy body anguish;
Thou in thy *feeling* feel'st thy force to languish.
Thou *feel'st* much woe and much calamity,
And many millions *feel* thy misery.
Thou *feel'st* the fearful *Plague*, the *Flux* and *Fever*,
Which many a soul doth from the body sever.                                 (230)
And I beseech *God* for our *Savior's* merit
To let thee *feel* the *Comfort* of his *Spirit*.
    Last, for the solace of the *smell*, or *scent*,[4]
Some in contagious rooms are closely pent,
Whereas corrupted Air they take and give
Till time ends or lends liberty to live.
One with a piece of tasseld well-*tarr'd Rope*
Doth with that nosegay keep himself in hope.
Another doth a wisp of wormwood pull
And with great Judgment crams his nostrils full.                            (240)
A third takes of his socks from's sweating feet,
And makes them his perfume alongst the street,
Whilst *Billets*, Bonfire-like, and *faggots* dry
Are burnt i'th streets, the Air to purify.
    Thou great *Almighty*, give them time and space,

---

[3]    [marginal note] *Smelling*. [the marginal notes mislabel "*Smelling*" for "*Feeling*"
and the reverse.]
[4]    marginal note] *Feeling*.

And purify them with thy heavenly *Grace*.
Make their repentance Incense, whose sweet savor
May mount unto thy throne and gain thy favor.
Thus every sense that should the heart delight
Are ministers and organs to affright.                    (250)
The Citizens do from the City run.
The country fears, the citizens do shun.
Both fear the *Plague*, but neither fears one jot
Their evil ways, which hath the plague begot.
This is the way this sickness to prevent:
Fear to offend more than the punishment.
     All trades are dead or almost out of breath,
But such as live by sickness, or by death:
The Mercers, Grocers, Silk-men, Goldsmiths, Drapers,
Are out of season, like noon-burning Tapers.             (260)
All functions fail almost, through want of buyers
And every art and mystery turn *Dyers*.
The very *Watermen* give over plying;
Their rowing trade doth fail; they fall to *dying*.
Some men there are that rise by other's falls:
Prophetic Augurists in urinals,[5]
Those are right watermen, and row so well,
They either land their *fares* in Heav'n or *Hell*.
But this much (Reader) you must understand,
They commonly are paid before they land.                 (270)
Next unto him, th' *Apothecary* thrives
By Physic bills and his preservatives;
Worm eaten *Sextons*, mighty gains do win,
And nasty *Gravemakers*, great comings in,
And *Coffin makers* are well paid their rent
For many a woeful wooden tenement.
The *Searchers* of each *corpse* good gainers be,
The *Bearers* have a profitable fee,
And last, the *Dog-killers*, great gain abounds,
For Braining bawling curs and foisting hounds.[6]        (280)
These are the *grave* trades, that do get and save,
Whose gravity brings many to their *grave*.
     Thus grieved *London*, fill'd with moans and groans
Is like a *Golgotha* of dead men's bones,

---

[5]   *The very Waterman ... urinal.* Poking fun at his own profession as a Thames
waterman, Taylor suggests that in plague-time, waterman take to examining urine to predict
people's health: only plague-related trades thrive.

[6]   *Braining bawling ... hounds.* For killing or otherwise removing yelping dogs.

The field where death his bloody fray doth fight,
And kills eight hundred in a day and night.
Fair houses that were late exceeding dear
At fifty or an hundred pounds a year,
The Landlords are so pitiful of late,
They'll let them at a quarter of the rate.                    (290)
So he that is a mighty, moneyed man
Let him but thither make what haste he can,
Let him disburse his gold and silver heap
And purchase *London*—'tis exceeding cheap.
But if he tarry but one-half year more,
I hope 'twill be as dear as 'twas before.
A Country cottage that but lately went
At four marks or at three pounds yearly rent,
A Citizen, whose mere necessity
Doth force him now into the country fly,                    (300)
Is glad to hire two Chambers of a Carter
And pray and pay, with thanks, five pounds a quarter—
Then, here's the alteration of this year:
The City's cheapness makes the Country dear.
     Besides another mischief is, I see,
A man dares not be sick although he be.
Let him complain but of the *stone* or *gout*
The plague hath struck him, presently they doubt.
Myself hath been perplexed now and then
With the wind Colic, years above thrice ten.                    (310)
Within the country, I durst not repeat [this],
Although my pangs and gripes and pains were great,
For, to be sick of any kind of grief,
Would make a man worse welcome than a thief.
To be drunk sick, which erst did credit win,
Was fear'd infectious and held worse than sin.
This made me, and many more beside,
Their griefs to smother and their pains to hide,
To tell a merry tale with visage glad,
Whenas the Colic almost made me mad.                    (320)
Thus, mere dissembling, many practis'd then,
And mid'st of pain, seem'd pleasant amongst men,
For why, the smallest sigh or groan or shriek
Would make a man his meat and lodging seek.
     This was the wretched *Londoner's* hard case,
Most hardly welcome into any place,
Whil'st Country people, where soe're they went
Would stop their noses to avoid their scent,

Whenas the case did oft most plain appear
'Twas only they themselves that stunk, with fear!                    (330)
*Nature* was dead (or from the country run):
A *Father* durst not entertain his son;
The *Mother* sees her daughter and doth fear her,
Commands her, on her blessing, not come near her.
Affinity nor any kind of kin
Or ancient friendship, could true welcome win.
The Children scarcely would their Parents know,
Or (if they did) but slender duty show.
      Thus *fear* made *nature* most unnatural,
Duty undutiful, or very small,                                      (340)
No friendship, or else cold and miserable,
And generally all uncharitable.
Nor *London* letters little better sped;
They would not be received (much less be read),
But cast into the fire and burnt with speed,
As if they had been *Heretics* indeed.
And late I saw, upon a Sabbath day,
Some Citizens at Church, prepar'd to pray,
But (as [if] they had been excommunicate)
The good Church wardens thrust them out the gate.                   (350)
Another country virtue I'll repeat,
The people's charity was grown so great
That whatsoever *Londoner* did die,
In Church or Churchyard should not buried lie.
Thus were they scorn'd, despised, banished,
Excluded from the Church, alive and dead.
Alive, their bodies could no harbor have,
And *dead*, not be allow'd a Christian *Grave*.
Thus was the country's kindness cold and small:
No house, no Church, no Christian burial.                           (360)
      Oh thou that on the winged winds dost sit
And seest our misery, remedy it.
Although we have deserv'd thy vengeance hot,
Yet in thy fury (Lord) consume us not,
But in thy mercies sheath thy slaying sword.
Deliver us, according to thy word.
Shut up thy Quiver; stay thy angry rod,
That all the world may know thou art our God.
Oh, open wide the gate of thy compassion.
Assure our souls that thou art our Salvation.                      (370)
Then all our thoughts, and words and works, we'll frame
To magnify thy great and glorious name.

The ways of God are intricate, no doubt
Unsearchable and past man's finding out.
He at his pleasure worketh wondrous things
And in his hand doth hold the hearts of kings,
And for the love, which to our *King* he bears,
By sickness, he our sinful country clears,
That *he* may be a patron and a guide
Unto a people purg'd and purifi'd.                                    (380)
This by a precedent is manifest,
When famous late *Elizabeth* deceast:
Before our gracious *James* put on the crown.
God's hand did cut superfluous branches down.
Not that they then that were of life bereft
Were greater sinners than the number left,
But that the *Plague* should then the kingdom clear
The good to comfort and the bad to fear,
That as a good king, God did us assure,
So he should have a Nation purg'd and pure.                           (390)
And now that Royal *James* entombed lies
And that our gracious *Charles* his room supplies,
As *He* did for his Father formerly,
A sinful nation cleanse and purify,
So *God* for him these things to pass doth bring,
And mends the *subjects* for so good a *King*,
Upon whose Throne may peace and plenty rest,
And he and his Eternally be blest.
AMEN

\*

# Abraham Holland,
## *A Description of the Great, Fearful, and Prodigious Plague*

Holland's plague epic, *A Description of the Great, Fearful, and Prodigious Plague* first appeared in 1626 as part of his posthumous oeuvre, *Hollandi posthuma. A funeral elegy of King James: with a congratulatory salve to King Charles. An elegy of the magnanimous Henry Earle of Oxford. A description of the great, fearful, and prodigious plague: and diverse other pathetical poems, elegies, and other lines, on diverse subjects. The posthumes of Abraham Holland, sometimes of Trinity-College in Cambridge. The author's epitaph, made by himself.* Of the three nearly identical versions of the posthumous work (STC 2nd eds. 13579, 13579.3, 13579.5), the edition used as the basis for transcription here is the one most clear in its print, 13579.5. Copies are held at the Cambridge University; British; Cambridge University St. John's College; Oxford University Balliol College; University of Illinois; Union Theological; and Folger Shakespeare Libraries. Four years later, *A Description* was retitled *London look-back* and appeared in another larger collection from 1630, *Salomon's pest-house, or tower-royal. Newly re-edified and prepared to preserve Londoners with their families, and others, from the doubted deluge of the plague. Item, a laudable exercise for those that are departed or shall depart out of the city into the country, to spend their time till they return, a handful of holy meditations useful and requisite for Gods people, men and women, of all estates and degrees, in these doubtful days, whether troubled in body or mind, and whether Gods visitation of the plague increase or decrease. By the reverend, learned and godly divine I.D. preacher of God's word, whereunto is added Mr. Holland's admonition, and Mr. Phayer's prescription for bodily physic. Also London look-back: a description or representation of the great and memorable mortality ann. 1625. in heroic matchless lines by A[braham] H[olland] of Tr[inity]. College in Cambridge.* Two editions of the 1630 collection appeared with slight variation (STC 2nd ed 6175 and 6176), and the work was reprinted again in 1636 (STC 2nd ed. 6176.5).

*A L'envoy to my endeared Friends*
*Mr. R.T., Mr. W.H., Mr. T.C. and others being in the Country,*
*Serving for an Introduction to the Description*
*of The Plague*

Do you not wonder that in this sad time
I still have leisure to compose a rhyme,
When, as a Christian, care forbids me now
The help of Poetry, that my hot brow
Should sweat with active Wine, or that my heart
Should be so free from passion to use Art
Unto my wild expressions? The mirth
That entertains a Muse and gives a Birth
To happy lines is far more fit for you,
Who in your Country's happiness do view                    (10)
Our slaughters from afar, as men in sight
That stand remote from spectators of a Fight.
Yet I would have both you and all suppose
Sorrow can speak as well in verse as pros—
In this *great Year* of *Elegies*, indeed—
Not with that life, that flame, and active speed,
As when Security did bid me play
With the smooth tresses of Asteria
And wander in her eyes; alas that theme
Is quell'd in grief and drowned in the Stream          (20)
Of the time's sorrow, those Heroic lays
That were begun have thrown away their bays
And cloth'd themselves in Cypress, and my brow
Expects a Night-cap more than Laurel now.
     Sirs, you perhaps are chasing o're the Fields
The Hare, the Deer, or what the season yields,
Do Imp your Falcon's wings, making it fly,
A subtle ambusher about the Sky.
We are the Prey of Death and each night stay
The call of Fate, until the Morning say                    (30)
We may draw forth a Noon, and so at Night,
Lie down again not sure of other light,
Till the great Resurrection, for [it] may be
Death hath his Writ this Night to serve on me.
Do you inquire whether we be afraid
Of Death or no? Which so soon doth invade,
So surely Kill? I answer, "No." That man
That liveth now and views the storm and can
Still be afraid of Death, I must surmise

A Renegade or full of Cowardice.                                     (40)
No Penitent can fear, and he that still
Retains a heart unbroken acts more ill
Than all his life before: that soul is Steel
Which doth not bleed; that hell, which doth not feel
The present blow—it is with us, who here
Hourly view death, as when, exempt of fear
At an Ostent or such a Siege to die,
The Soldiers thought it a Necessity
And so did slight it when each hour were shown
So many other's Deaths t'assure their own.                          (50)
    Endeared Friends, I am well and better much
And in more sweet security than such
Who think of a long life, by these deaths here
Being freed from what is worse than death, the Fear.
Seldom is Christian Valor better gain'd
Than when 'tis by such misery obtain'd.
    I doubt not but that Fame, which still doth use
To spread abroad more large than certain news,
Hath blaz'd our State, and haply doth assure,
As you suppose, far more than we endure                             (60)
Thus far; let me your doubts herein suffice:
Rumor itself can scarce Hyperbolize
Our Real woe. Fear itself cannot vow
There is more Mischief than we suffer now.
If you shall hear of Streets wherein the Grass
Doth grow for want of men that use to pass,
Or *Smithfield* turn'd a meadow or a plain
Wherein the Horses, Kine, and Sheep again
May feed rather than sell; or of poor men
That in their Graves together lie by ten                            (70)
By twenties or by more; or sudden Fates
Of people dying in the streets and gates—
Do not suppose it false. We wretches try
What other Ages shall hold Poetry.
    A March in midst of August, and the Star
That reigneth now, far from Canicular;
In all but the effects, not cloth'd in bright
And scorching Sunshine but in midst of Night,
And Winter storms, as if the Plague did fly
Wrap't in those clouds to fright the troubled Sky                   (80)
And blast mortality; the air the while
Scarce in a Month strikes forth one pleasing smile,
Muffled in damps so close that, from beneath,

We deem it hard by any way, but Death,
To see bright Heaven again. The Rural Swains
Begin to doubt the Usury of their pains
And Prophesy a *Famine*, and the Earth
Choked with Carcasses threatens a *Dearth*
As a Revenge; the Skies the while do shower
Down poisonous tempest to augment the power                    (90)
Of her pretended Malice, while the breath
Of black contagious winds do transport Death
Through the envenom'd air—Earth, Air, and Sky
Conspiring to our great Calamity.
    In what a case poor London stands! To show
Would ask a Pen and Muse that only know
How to write grief. Alas, it is become
A Theatre of Tragedies, where some
Dy'd i'th' first acts, and, many slaughters pass'd,
God knows what murder shall be in the last!                    (100)
    I live not in it but in Chelsea air,
Where Death but in his Outroads doth repair,
And thence do only hear the murmuring Bells
Disclose the slaughter by the frequent Knells.
Yet, as a tender Mother, though she have
A Child interr'd and sleeping in the grave,
Yet will she oft go see the tomb and dew
His dust with pious tears and oft renew
His Posthume exequies, so sometimes I
Go to behold the City and espy                    (110)
As I do walk along the widow'd streets
Nothing but sorrow in each face that meets,
In the Large ruin, nothing but a grief
That speaks itself in silence, true and brief.
Ah dear Sirs, it is changed from the Place
Ye knew it once, whenas the beauteous face
Of Gallantry enriched the Streets, and Eyes
Of frequent beauty made it a Paradise
And the Delight of Nations, whose concourse
Thither and the Reflux as from the Source                    (120)
Of humankind did make it seem to be
The Center of the World, the World's Epitome.
Death now, alas, hath not begun but led
His Triumph through the Town and largely spread
His gloomy wings in circuit o're the Walls,
Attended by ten thousand Funerals,
As if those Pageants—raised to renown,

Our dear Queen's Welcome and great Charles, his Crown—
Had been of purpose made a Woeful throne
For Death and Fate to sit spectators on.                                    (130)
       When I see these, think you I can forbear
But praise that God, who lets me still be here
And makes me not a Spectacle, as they
That now are mine and liv'd but yesterday?
Dear Friends, it is not *London* but the shade
And Carcass of that place in ashes laid,
Where you shall see instead of sport and play,
A false, yet as it seems, a Holiday—
The Doors shut up and all the Streets about,
But here and there a Passenger walk out,                                    (140)
So solemn silence that a man would say
'Twere a light Night or Service-time all Day.
The Bells as frequent as when oft they sound
When a young Prince is born or a new King crown'd,
Which heard, a Stranger might be brought to swear
The Fifth of August or November[1] there
Were Solemnized now, which to assure
The Bonfires almost every night procure
A Shade of Joy, which if you right will Know,
As funeral Piles, not solemn Bonfires, glow.                                (150)
The Bells in their sad language almost tell
They ring no Holiday, but speak a Knell.
The Doors so shut that one in them might doubt
Whether it were to keep Death in or out.
       What Muse shall I invoke t'indite a rhyme
That may express our miserable time:
Where the pale Visages of men express
Far above Poetry in the Heaviness
Of God's sharp Scourge; where the Red wand affrights
The Starting Passenger, and troubled Nights                                 (160)
Are spent in Burials; when whate're we see
Is but an Argument of Misery;
The Wormwood Nosegays and the trembling Pace
Of them that pass, though they have Herb of Grace
And curious Boxes to repel the air,
Which might assault them, seeming to out-dare
The will of Destiny? Nor can I blame

---

[1]    *Fifth of August or November.* English holidays commemorating the safe deliverance
of King James I from treasonous plots (the first in 1600 while he was King of Scotland and
the second in 1605, known as the Gunpowder Plot).

Our weak Mortality, which thinks no shame
To show a frailty, deeming perhaps that Fate
Can yield to Sovereign *Bezoar*, Mithridate                    (170)
Or such Death-killers; let us think so still,
So we root out that weed of Sin and ill,
Which taints our souls so; though for many years
It have prevail'd, we'll drown it in our tears
And Kill this Giant Plague, which through the town
As an unloosed Lion beareth down,
Whate're it meets, making no doubt to strike
The cloudy Cedar and low Shrub alike.
So quick and fast that it makes men to say
"'Twill not be long until the Judgment Day."                    (180)
Absolve the Massacre; Death so doth shrine[2]
To bring the Universe to light again.
So few are born to life; so many Die;
Lucina doth not Tithe Mortality.[3]
As if Death would not leave, until, for all,
Doomsday do make one fire, one funeral.
When now the Week-bills almost reach unto
The sum which that of th'year had wont to do.
    If from the Town a Stranger should but spy
How the affrighted People haste to fly                         (190)
In trembling heaps, he could not but suppose
The ransack'd City taken by the Foes,
And now possess'd, and the remaining rout
On a strict composition flying out.
Enter the City, you shall meet with there
A fearful Valor and audacious Fear,
Where men do think't so difficult to scape
That they expose themselves unto the rape
While they yet tremble, as if thence to fly
Were to give wings to Death and haste to die.                  (200)
    A Noon in *Fleet Street* now can hardly show
That Press which Midnight could not long ago.
No Proclamation needs, the Gentry hast[e]
Unto their Homes; they do it now too fast,
While the poor Starved rout are taken hence
Alike by Famine and by Pestilence.
    Walk through the woeful Streets (whoever dare

---

[2]   *Shrine*. Enshrine, entomb.
[3]   *Lucina doth not Tithe Mortality* Lucina, the Roman goddess of childbirth, does not
pay back in new births a tenth of the population killed by plague.

Still venture on the sad infected air)
So many marked houses you shall meet
As if the *City* were one *Red-Cross street*.                    (210)
The Plague hath spread itself so vast and far
They need not set Marks in Particular
On every Door, but to express the Loss
Not guild but red the Public City cross,
And, brief, for all to show the wrath of Fate,
Set "Lord Have Mercy On's" on every Gate.
Alas, the little house hath lost the Name
While wretched London may the Title claim
Of "the great Pest-house," where are buried more
Than we had thought it had contain'd before,                    (220)
That in our Judgments it may well appear
Turn'd from a City to a Sepulcher.

## The Description of the late great memorable and prodigious Plague. 1625.

Good God! What poison lurkd in that first fruit,
Whose surfeit left us wretches prostitute
To such a world of sorrow? Not confin'd
Only to tear and cruciate the mind
With sad remembrance of the bliss, wherein
We might have liv'd, but see the cruel Sin
Spares not our souls' weak houses but doth spread,
From viler parts unto the nobler head,                    (230)
As thousand Maladies, which now, alas,
Through each small Inlet of the Body pass
Remorseless Enemies, and batter down
The clayie bulwarks of our Mud-wall'd town.
    Our throat is like that vast breach, which doth bring
In like the *Trojan* Horse, dire surfeiting.
When in the Stomach, like the Market-place,
The foes let loose are spread themselves and trace
Through all the City; some are ready first
To break the Sluices, which do raging burst                    (240)
And drown low buildings; some with flaming brands
Fire holy Temples; some with Swords in hands
Sharp-pointed-Javelins, Mauls, and poisonous darts
Make Massacres through all the trembling parts
Of the distressed fabric; no control
Can bar 'em but they will assault the Soul
Itself almost, while each small-breathing Pore,

Betrays unto the foe, a Postern Door
To enter in at; every crawling vein
Affords him harbor and doth Entertain                    (250)
The bloody Enemy; each Muscle, Nerve
And Film makes him a Fortress to preserve
His longer durance, till the guest at last
With ruin pays his Host for all that's pass'd.
How many such foes, think you, Secret lie,
When hundreds of them ambush in one Eye,
Which is the Lantern and the Watch and Light,
Keeps Century,[4] for all the Body's Night?
          As soon may I exactly number all
The fainting leaves that in an Autumn fall,               (260)
The Creatures of the Summer or the Store
Of wilder insects, which old Nilus' shore
Each year produceth, as with Judgment show
How many fierce and bold diseases flow
Upon this wretched Carcass, when each year
New troops of raging Fevers domineer
That know no name. Each boy can nigh express
Diseases now to Pose *Hippocrates.*
          Happy that age of gold, not only 'cause
It had no vice and so no need of Laws,                    (270)
When Nature was their Solon, and the want
Of Knowledge to do ill did make them Ignorant
Of the Redress—not bless'd alone in this
Although the air and earth increas'd their bliss,
But that an able body was combin'd
In a sweet friendship with a harmless mind.
They knew no Physic (though their drugs did grow
Then in full virtue, able to bestow
Health on this age) because they Knew not how
To get those Sicknesses which men Know now:               (280)
The Ague with a hundred names; the Aches
More than the Joints; the Palsy that attacks
The limbs with Dissolution; the wild
And Bedlam Frenzy: the Vertigo, styled
Because it whirls the giddy brains about;
The swerving Megrim, and the racking Gout;
The cruel Stone; the torturing Colic fierce,
And wringing winds, which through the limbs dispense
Their airy torments, lingering, dispense

---

4    *Keeps Century.* That stands as sentry, so spelled to achieve meter.

Of pale Consumptions, which besot the sense;                (290)
The Deluges of a Dropsy. When shall I
Run through 'em all? The sleepy Lethargy;
Quick-murdring Apoplexy, which doth Kill
E're it makes Sick; the piteous Falling-Ill;
The Elephant-skin'd Leprosy; Jaundice stain;
Ambush'd Impostumes, which surprise the brain
With heart-assaulting Pleurisies; the tough
And cluttered Phlegm, and Rheum that breeds the cough;
Strappado Cramp; the sudden pricking Stitch;
The Nightmare which the people think a Witch;                (300)
Th'all-conquering Pox, to which compar'd the rest
Are Lady Sick-fits—this is that foreign guest
The Devil-instructed *Indies* to us sold
To recompense the filching of their Gold.[5]
    All these and more innumerable powers
Lay siege unto this weak-wall'd Fort of ours,
And oft surprise an Outwork; yea, sometime
In desperate malice ready are to climb
The walls themselves, till that the heart, much like
A strong Defendant, maketh good the Dike                    (310)
And gives 'em a repulse; yet oft, alas,
This noble Champion stains the conquer'd Mass
With dying blood, for Sickness is a Fight:
The victory doubtful, chances infinite.
    But, hath that power, who is all Mercy, still
More and more cruel Punishments to Kill
Minute-liv'd man? Yea, though you add to these
Pale meager Famine, Murders of the Seas,
And War's vast Slaughters, you shall find one more
That may affright the rest, we nam'd before:                (320)
The *Plague*, whose very naming seems t'affright
My trembling Quill, as it doth haste to write,
Lest as it raging flies about the land
This Instant it might seize upon my hand.
The Plague a dreary Punishment, Heaven's curse,
That fatal Engine of Destruction, worse
Than we can well imagine, which doth bring
Terror on mortals, Death on everything,
And Desolation unto Cities: O
Whatere thou art, dire Ill, whether thou dost flow          (330)

---

[5]   *this is ... Gold.* Seventeenth-century belief that smallpox came from Indians (of the Americas).

From powerful Influence of the Star or rather
Dost thy vast malice and contagion gather
From poisonous Southern winds, which have prevailed
Upon the sickly air, or Steams Exhal'd
From th'Earth's envenom'd womb, or whether't be
Our Bodies' Constitutions, which agree
With the malicious air and so contract
The quick Infection, whether't be the Pact
Of Fate and will of Heaven which doth stand,
Or God's immediate angry moved hand—                    (340)
As 'tis, O pull it in, thou Gracious Power,
And let not this blind Enemy devour
The Grace of England. CHARLES implores; we
With him in Zealous Orisons agree.
Hear him, for us and us for him, and stay
Thy dreadful vengeance which doth now display
Horror through all thy People and begins
To show the ugly portrait of our sins,
Which have pull'd down thy wrath. O, let suffice
That world of blood in foreign Air that lies            (350)
Of noble English souls, whose carcasses
The brutish Shores, wild Fields, and greedy Seas
Expose to Dogs, to ravenous Fowls and Fishes,
Ah, little answering to the tender wishes
Of their poor mothers, who at home the while
Gape at their childrens' Honors and beguile
Their early fears with too late hopes. Alas,
They little think that now the soiled Grass
Usurps their dear embraces, and grim Fate
Sits pale upon those Beauties, which of late           (360)
They made their Age's comforts, who now shall
Ah! be bound to them for a Burial.
      O call to mind this Fatal Year, wherein
Thy Justice hath been equal to our Sin—
Both great.[6] O let thy blessed Goodness still,
As it is wont to do, surpass our Ill.
Those men whom we did love, whom we did trust
Should be our Shields, are turn'd to Shades, to Dust.
Let the enthroned Soul of JAMES implore
That after Him, thou punish His no more.                (370)
Let the great Sprite of Oxford, which hath pass'd
The Sentence of thy Anger, be the last

---

6    [marginal note] Equally and justly sent.

Thou plaguest us withal, and let us know
That still thou pitiest us, poor men, below.
    But never let this Land endure again
That woeful solitude, which once did reign
In our fair Cities, which neglected left
In a deplored ruin, show'd the theft
Of angry Fate, when scarce a tenant Mouse
Was left in many a fair unpeopled house,          (380)
But the sad Owls and Night-Ravens aloof
Did keep their Revels on the silent roof;
When at high Noon one passing by should meet
A Midnight Dark and silence in the street;
When in the ways well-pav'd and worn before
By frequent steps of men, there now grew store
Of uncouth Grass, and Harvests now apace
Grew where they once were sold i'th'Market-place;
Whenas no Merriments, no Sports, no Plays
Were known at all, and yet all Holy-days.          (390)
No Papers then over the doors were set,
With "Chambers ready furnish'd to be let,"
But a sad, "Lord have mercy upon us," and
A bloody Cross, as fatal marks did stand,
Able to fright one from the Prayer. The time
Then held it an inexpiable Crime
To visit a sick friend; strange Store, wherein
Love was a fault and Charity a sin;
When Bad did fear infection from the Good,
And men did hate their cruel Neighborhood.          (400)
    'Twas a deplored time, wherein the Skies
Themselves did labor and let fall their eyes;
When one might see the Sun, with sallow hair
And languishing complexion, dull the air
Looking ev'n so, as when, at *Chryses'* Plaint,
He went like Night, the *Grecian* troops to taint
With sad Infection; when his dire shafts cast
Kill'd more than *Hector* in the nine years pass'd.[7]
The Heavens were cloth'd with bleak mists, and the air
With the thick Damp was struck into despair          (410)
Of future clearness or serener day,
But that the Clouds for fear ran oft away.
The Night, whose dewy shade had wont to tame
The sultry relics of the Midday flame,

---

[7]    The "he" here, who "went like Night," is Apollo, god of sun, music, and plague.

Distill'd no Crystal pearls upon the ground,
But wrapt in vaporous smoke, and cloth'd around
With poisonous Exhalations, did affright
The trembling Moon, whose dim and paler light
Look'd with that countenance, as if again
Her silver horns should ne're escape the Wane        (420)
So to renew her Circuit. The dull Choir
Of sickly Stars show'd now no smiling fire,
But shone like un-snuff'd Tapers: as if Fate
Did give them leave now to prognosticate
Their own estate, not others, and apply
Themselves at last to sad Astrology.
The poison-clutter'd Springs, with *Plague* infus'd,
Ran not with Crystal torrents, as they us'd,
But in dull streams, as them dire influence fills
With fainting pace, scarce reach'd unto their rills,        (430)
And languid Rivers, which before did pass
The Crystal with their clearness, now, alas,
Look muddy without stirring, and their streams
That wont to be all spangled with the beams
Of the blithe sun, now in a weltering flood,
Ran not with water but prodigious blood.

    Those Trees whereof the Ancients us'd to raise
Their funeral Piles, might in these fatal days
Burn at their own Deaths, which, in sad despair,
Spread not their leafy beauties through the air        (440)
But suffer'd Autumn in the spring. Forlorn
And several Cypress now had cause to mourn.
Poppies themselves in this time in death did sleep,
And the Myrrh tree had reason here to weep
A funeral Perfume. Those gaudy flowers,
Which wont to make Garlands for Paramours,
Mourn'd in their drooping bravery and spread
The ground at their own deaths, as for the dead.
The Corn grew not, as if it meant t'undo
Men not with *Plague* alone but *Famine* too.        (450)
Herbs, Physic's Sovereigns, here infected die,
And for themselves could find no remedy.

    The brute Beasts now, which Nature to bestow
The Excellence on Man did make with low
Down-looking Postures, first did feel the rage
Of th'Earth-born *Plague* and died before their age.
The long-liv'd Hart this time to die began
Before it reach'd unto the age of Man.

The faithful spaniel by his death did try
The mischief of his well-nos'd Faculty,                           (460)
And ranging with quick Scent did soonest prove
Th'infectious malice of the Dog above.[8]
The lusty Steed, scouring in's Game apace,
Lights on Death's Goal in middle of his Race.
The nimble Fowl, as th'air it flies around,
Flags his sick wings and sinks unto the ground,
Not long before, to the remorseless Sky
In silly Notes, have sung his Elegy.
The luckless Night-Ravens, which us'd to groan
The death of others, now might Dirge their own.                  (470)
The Snow-plum'd Swan, as it did gently ride
Upon the silver Stream sung forth and died.
    Anon the Damp dares break into the Walls,
Making a way by thousand Funerals.
Who can express th'astonishment and fear,
Which doth at entrance of a *Plague* appear?
    Even so, the fleeced Herd doth tremble when
An Auburn Lion, hungry from his Den,
Breaks in among 'em; then, you may behold
The pale-look'd Shepherd gaze upon his Fold                      (480)
With helpless pity; the poor Lambkins creep
Under their Dams; the silly trembling Sheep
Stand full of cold amazement at the sight—
Small hope for mercy and less hope in flight—
Expecting only which of all shall scape
The ready horror of the Lion's rape.
    Other Diseases warning give before,
That we may reckon and acquit the Score
Of our sins' Prodigality; in this,
We scarce can be resolved wherewith 'tis                         (490)
Sickness or Death itself, so quick it tires
The strength of Nature; so soon poor Man dies,
That many to repose in th'Evening laying
Have made their sleep true kin to Death by dying
Before the Morn. Ah! Who would then defer
A preparation for this messenger
Of bless'd or curs'd Eternity? What man
Would still presume to sin that knows the span
Of short, uncertain Life? Ye gracious Powers
That measure out the minutes and the hours                       (500)

---

   [8]   *the Dog above.* The Dog star, Sirius, associated with hot months known as the dog days.

Of this our wandering Pilgrimage, restrain
These sudden slaughter-men, or, good God, wain
Us from our sins that we may neither fear
The rape of Death nor covet to be here.
    O curb this raging sickness, which with sense
Bereaves us of the means of Penitence.
When a dire Frenzy seizeth on the Brain,
Full of resistless flame and full of pain,
That Madness which no cure can well appease,
Is but a Symptom unto this Disease,                                    (510)
Our blood, all fire, as if it did portend
We were not here to stay but soon ascend,
When streams of sulfur through our veins do glide,
And scarce the sense of sorrow doth abide—
This time how miserable may we guess,
Where want of sense is chiefest happiness,
When the distracted Soul can scarce devise
How to supply the weakest Faculties
Of the disturbed Body, but presents
Unto the eye strange objects, strange portents,                        (520)
And antique shadows; when the feverish rage
Sets us on Journeys oft and Pilgrimage,
And entertains our wild and wandering sight
With monstrous Landships able to affright
A man in's wits; when the deceived Ears
Do apprehend whatere the Fancy fears:
The groans of Ghost and whispering of Sprites,
The silken tread of Fairies in the Nights,
The language of an airy Picture howls
Of funeral Dogs and warnings of sad Owls.                              (530)
The taste distasteth all things, and the same
Is sweet and bitter when the inward flame
Furs the swollen Tongue and the quick Feeling marr'd,
Knoweth no difference between soft and hard.
Such a confused Error doth distract
The laboring Senses, so is the Fancy rackt
By the dire sickness, when from place to place
The Body rolleth and would fain embrace
Some Icy cooler, but alas the heat
Assuaging there ensues a Marble sweat.                                 (540)
'Twixt Death and Nature wrestling, then appear
Those deadly Characters, which th'Ensign bear
Before approaching Fate, which notice give:
None spotless die, however they did live.

A sickness comfortless, when we do fear
To see those friends whom we do love most dear.
The minister's Devotion here doth stick,
By leaving Visitation of the sick,
Making the Service-Book imperfect; when
We see a crossed Door as 'twere a Den                                    (550)
Of Serpents or a Prodigy, we shun
The poor distressed Habitation.
　　　The Death as comfortless, where not appears
One friend to shed some tender funeral tears.
Black Night's the only Mourner. No sad Verse,
Nor solemn flowers do deck the dreary Hearse.
Some few old folk perhaps, for many a year
Who have forgot to weep, attend the Bier,
Such whose dire age hath made most fit to keep
Th'infected without fear, but not to weep,                               (560)
Whose kin, to death, made them not fear to die,
Whose deafness made them then fit company
Unto the sick, when they were speechless grown—
A miserable Consolation.
　　　But had you look'd about, you might have seen
Death in each corner and the secret teen
Of angry Destiny. No sport dispels
The mists of sorrow. A sad silence dwells
In all the streets, and a pale terror seizes
Upon their faces who had no Diseases.                                    (570)
So usual 'twas, before the Morn to die,
That when at Night two friends left company
They would not say, "*Good Night*," but, thus, alone:
"God sends a joyful Resurrection."
　　　If two or three days interpos'd between
One friend by chance another friend had seen,
It was strange and joyful, as to some
When a dear friend doth from the Indies come.
Through the nak'd town, of death there was such plenty,
One Bell at once was fain to ring for twenty.                            (580)
No Clocks were heard to strike upon their Bells,
Cause nothing rung but death-lamenting Knells.
Strange that the Hours should fail to tell the Day,
When Time to thousands ran so fast away.
Time was confus'd and kept at such a plight,
The Day to thousands now was made a Night.
　　　Hundreds that never saw before but, dy'd
At one same time, in one same Grave abide,

That our weak Fancies, if we did not hold
It Profanation, here to be too bold,                                    (590)
Might wonder what, being strangers, they would say
To one another at the Judgment Day.
Some, by their fear to go to church, debarr'd,
Anon are carried dead unto the Yard.
The Churchyards groan'd with too much death opprest,
And the Earth rests not, 'cause so many rest.
And Churches now with too much burial fed
Fear'd they should have no meetings but of Dead.
Death fell on death, and men began to fear
That men would want[9] to carry forth the Bier.                         (600)
The Bearers, Keepers, Sextons that remain
Surpass in number all the town again.
Friends here kill'd friends, womb-fellows Kill their Brothers,
Fathers their Sons, and Daughters kill their Mothers.
By one another (strong!) so many dy'd
And yet no murder here, no Homicide.
    A Mother great with Child by the Plague's might
Infects to Death her child not born to light.
So killing that which yet ne're liv'd, the womb
Of th'alive Mother, to th'dead Child was tomb,                          (610)
Where in the fleshy grave the still Babe, lying,
Doth kill his Mother by his own first dying.
Her travail here on Earth she could not tend
But finishes in heaven her Journey's end.
    To others—frolic, set unto their meals,
Secure of death—sly Death upon them steals
And strikes among' 'em, so that thence in speed
With heavy Cheer th'are borne, the worms to feed.
To some at work to others at their play
To thousands death makes a long Holy-day.                               (620)
    Death all conditions equally invades,
Nor riches, power, nor beauty here persuades.
Old die with young, with women men; the rage
Of the dire Plague spares neither sex nor age.
    Most powerful Influence of ruling Stars,
Which with blind darts Kill more than bloody Wars,
Resistless Famine, greedy Time, or when
The threatful hand of Tyrants striketh men
Into pale terror—more than all diseases—
Ah, happy he who heaven least displeases.                               (630)
FINIS

---

[9]   *Want.* Be wanting; lack.

\*

# George Wither,
## *Britain's Remembrancer*

More than three dozen copies of this eight-canto poem from 1628 (STC 2nd ed 25899) exist in as many libraries around the world. Preceding the poem are two other brief poems, "The meaning of the Title page" and a dedication "TO THE *KING'S* MOST EXCELLENT MAJESTY," as well as a prose section called, "A Premonition." Following the eight cantos, Wither offers a lengthy verse conclusion. In 1633, *Britain's Remembrancer* appeared as the second full volume of the two-volume, *Juvenilia, A collection of those poems heretofore imprinted, and written by George Wither* (1633; STC 25912.5); and in 1643, it was printed in abbreviated form as *Mr. Wither his prophesy of our present calamity, and (except we repent) future misery. Written by him in the year 1628* (1643; Wing [CD-Rom, 1996], W3182 and W3186; 1680; Wing [CD-ROM, 1996], W3172B). Due to its length, the 1628 *Britain's Remembrancer* is here represented by its full fourth canto, which in many ways performs the function of a brief plague epic unto itself.

BRITAIN'S REMEMBRANCER
Containing
A *Narration* of the Plague lately pass'd,
A *Declaration* of the Mischiefs present,
And a *Prediction* of Judgments to come
(If *Repentance* prevent not)
It is *Dedicated* (for the glory of God)
to POSTERITY and to *These Times* (if they please)
by GEORGE WITHER


Job 32.8, 9, 10, 18, 21, 22
Surely, there is a spirit in man, but the inspiration of the
Almighty giveth understanding.
Great men are not always wise; neither are the aged
always understood in judgment.
Therefore, I say, hear me, and I will show also my opinion.
For I am full of matter, and the spirit within me compelleth me.
I will not accept the person of man, neither will I give flattering titles to man,
For I may not give flattering titles, lest my maker take me away suddenly.


Read all, or censure not,
For He that answereth a matter before he hear it
It is shame and folly to him. PROVERBS 18.13


Imprinted for *Great Britain* and are to be sold by JOHN GRISMOND
in *Ivy-Lane*, MDCXXVIII


**The fourth *Canto***
Our *Muse* in this fourth Canto writes
Of melancholy thoughts and sights,
What changes were in every place,
What Ruins in a little space,
How *Trades* and how provisions fail'd,
How sorrow thriv'd, how *Death* prevail'd,
And how in triumph he did rise
With all his horrors, by his side.
To LONDON, then, she doth declare
How suiting her afflictions were                                    (10)
To former sins, what good and bad
Effects this *Plague* produced had,
What friendly *Champions* and what *Foes*
For us did fight or us oppose,
And how the greatest *Plague* of all
On poor *Artificers* did fall.

Then, from the *Fields*, new grief she takes,
And useful Meditations makes,
Relates how slowly *Vengeance* came,
How God forewarn'd us of the same,                    (20)
What other *Plagues* to this were joined,
And here and there are interlined
Upbraidings, warnings, exhortations,
And pertinent *expostulations*.

    When *Conscience* had allowed my *Commission*
For staying, and declar'd on what condition,
I did not only feel my heart consent
To entertain it with a full content,
But also found myself prepared so
To execute the work I had to do,                    (30)
That without pain (methought) I was employ'd,
And all my *Passions* to good use enjoy'd.
    For though God freed my soul from slavish *fear*,
Yet so much awe he still preserved there,
As kept within my heart some natural sense
Of his displeasure and of penitence.
He gave me *Joys*, yet left some *Grief* withal,
Lest I into security might fall,
Or lose the fellow-feeling of that pain,
Whereof I heard my neighbors to complain.                    (40)
He lent me *health*, yet ev'ry day some twitches
Of pangs unusual; many qualms and stitches
Of short continuance, my poor heart assailed,
That I might heed the more what others ailed.
He kept me hopeful, and yet now and then,
His rods (wherewith, in love, he scourgeth men)
Did make me smart, lest else I might assume
The liberty of *Wantons,* and presume
My ordinary means was made their prey,
Who seek my spoil, and lately took away.                    (50)
Yet me with plenties daily did he feed,
And I did nothing want which I could need,
Which God vouchsafed to assure to me
That when unusual works required be,
He will (e're we shall want what's necessary)
Supply us by a means not ordinary.
    By many other signs unmention'd here,
God's love and providence did so appear,
And so, methought, engage[d] me to remove

Whatever to his work a let[1] might prove,                              (60)
That (so far forth as my frail nature could
Admit, and things convenient suffer would)
My own *Affairs* aside a while I threw
And bent myself with heedfulness to view
What worth my notice in this *Plague* I saw,
Or what good uses I from thence might draw.
  But far I needed not to pace about,
Nor long enquire to find such *Objects* out,
For ev'ry place with sorrows then abounded,
And ev'ry way the cries of *Mourning* sounded.                          (70)
Yea, day by day, successively till night,
And from the evening till the morning light,
Were *Scenes* of Grief with strange variety
Knit up, in one continuing *Tragedy*.
No sooner wak'd I, but twice twenty knells,
And many sadly-sounding *passing-bells*
Did greet mine ear, and by their heavy tolls,
To me gave notice that some early souls
Departed whilst I slept, that other some
Were drawing onward to their longest home,                             (80)
And seemingly, presag'd, that many a one
Should bid the world *good-night* e're it were *noon*.
  One, while the mournful *Tenor* in her tones
Did yield a sound as if in deep-set groans,
She did bewail the sorrow which attends
The separation of those loving friends,
The Soul and Body. Other while, again,
Methought, it call'd on me and other men
To pray that God would view them with compassion,
And give them comfortable separation.                                  (90)
(For we should with a fellow-feeling share
In ev'ry sorrow which our brethren bear.)
Sometime my Fancy tuned so the Bell,
As if her *Tollings* did the story tell
Of my mortality and call me from
This life by oft and loudly sounding, "*Come*."
  So long the solitary nights did last
That I had leisure my accounts to cast
And think upon and over-think those things,
Which darkness, loneliness, and sorrow brings                          (100)
To their consideration, who do know,

---

[1] *a let.* Hindrance, stoppage, obstruction.

From whence they came, and whither they must go.
    My Chamber entertain'd me all alone,
And in the rooms adjoining lodged none.
Yet through the darksome silent night did fly
Sometime an uncouth noise, sometime a cry,
And sometime mournful callings pierc'd my room,
Which came I neither knew from whence nor whom.
And oft betwixt awaking and asleep,
Their voices who did talk or pray or weep           (110)
Unto my listning ears a passage found,
And troubled me by their uncertain sound.
For though the sounds themselves no terror were,
Nor came from anything that I could fear,
Yet they bred *Musings*, and those musings bred
*Conjecturings* in my half sleeping head.
By those Conjectures into mind were brought
Some real things, before quite out of thought;
They diverse Fancies to my soul did show,
Which me still further and still further drew      (120)
To follow them, till they did thoughts procure
Which human frailty cannot long endure,
Ev'n such as when I fully was awake,
Did make my heart to tremble and to ache.
And when such frailties have disheartned men,
Oh! God, how busy is the Devil then?
    I know in part his malice and the ways
And times and those occasions which he lays
To work upon our weakness, and there is
Scarce any which doth show him like to this.      (130)
I partly also know by what degrees
He worketh it, how he doth gain or lease
His labors, and some sense I have procur'd,
What pangs are by the soul that while endur'd.
    For though my God in mercy hath indu'd
My Soul with Knowledge and with Fortitude
In such a measure that I do not fear
(Distractedly) those tortures which appear
In solitary darkness, yet some part
Of this and of all frailties in my heart        (140)
Continues he, that so I might confess
His mercies with continual thankfulness,
And somewhat (evermore) about me bear,
Which unto me my frailties may declare.
Yea (though without distemper, now it be)

So much of those grim fears are showed me,
Which terrifi'd my childhood and which make
The hearts of aged men sometimes to quake,
That I am sensible of their estate
And can their case the more compassionate,[2]                    (150)
Who on their beds of death do pained lie,
Exil'd from comfort and from company,
When dreadful *Fancies* do their souls affright,
Begotten by the melancholy night.
   Glad was I when I saw the Sun appear,
(And with his Rays to bless our Hemisphere)
That from the tumbled bed I might arise
And with more lightsomeness refresh mine eyes,
Or with some good companion read or pray
To pass, the better, my sad thoughts away.                       (160)
For though such thoughts oft useful are and good,
Yet knowing well I was but flesh and blood,
I also knew man's natural condition
Must have in joys and griefs an intermission,
Lest too much joy should fill the heart with folly,
Or too much grief breed dangerous melancholy.
   But when the Morning came, it little shewed,
Save light, to see discomfortings renewed,
For if I stayed within, I heard relations
Of naught but dying pangs and lamentations.                      (170)
If in the Streets I did my footing set,
With many sad disasters there I met.
And objects of mortality and fear,
I saw in great abundance ev'rywhere.
   Here one man stagger'd by with visage pale;
There lean'd another, grunting on a stall.
A third, half dead, lay gasping for his grave;
A fourth did out at window call and rave.
Yon came the *Bearers*, sweating from the *Pit*,
To fetch more bodies to replenish it.                            (180)
A little further off, one sits and shows
The *spots* which he *Death's tokens* doth suppose
(E're such they be) and makes them so indeed,
Which had been *signs of health*, by taking heed.
For those *round-purple-spots*, which most have thought
*Death's* fatal tokens (where they forth are brought),
May prove *Life tokens*, if that ought be done,

---

[2]   *compassionate.* Here the word is used as a verb.

To help the work which *Nature* hath begun;
Whereas, that fear, which their opinion brings
Who threaten *Death*, [is] the want of cordial things                    (190)
To help remove that poison from the heart
(Which *Nature* hath expelled thence in part).
And then the *Sickman's* liberty of having
Cold drinks and what his appetite is craving
Brings back again those humors pestilent,
Which by the vital pow'rs had forth been sent.
So, by recharging him that was before
Nigh spent, the fainting Combatant gives o're,
And he that cheerfully did raise his head
Is often, in a moment, strucken dead.                    (200)
*Fear* also helps it forward. Yea, the terror
Occasion'd by their fond and common error,
Who tell the *sick* that markt for Death they be,
(When those *blue spots* upon their flesh they see)
Ev'n that hath murd'red thousands who might here
Have lived else among us many a year.
    For if the *Surgeons*, or the *Searchers*, know
Those *marks*, which for the marks of death do go,
From *common-spots*, or *purples* (which we must
Confess, or else all kind of spots distrust)                    (210)
Then, such as we "*Death-tokens*" call, were seen
On some that have long since, recover'd been.
    Before I learned this, I fixt mine eyes
On many a private man's calamities,
And saw the Streets (wherein a while ago
We scarce could pass, the people fill'd them so)
Appear nigh desolate, yea, quite forlorn
And for their wonted visitants to mourn.
    Much peopled *Westminster*, where late I saw
So many rev'rend *Judges* of the Law                    (220)
With Clients and with Suitors hemmed round,
Where *Courts* and *Palaces* did so abound
With businesses and where together met
Our Thrones of Justice and our Mercy-seat—
That place was then frequented, as you see
Some *Villages* on *Holy-days* will be,
When half the Township and the Hamlets nigh
Are met to revel at some Parish by.
Perhaps the wronging of the Orphan's cause,
Denying or perverting of the Laws                    (230)
There practiced did set this *Plague* abreeding,

And sent the *Term* from *Westminster* to *Reading*.
Her goodly *Church* and *Chapel* did appear
Like some poor *Minster*, which hath twice a year
Four visitants, and her great *Hall*, wherein
So great a *Rendezvous* had lately bin,
Did look like those old *Structures*, where long since
Men say King *Arthur* kept his residence.
    The *Parliament* had left her to go see
If they could learn at *Oxford* to agree,                                        (240)
Or if that air were better for the health
And safety of our English *Commonwealth*.
But there some did so counsel and so urge
The Body politic to take a purge,
To purify the parts that seemed foul.
Some others did that motion so control,
And plead so much for Cordials and for that
Which strengthen might the sinews of the *State*,
That all the time, the labor, and the cost,
Which had bestowed been was wholly lost.                                          (250)
And here, the empty House of *Parliament*
Did look as if it had been discontinent
Or griev'd (methought) that *Oxford* should not be
More prosperous. Yet nor could I any see
Resort to comfort her, but there did I
Behold two *Traitors'* heads, which perching high,
Did show their *teeth*, as if they had been grinning
At those Afflictions which are now beginning.
Yea, their wide *eyeholes*, star'd, methought, as though
They lookt to see that *House* now overthrow                                      (260)
Itself, which they with Powder up had blown,[3]
Had God, their snares, and them, not overthrown.
    *White Hall*, where not three months before I spy'd
Great *Britain* in the height of all her pride,
And *France* with her contending, which could most
Outbrave old *Rome* and *Persia* in their cost
On *Robes* and *Feasts*—ev'n that lay solitary,
As doth a quite-forsaken *Monastry*
In some lone Forest, and we could not pass
To many places but through weeds and grass.                                       (270)
Perhaps the sins of late committed there,
Occasions of such desolation were.

---

[3]   *Traitors' heads ... blown.* A reference to the traitors executed for their role in the Gunpowder Plot of 1605.

Pray God there be not others in the *State*
That will make all, at last, be desolate.
    The *Strand*, that goodly thoroughfare between
The *Court* and *City* (and where I have seen
Well nigh a million passing in one day),
Is now, almost, an unfrequented way:
And peradventure, for those impudencies,
Those riots and those other foul offences,                            (280)
Which in that place were frequent, when it had
So great resort, it is now justly made
To stand unvisited. God grant it may
Repent, lest longer and another way
It stand unpeopled, or some others use
Those blessings which the owners now abuse.
    The *City-houses* of our English *Peers*,
Now smoakt as seldom as in other years.
Their *Country-palaces* and they perchance
Much better know than doth my ignorance                               (290)
Why so it came to pass, but wish I shall
That they their ways to mind would better call,
Lest both their Country and their City-piles
Be smoking seen and burning many miles.
    The *Inns of Court* I entred and I saw
Each Room so desolate, as if the *Law*
Had outlaw'd all her *Students* or that there
Some fear'd arrestings where no *Sergeants* were.
    Most dream that this great fright was thither sent
Not purposely but came by accident,                                   (300)
And so but little use is taken from
God's *Judgments* to amend the times to come.
Yet I dare say it was a warning given
Ev'n by appointment and decreed in heaven,
To signify that if our *Lawyers* will
In their abusive ways continue still,
The cause of their profession quite forgetting
And to their practices no limits setting,
Till they (as heretofore the Clergy were)
Are more in number than the *Land* can bear—                         (310)
Their goodly *Palaces* shall spew them forth,
As excrements that have nor use nor worth,
And be disposed of, as now they see
The Priories and Monasteries be.
    It griev'd me to behold this woeful change,
And places so well known appear so strange.

But oh poor *LONDON!* when I lookt on thee,
Remembring therewithal thy jollity
Erewhile, and how soon after I did meet
With grief and sad complaints in ev'ry street,                    (320)
When I did mind how thronged thy Gates have bin
And then perceiv'd so few pass'd out or in.
When I consider'd that abundant store
Of wealth, which thou discover'dst heretofore,
And looking on thy many empty *stalls*,
Beheld thy *shops* set up their wooden-walls,
Methought thou shouldst not be that *London*, which
Appear'd of late so populous and rich,
But some large *Borough*, either falling from
Her height or not unto her greatness come.                       (330)
If to thy *Port* I walkt, it mov'd remorse
To see how greatly Trade and Intercourse
Decayed there and what depopulations
Were made in thy late peopled habitations.
　　Thy *Royal Change,* which was the Rendezvous
Wherein all Nations met the whole world through,
Within whose princely walls we heard the sound
Of ev'ry Language spoke on Earth's vast *Round*,
And where we could have known what had been done
In ev'ry foreign *Coast* below the Sun—                          (340)
That *Place* the City-Merchant and the Stranger
Avoided as a place of certain danger
And feared (as it seems) they might have had
Some bargain there that would have spoild their trade.
　　Thy large *Cathedral*, whose decaying frame
Thou leavest unrepaired to thy shame,
Had scarce a *Walker* in her *middle Aisle*,
And ev'ry Marble of that ancient *Pile*
Did often drop and seem to shed forth tears
For thy late ruin, though thou slightest hers.                  (350)
The time hath been that once a day from thence,
We could have had a large intelligence
Of most occurrences that public were.
Yea, many times we had relations there
Of things whose foolish actors never thought
Their deeds to open scanning should be brought.
There heard we oft made public by report,
What *Secrecies* were whisper'd in the *Court*,
The *Closet-Counsels*, and the Chamber work,
Which many think in privacy doth lurk.                          (360)

There heard we what those *Lords* and *Ladies* were
Who met disguised; they know when and where.
There heard we what they did and what they said,
And many foolish plots were there bewray'd.
There heard we reasons why such men were made
Great *Lords* and *Knights*, who no deserving had
In common view, and how great *Princes'* eyes
Are dazzled and abus'd with fallacies.
There heard we for what *Gifts* most *Doctors* rise
And gain the *Church's* highest dignities.                    (370)
The truest causes also there were known,
Why men advanced are or pulled down.
Why *Officers* are changed or displaced,
Why some confined are and some disgraced,
And what among the wise those men do seem,
That are great *Statesmen* in their own esteem.
There we have heard what Princes have intended
When they to do some other thing pretended,
What *Policies* and *Projects* men pursue
With public aims and with a pious shew.                    (380)
Why from the *Counsel* one is turned out,
What makes another counterfeit the gout,
And many other mysteries beside,
Which hardly can the mentioning abide.
     But those *Athenian* Merchantmen were gone,
Who made exchange of News, and few or none
To hear or make reports remained there.
Yea, they who scarce a day (as if they were
Of *Paul's* the walking *Statues*) stayed from thence
Since *LONDON* felt the last great *Pestilence*—                    (390)
Ev'n they were gone, and those void *Aisles* did look
As if some *properties* had them forsook.
     Our Theaters, our Taverns, Tennis-courts,
And *Gaming houses*, whither great resorts
Were wont to come, then seldom were frequented,
Not that such vanities we much repented.
But lest those places which had follies taught us
Might some reward, unlooked for, have brought us,
Where we, with Pestilences of the soul,
Each other had polluted and made foul,                    (400)
Our bodies were infected, and our breaths—
Which had endanger'd our eternal deaths
(In former times) by uttring heresies,
By scandals, and by basest flatteries,

Or wanton speeches—putrefied the Air.
The blood ev'n at the fountain did impair
To cool our lust, and they that were the blisses[4]
Of some men's lives did poison them with kisses.
    The Markets, which a while before did yield
What air, seas, rivers, garden, wood, or field,             (410)
To furnish them afforded, now had naught
But what some few in secret thither brought.
For (as aforesaid) it was ordred so,
That none should with provisions come or go.
    So, like a Town beleaguer'd, thou didst fare
In some respect, and but that God had care
By making others feel necessities
Which forced them to minister supplies,
Thou hadst been famisht or been fain to bring
Provisions in by way of foraging,                  (420)
And then their foolishness had brought upon
Those men two mischiefs, who did fear but one.
    Hereafter, therefore, practice well to use
Those plenties thou didst heretofore abuse,
Lest God again bereave thee of thy store,
And never so enlarge his bounty more.
For to correct thy *Surfeits* and *Excess*,
Thy slighting of the poor, thy thanklessness,
And such like sins, God worthily restrained
Those plenties which thy pride and lust maintained.    (430)
Thy Dwellings—from whose windows I have seen
A thousand Ladies that might Queens have been
For bravery and beauty, and some far
More fair than they that fam'd in *Legends* are—
Those stood unpeopled as those houses do,
Which *Sprites* and Fairies do resort unto;
None to their closed wickets made repair;
Their empty casements gaped wide for air;
And where, once, footcloths and Carriages were
Attending, now stood *Coffins* and a *Bier*.            (440)
Yea, Coffins oftner pass'd by ev'ry door,
Than Coaches and Carriages heretofore.
    To see a country Lady or a Knight
Among us then had been as rare a sight
As was that *Elephant* which came from Spain,

---

    [4]   *The blood ... lust* Likely a reference to menstrual blood, as in Mark 5.29 and
Leviticus 20.18.

Or some great Monster spewd out of the *Main*.
If by mischance the people in the street,
A *Courtier* or a Gentleman did meet,
They with as much amazement him did view,
As if they had beheld the wandring *Jew*.[5]                    (450)
And many, seeing me to keep this place,
Did look as if they much bewaild my case,
And half believ'd that I was doomed hither,
That (since close-prison, half a year together,
Nor private wrongs, nor public disrespect,
Could break my heart, nor much the same deject)
This *Plague* might kill me, which is come to whip
Those faults which heretofore my pen did strip.
    But here I walkt in safety to behold
What changes, for instruction, see I could.                    (460)
And as I wandred on, my eye did meet
Those half built *Pageants* which, athwart the street,
Did those triumphant Arches counterfeit,
Which heretofore in ancient *Rome* were set,
When their victorious *Generals* had thither
The spoil of mighty kingdoms brought together.
The loyal Citizens (although they lost
The glory of their well-intended cost)
Erected those great Structures to renown
The new receiving of the Sov'reign Crown                       (470)
By hopeful CHARLES (whose royal exaltation,
Make thou, oh! God, propitious to this Nation.)
    But when those works, imperfect, I beheld,
They did new causes of sad musings yield,
Portending ruin, and did seem, methought,
In honor of Death's trophies to be wrought,
Much rather than from purposes to spring,
Which aimed at the honor of a King.
For their unpolisht form did make them fit
For direful *Shows*, yea, *DEATH* on them did sit.             (480)
His Captives passed under every *Arch*.
Among them, as in *Triumph* he did march.
Through ev'ry Street, upon men's backs were borne
His Conquests. His black Liveries were worn
In ev'ry House almost. His spoils were brought
To ev'ry Temple. Many Vaults were fraught

---

5    the *wandering Jew*. Imaginary figure of legend said to have been cursed to walk the
earth forever for having refused Jesus a place to rest on his way to crucifixion.

With his new prizes, and his followers grew
To such a multitude that half our Yew,
And all our Cypress trees could hardly lend him
A branch for ev'ry one who did attend him.                    (490)
        My Fancy did present to me that hour
A glimpse of *DEATH* ev'n in his greatest power.
Methought I saw him, in a Charet ride,
With all his grim companions by his side,
Such as *Oblivion* and *Corruption* be.
Not half a step before him rode these three,
(On Monsters backt): *Pain*, *Horror*, and *Despair*,
Whose fury—had not *Faith*, and *Hope*, and *Pray'r*,
Prevented, through God's mercy—none had ever
Escap'd Destruction by their best endeavor.                   (500)
For next to *Death*, came *Judgment*; after whom,
*Hell* with devouring jaws did gaping come
To swallow all, but she at *One* did snap,
Who now, for many, hath made way to scape
*Death*'s Car, with many chains, and ropes, and strings,
And by a multitude of several things,
As *Pleasures*, *Passions*, *Cares*, and such as they,
Was drawn along upon a beaten way,
New gravell'd with old bones, and *Sin* did seem
To be the foremost *Beast* of all the *Team*,                 (510)
And *Sickness* to be that which haled next
The *Charet wheel*, for none I saw betwixt.
*Time* led the way, and *Justice* did appeal,
To sit before and play the *Charioteer*,
For since our *Sin* to pull on *Death* begun,
The whip of *Justice* makes the Charet run.
There was of Trumpets and of Drums the sound,
But in loud cries and roarings it was drown'd.
Sad *Elegies* and songs of *Lamentation*
Were howled out, but moved no compassion.                     (520)
Skulls, Coffins, Spades, and Mattocks placed were
About the Charet. Crawling *Worms* were there
And whatsoever else might signify
*Death's* nature and weak man's mortality.
        Before the Charet, such a multitude
Of ev'ry Nation in the world I view'd,
That neither could my eye so far perceive,
As they were thronging, nor my heart conceive
Their countless number, for all those that were
Since *Abel* dy'd, he drove before him there,                 (530)

And of those thousands, dying long ago,
Some here and there, among them, I did know,
Whose Virtues them in death distinguished
(In spite of *Death*) from others of the dead.
I saw them stand, methought, as you shall see
High spreading *Oaks*, which in fell'd Copses be,
O're-top the shrubs, and where scarce two are found
Of growth within ten thousand rod of ground.
    Of those who dy'd within the Age before
This year, I scarce distinguished a score                          (540)
From Beasts, and Fowls, and Fishes, for *Death* makes
So little difference twixt the flesh he takes,
That into dust alike he turns it all.
And if no virtue make distinction shall,
Those men who did of much in lifetime boast,
Shall dying in the common heap be lost.
    But of those *Captives* which my fantasy
Presented to my apprehension's eye
To grace this *Monarch's* Triumph, most I heeded
Those troops which next before the *Car* proceeded—               (550)
Ev'n those which in the circuit of this year
The prey of *Death* within our Island were.
It was an *Army royal*, which became
A King, and lo, King *JAMES* did lead the same.
The Duke of *Richmond* and his only brother,
The Duke of *Lennox*, seconded each other.
Next them in this attendance follow'd on
That noble *Scott*, the Marquis *Hamilton*;
Southampton, Suffolk, Oxford, Nottingham,
And *Holderness*, their Earldoms leaving, came                    (560)
To wait upon this Triumph. There I saw
Some rev'rend *Bishops*, and some men of *Law*,
As *Winchester* and *Hubbard*, and I know not
Who else, for to their memories I owe not
So much as here to name them, nor do I
Upon me take to mention punctually
Their order of departing, nor to swear
That all of these fell just within the year.
For of the time, if somewhat I do miss,
The matter sure, not much material is.                            (570)
    Some Barons and some Viscounts, saw I too,
Zouch, Bacon, Chichester, and others more,
Whose Titles I forget. There follow'd then
Some Officers of note, some Aldermen,

Great store of Knights, and Burgesses with whom
A couple marcht that had the *Sheriffdom*
Of London that sad year: the one of which
In Piety and Virtue dy'd so rich,
(If his surviving fame may be believed)
That for his loss the City much hath grieved.                                         (580)
To be an honor to him, here, therefore
I fix the name of *Crisp*, which name he bore,
And I am hopeful it shall none offend,
The Muses do this right unto their friend.
Some others also of great state and place,
To me not known by office, name, nor face,
Made up the concourse, but the common Rabble
To number or distinguish, none was able.
For rich and poor, men, women, old and young,
So fast and so confusedly did throng,                                                 (590)
By strokes of *Death*, so markt, so ghastly wounded,
So thrust together, and so much confounded
Among that glut of people, which from hence
Were sent among them, by the *Pestilence*,
That possible it was not to descry
Or who or what they were who passed by.
Yet, now and then, methought, I had the view
Of some who much resembled those I knew.
And fain I would the favor have provided
To keep their Names from being quite obscured                                        (600)
Among the multitude, but they were gone
Before the means could well be thought upon,
And as they must, for aye, unknown of me,
For this was but a waking Dream, I see.
      These *Fancies,* Melancholy often bred.
Yea, many such like *Pageants* in my head
My working apprehension did beget,
According to those objects which I met—
Some full of comfort, able to relieve
The heart, whom dreadful thoughts did over-grieve;                                   (610)
Some full of horror, such as they have had
(If I mistake not) that grow desp'rate mad;
Some, like to their illusions, who instead
Of being humbled in this place of dread,
Are puffed up by their deliverance,
And being full of dangerous arrogance,
Abuse their souls with vain imaginations,
Ill-grounded hopes, suggested revelations,

And such-like toys, which in their hearts arise
From their own Pride and Satan's fallacies.                    (620)
    Some such as these I had, and other some,
Which cannot be by words expressed from
My troubled heart, and if I had not got
God's hand to help untie their *Gordian-knot*,
His presence, my bold reas'nings to control,
To curb my passion, to inform my soul,
My faith to strengthen, doubtings to abate,
And so to comfort, and to arbitrate,
That I might see I was of him beloved,
(Though me with many secret fears he proved)                  (630)
Sure, in myself, some *Hell* I had invented,
Where endless thoughts, and doubts, had me tormented.
But God those depths hath show'd me, that I might
See what we carry in ourselves to fright
Ourselves withal, and what a hell of fear
Is in our very souls, till he be there.
Ev'n when I had the brightness of the day
To chase my melancholy thoughts away,
I was to musings troublesome disposed,
As well as when the darkness me enclosed,                      (640)
That, by experiments, which real are,
Those horrors which to others oft appear
(And are not demonstrable) might in part
Be felt in me, to mollify my heart,
To stir up hearty thankfulness and make
My soul, in him, the greater pleasure take.
For from those prospects, and those thoughts that grieve me,
I, those extractions make that much relieve me.
And when my inward combatings are pass'd,
It giveth to my joys the sweeter tast[e].                       (650)
    But, leaving this, I will again return
To that for which the people soonest mourn:
I lookt along the Streets of chiefest trade,
And there, perpetual *Holiday* they made.
They that one day in sev'n could not forbear
From trading, had not one in half a year.
And all which some had from their childhood got,
The charges of their flight defrayed not
To make the greedy *Cormorant* regard
The *Sabbath* more and of ill gains affear'd.                   (660)
False wares, false oaths, false measures, and false weights,
False promises, and falsified lights,

Were punisht with false hopes, false joys, false fears,
False servants, and false friends, to them, and theirs.
These who of late their neighbors did contemn,
Had not a neighbor left to comfort them.
When neighborhood was needful, such as were
*Self-lovers*, by themselves remained here,
And wanted those contentments, which arise
From Christian *Lover* and mutual Amities.                    (670)
    Most *Trades* were tradefaln, and few Merchants thriv'd,
Save those men, who by *Death* and *Sickness*, liv'd.
The *Sextons*, *Searchers*, they that *Corpses* carry,
The Herb-wife, Druggist, and Apothecary,
Physicians, Surgeons, Nurses, Coffin-makers,
Bold *Mountebanks*, and shameless undertakers—
To cure the *Pest* in all, these, rich become,
And what we pray to be delivered from
Was their advantage. Yea, the worst of these
Grew stout and fat and proud by this disease.                 (680)
Some vented refuse wares at three times more
Than what it best was prized at before.
Some set upon their labors such high rates
As passed Reason, so, they whose estates
Did fail of reaching to a price so high,
Were fain to perish without remedy.
Some, wolfishly, did prey upon the quick.
Some, thievishly, purloined from the sick.
Some robb'd the dead of sheets; some of a grave
That there another guest may lodging have.                    (690)
Yea, Custom had so hardned most of them,
That they God's Judgments wholly did contemn.
They, so hard-hearted and so stupid grew,
So dreadlessly their course they did pursue;
Yea, so they flouted and such jests did make
At that, for which each Christian heart did ache,
That greater were the Plague their mind to have,
Than of the *Pestilence* to lie and rave.
    Now, muse I not at what *Thucydides*
Reporteth of such wicked men as these,                        (700)
When *Athens* was depopulated nigh
By such a Pestilence. Nor wonder I
That when the *Plague* did this time sixty year[s]
Oppress the Town of *Lyon*, that some there
Were said to ravish women, ev'n when death
Was drawing from them their last gasp of breath,

And when infectious Blains on them they saw,
Which might have kept their lustful flesh in awe.
For man once hardned in impenitence
Is left unto a reprobated sense.                                    (710)
     Till God shall sanctify it, weal nor woe
Can make us fear him as we ought to do.
His love made wanton *Isr'el* spurn at him;
His plagues made *Phar'oh* his sharpst rod contemn,
And as the Sun from dunghills and from sinks
Produceth nothing but rank weeds and stinks,
Yet makes a Garden of well-tilled ground
With wholesome fruits and fragrant flowers abound,
Or, as in bruising, one thing scenteth well,
Another yields a loathsome, stifling smell—                        (720)
So, *Plagues* and *Blessings*, their effects declare,
According as their sev'ral objects are.
     Indeed, my young experience never saw,
So much security and so much awe
Dwell both together in one place, as here
In this mortality there did appear.
I am persuaded, time and place was never
In which afflicted men did more endeavor
By tears, vows, prayers and true penitence,
To pacify God's wrath for their offence.                           (730)
Nor ever was it seen, I think, before,
That men in wickedness presumed more.
     Here you should meet a man with bleared eyes,
Bewailing our increasing miseries.
Another there quite reeling drunk or spewing,
And by renewed sins our woes renewing.
There sat a *piece of shamelessness*, whose flaring
Attires and looks did show a monstrous daring,
For in the postures of true impudence,
She seem'd as if she woo'd the *Pestilence.*                       (740)
Yon talkt a couple, matter worth your hearing.
Hard by were others telling lies or swearing.
Some streets had *Churches* full of people, weeping;
Some others *Taverns* had, rude-revel keeping.
Within some houses, *Psalms* and *Hymns* were sung.
With railings and loud scoldings others rung.
More *Charity* did never yet appear,
Nor more maliciousness than we had here.
True piety was eminently known.
Hypocrisy as evidently shown.                                      (750)

More avarice, more gapers for the wealth
Of such as dy'd, no former times of health
Afforded us, nor men of larger heart,
Things needful for their brethren to impart.
Their masters' goods, some servants lewdly spent
In nightly feastings, foolish merriment
And lewd uncleanness. Other some again
Did such an honest carefulness retain,
That their endeavors had a good success,
And *Man* and *Master* met with joyfulness.                    (760)
    Yea, *Good* and *Evil*, penitence and sin,
Did here so drive each other out and in,
That in observing it, I saw, methought,
In sight of Heav'n, a dreadful *Combat* fought
Concerning this whole *Island*, which yet lies
To be God's purchase, or the Devil's prize.
    *Vice* wounded *Virtue*; *Virtue* oft compeld
The strongest *Vices* to forsake the field.
*Distrust* rais'd up a storm to drive away
*Sure-help*, our ship, which at *Hope's* anchor lay,          (770)
And brought supplies with ev'ry wind and tide,
Whereby this Land was fed and fortified.
The *Fort* of *Faith* was play'd on by *Despair*,
But then the gun-shot of *continual-Pray'r*
(Well aim'd at *Heav'n*) *Devotion* so did ply
That he dismounts the *Foe's Artillery*.
The *Spirit* and the *Flesh* together strive,
And oft each other into peril drive.
Presumption, huge, high, Scaling ladders reared,
And then the taking of our *Fort* was feared.                 (780)
But *awful Reverence* did him oppose,
And, with *Humilities*, deep *Trench* enclose
The *Platform* of that Fortress, from whose Towers
We fight with *Principalities* and *Pow'rs*.
    Suggestion lay perdu by Contemplation
And sought to disadvantage *Meditation*.
The *Regiment* of *Prudence* was assailed,
By headstrong *Ignorance*, who much prevailed
Where *Temperance* was quarter'd; there I saw
*Excess* and *Riot*, both together draw                        (790)
Their troops against her, and I some espy'd
To yield and overcome on either side.
    The place that valiant *Fortitude* made good,
*Faint-heartedness* (though out of sight he stood)

Did cowardly oppose and courses take,
Which otherwhile his Constancy did shake,
For *Carnal policy* her Engineer,
Had closely sunk a *Mine* which had gone near
To blow all up, but *Providence* divine
Did soon prevent it by a *Counter-mine*.                    (800)
Yet Moral-Justice (though a Court of Guard
Was plac'd and oft relieved in her *Ward*)
Had much ado to make a strong defense
Against her *Foes*, for *Fraud*, and *Violence*,
Respect of persons, Fear, Hate, Perjury,
Fair-speaking, and corrupting Bribery,
Did wound her much, though she did often take
Avengement and, of some, examples make.
    Some *Vices*, there, I saw themselves disguise
Like *Virtues*, that their Foes they might surprise;        (810)
As do the Dunkirks, when aboard to lay
Our ships, an *English* flag they do display:
*Pride* went for *Comeliness*; profuse *Excess*,
For Hospitality; base Drunkenness
Was call'd *Good fellowship*; blunt *Rashness* came
Attir'd like *Valor*; *Sloth* had got the name
Of *Quietness*; accursed *Avarice*,·
Was term'd *Good husbandry*; mere *Cowardice*
Appear'd like prudent *Wariness*, and might
Have passed for a very valiant wight.                       (820)
Yea, ev'ry *Vice*, to gain his purpose had
Some masks of virtue-like disguises made.
And many times, such hellish plots were laid,
That diverse moral *Virtues* were gainsaid,
Defam'd, pursu'd, and wounded by their own,
Whose glory had not else been overthrown.
    *Fast-dealing* hath been took for *Cruelty*;
*Pure-love* for *Lust*; upright *Integrity*
For cunning *Falsehood*; yea, divinest *Graces*
Have been at variance brought in diverse Cases,            (830)
(By wicked *Stratagems*) that vain Inventions,
Might frustrate pious works and good intentions.
    To further strife, great *Quarrels* broached are,
Twixt *Faith* and *Works*. There is another jar
Begun erewhile, betwixt no worse a pair
Than *Preaching* and her blessed Sister *Pray'r*.
God grant they may agree, for I ne're knew
A quiet Church but where they kept one Pew.

*Faith* and *Repentance* also are, of late,
About their *Birthright* fallen at debate.                    (840)
But by the *Church-books,* it appears to me,
Their *Births* and their *Conceptions* mention'd be,
Without such nice regard to their proceedings,
As some have urged in their needless pleadings.
And so it pleas'd the *Father*, *Son,* and *Spirit*,
Because that *Law* by which they shall inherit
The promist meed doth never question move,
How soon or late, but how sincere they prove.
    Moreover, in this *Battle* I espy'd
Some *Ambodexters* fight on either side.                      (850)
The *Moralist*, who all Religion wants,
Church-Papists, Time-observing Protestants,
All Double-dealers, Hypocrites, and such
Base *Neutrals*, who have scandalized much,
And much endanger'd those who do contend
This *Isle* from desolation to defend.
    Beside these former *Combatants*, which fought
Against or for us, I perceiv'd, methought,
Both good and evil *Angels* fighting too,
The one, to help, the other, harm to do.                     (860)
And though this battle yet appeareth not
To common view so cruel nor so hot
As I conceive it, yet it will appear
To all in time, with comfort or with fear,
For full and ev'ry day those enemies
Stand arm'd and watching opportunities
To seize us, and will seize us if these times
Shall make complete the measure of our Crimes,
Or our continuing Follies drive away
Our Angel Guard, which doth our fall delay.                  (870)
Oh stay them Lord! and make that side the stronger,
For whom this Land shall yet be spared longer.
    And let us, my dear Countrymen, with speed
Of that which so concerneth us, take heed.
Observe, thou famoust City of this Land,
How heavily on thee God lays his hand.
The very rumor of this *Plague* did make
The farthest dwellers of this *Isle* to shake,
And such a scent of *Death* they seem'd to carry,
Who in or near about thy Climate tarry,                      (880)
That from the *Mount* to *Barwick* they were hated
Or shunn'd, as persons excommunicated.

And three weeks airing on old *Sarum* plain, [6]
Would scarce a lodging for a brother gain.
    Yea, mark, mark *London*, and confess with me,
That God hath justly thus afflicted thee,
And that in ev'ry point this *Plague* hath bin
According to the nature of thy sin.
In thy prosperity, such was thy pride,
That thou the *Country's* plainness didst deride.          (890)
Thy wanton Children would oft straggle out,
At honest husbandmen to jeer and flout.
Their homely garments did offend thine eyes.
They did their rural Dialects despise.
Their games and merriments (which for them be
As commendable as are thine for thee)
Thou laughedst at; their gestures and their fashions,
Their very diet and their habitations
Were sported at; yea, those ungrateful Things,
Did scoff them for their hearty *Welcomings*,          (900)
And taught ev'n those that had been country-born
The wholesome places of their birth to scorn.
    And *see*, now *see*, those thankless ones are fain
To seek their fathers' thatched Roofs again
And asked those *good old women* blessing, whom
They did not see since they did rich become,
And never would have seen, perhaps, unless
This *Plague* had whipped their ungratefulness.
Yea, thine own natural Children have been glad
To scrape acquaintance where no friends they had,          (910)
To praise a homely and a smoky *Shed*,
A dark low *Parlor*, an uneasy *Bed*,
An ill drest diet, yea, perchance, commend
A churlish Landlord for an honest Friend,
Yet be contented both to pray and pay,
That they may leave obtain with him to stay.
    And, peradventure, some of those who played
The scoffers heretofore, were fully paid.
Then, *Citizens* were sharkt and prey'd upon,
In recompense of wrongs before-time done          (920)
To silly Countrymen and were defeated
Of that whereof some Rustics they had cheated.

---

   [6]  *from the Mount to Barwick.* From St. Michael's Mount, on the tip of Cornwall in the southwest, to Barwick in Norfolk, in the northeast; essentially, from one end of the island to the other.

Moreover, for the *Country's* imitations
Of thy fantastic, vain, and fruitless fashions,
(Of thy apparel and of thy excess
In Feasts, in Games, in Lust, in Idleness,
With such abominations) some of those
Who came from thee, shall doubtlessly dispose
To ev'ry *Shire* a *Vial* of that wrath,
Which thy transgression long deserved hath,                    (930)
That thou and they, who sinners were together,
May Rods be made to punish one another,
And give each other bitterness to sup,
As you have jointly quaft of *Pleasure's* Cup.
      As to and fro I walked, that I might
On ev'ry ruthful *Object* fix my sight,
Upon those *Golgathas* I cast mine eye,
Where all the common people buried lie.
"Lie buried," did I say? I should have said,
"Where Carcasses to bury Graves were laid."                    (940)
      Lord! what a sight was there, and what strong smells
Ascended from among *Death's* loathsome Cells.
You scarce could make a little Infant's bed
In all those *Plots* but you should pare a head,
An arm, a shoulder, or a leg away
Of one or other who there buried lay.
One grave did often many scores enclose
Of men and women, and it may be those
That could not in two Parishes agree,
Now in one little room at quiet be.                            (950)
      Yon lay a heap of skulls, another there.
Here, half unburied did a Corpse appear.
Close by, you might have seen a brace of feet
That had kickt off the rotten winding-sheet.
A little further saw we othersome,
Thrust out their arms for want of elbow room.
A lock of woman's hair, a dead man's face
Uncover'd, and a ghastly sight it was.
Oh! here, here view'd I what the glories be
Of pamper'd flesh; here plainly did I see                      (960)
How grim those *Beauties* will e're long appear,
Which we so dote on and so covet here.
Here was enough to cool the hottest flame
Of lawless lust. Here, was enough to tame
The madst ambition. And all they that go
Unbetter'd from such objects, worse do grow.

From hence (for here was no abiding long)
Our *Allies* and our *Lanes*, I walkt among,
Where those *Artificers* their dwellings had,
By whom our idle *Traders* rich are made.                    (970)
The *Plague* rav'd there indeed, for who were they
Whom that *Contagion* fastest swept away,
But those whose daily lab'ring hands did feed
Their honest Families and greatly stead
This place by their mechanic industries?
These are the swarms of *Bees*, whose painful thighs
Bring *Wax* unto this *Hive* and from whose bones
The *Honey* drops that feedeth many *Drones*.
These are the *Bulwarks* of this senseless *Town*,
And when this *Wall of Bones* is overthrown,                (980)
Our stately Dwellings, now both fair and tall,
Will quickly, of themselves, to ruin fall.
Of these and of their households daily dy'd
Twice more than did of all sorts else beside,
And hungry *Poverty* (without reliefs)
Did much enrage and multiply their griefs.
The *Rich* could fly, or if they stayed, they had
Such means that their disease the less was made.
Yea, those poor, aged folks that make a show
Of greatest need did boldly come and go                    (990)
To ask men's Alms or what their Parish granted,
And nothing at this time those people wanted
But thankfulness, less malice to each other,
And grace to live more quietly together.
Their bodies, dry'd with age, were seldom struck
By this *Disease*. Their neighbors notice took
Of all their wants. Among them were not many
That had full families, or if that any
Of these had children sick, some good supplies
Were sent them from the general Charities.                 (1000)
　　　Moreover, common *Beggars* are a nation,
Not always keeping in one habitation.
They can remove as time occasion brings.
They have their progresses as well as King,
And most of these, when hence the rich did go,
Remov'd themselves into the Country too.
The rest about our streets did ask their bread,
And never in their lives were fuller fed.
　　　But those good people mentioned before,
Who, till their work did fail them, fed the poor           (1010)

As well as others, and maintained had
Great families by some laborious trade—
Ev'n those did suffer most, for neither having
Provision left them, nor the face of craving,
Nor means of labor, first, to pawn, they sent
Their brass and pewter; then, their bedding went;
Their garments next or stuff of best esteem;
At length, ev'n that which should the rest redeem,
Their working Instruments. When that was gone,
Their Lease was pawned, if it might be done.                    (1020)
And peradventure, at the last of all,
These things were sold outright for sums but small,
Or else quite forfeited. For here were they
Who made of these poor souls a gainful prey.
And as one Plague had on the life a pow'r,
So did these other *Plagues* their goods devour.
When all was gone, afflicted they became
With secret griefs, with poverty, and shame.
And wanting cheerful minds and due refection,
Were seized on, the sooner, by *Infection*,                    (1030)
For hearts half broke and households famisht near,
Are quickly spent, when visited they are.
        The careful *Master*, though it would have saved
A servant's life to get him what he craved,
No kind of Med'cine able was to give him,
Nay scarce with bread and water to relieve him.
The tender-hearted Mother hath for meat
Oft heard her dearest child, in vain, entreat,
And had or four or five on point of dying
At once, for drink to ease their torment, crying.              (1040)
        The loving husband sitting by her side,
To save whose life he gladly would have dy'd,
Unable was out of his whole estate,
To purchase her a dram of *Mithridate*,
One mess of Cordial broth, or such like thing,
Although it might prevent her perishing.
        Sometime, at such a need, abroad they came
To ask for help, but then the fear of shame,
Of scorn, or of denial them withheld
To put in practice what their want compell'd.                  (1050)
        Upon an Evening (when the waning light
Was that which could be call'd nor day nor night)
I met with one of these, who on me cast
A ruthful eye, and as he by me pass'd,

Methought I heard him, softly, somewhat say,
As if that he for some relief did pray,
Whereat (he seeming in good clothes to be)
I stayed and askt him if he spake to me.
He bashfully replied that indeed,
He was asham'd to speak aloud what *Need*                              (1060)
Did make him softly mutter. Somewhat more
He would have spoken, but his tongue forbore
To tell the rest, because his eyes did see
Their tears had (almost) drawn forth tears from me,
And that my hand was ready to bestow
That help which my poor fortunes could allow.
    Nor his, nor all men's tongues, could more relate,
Than I myself conceiv'd of his estate.
Methought I saw, as if I had been there,
What wants in his and such men's houses were:                          (1170)
How empty and how naked it became;
How nasty *Poverty* had made the same.
Methought I saw how sick his wife might lie;
Methought I heard his half starv'd children cry;
Methought I felt with what a broken heart
He lookt upon them e're he could depart
To try if (by God's favor) he could meet
With any means of comfort in the street.
And *Lord, my God*, thou know'st that, when alone,
The griefs of such as these I mused on,                                (1080)
My pity I with watry eyes have shown,
And more bewail'd their sorrows than my own.
    But since those *Dews* are vain that fruitless be,
And since the share that is allotted me
Of this world's heritage will not suffice
To bring relief to these men's miseries,
Oh! let my tears (ye *rich men*) make your ground
With fruits of Charity the more abound.
Let me entreat you that when God shall bring
Upon this place another *Visiting*,                                    (1090)
You would remember some relief to send
To those who on their labors do depend
And have not got their impudence of face,[7]
Who idly beg their bread from place to place.
God, you the *Stewards* of his goods doth make,

---

[7]    *impudence of face*. Ability to protect themselves, to stand up aggressively in a face-off.

And how you use them, he account will take.
It will not be enough that you have paid
The public taxes on your houses laid,
Or that you now and then do send a sum
To be disposed to you know not whom,                              (1100)
But you yourselves must, by yourselves alone,
Those neighbors or acquaintance think upon,
Who likeliest are in such a time of need,
To want of that, wherein you do exceed,
And if you know of none, enquire them out,
Or leave some honest neighbor thereabout
To be your *Alm'ner* (when the Town you leave)
That you and they a *Blessing* may receive.
For if that ev'ry wealthy man would find
But one or two to cherish in this kind,                           (1110)
God's wrath would much the better be appeased,
And we should of our plagues be sooner eased.
   As I request the Richer men to take
This pious course, a suit, I likewise make
That our inferior *Tradesmen* would not so
Abuse their times of profit as they do.
For most of those do live at rates as high,
As all their gains (at utmost) will supply.
Yea, many times they mount above the tops
Of present fortunes and ensuing hopes,                            (1120)
That if a sickness or unlook'd-for Cross[8]
Or want of trade or any slender loss,
But for a *Year*, a *Quarter*, or a *Term*,
Befalls them, it soon maketh so infirm
Their over-strain'd Estates that Alms are needed,
Ere any failings are by others heeded.
   Of these, and other things I notions gained,
Whilst in our sickly *City* I remained,
And much I contemplated what I saw,
Some profitable uses thence to draw,                              (1130)
But feeling that my thoughts nigh tir'd were
With over-musing on those objects there,
I thought to walk abroad into the field
To take those comforts which fresh air doth yield,
And to revive my heart which heavy grew
With what the streets did offer to my view.
But little ease I found, for there mine eyes

---

[8]   *unlook'd-for Cross.* Unforeseen affliction, in this case causing economic hardship.

Discover'd *Sorrow* in a new disguise,
And in so many shapes himself he shewed,
That still my passion was afresh renewed.                    (1140)
Here, dead upon the *Road*, a man did lie
That was (an hour before) as well as I.
There sat another, who did thither come
In health but had not strength to bear him home.
Yon sprawl'd a third, so sick he did not know
From whence he came nor whither he should go.
A little further off, a fourth did creep
Into a ditch and there his *Obit* keep.
About the Fields ran one, who being fled
(In spite of his attendance) from his bed,                   (1150)
Lookt like a Lunatic from *Bedlam* broken,
And though of health he had no hopeful token,
Yet, that he ailed ought, he would not yield,
Till *Death* had struck him dead upon the field.
This way, a *Stranger* by his Host expelled.
That way, a *Servant* (shut from where he dwelled)
Came weakly stagg'ring forth and (crush'd beneath
Diseases, and unkindness) sought for Death,
Which soon was found, and glad was he, they say,
Who, for his *Death-bed*, gain'd a Cock of Hay.              (1160)
At this cross path were *Bearers* fetching home
A Neighbor, who in health did thither come.
Close by were others digging up the ground
To hide a stranger whom they dead had found.
Before me went with Corpses, many a one.
Behind, as many more did follow on.
With *running sores*, one begg'd at yonder gate.
At next Lane's end, another *Lazar* sate.
Some halted as if wounded in the wars.
Some held their necks awry; some show'd their scars.         (1170)
Some, met I, weeping for the loss of friends,
Some others for their swift approaching ends.
And ev'rything with sorrow was affected,
On whatsoe're it was mine eye reflected.
    The *Prospect* which was wont to greet mine eye
With shows of pleasure in variety
(And lookt, as if it cheerfully did smile,
Upon the bordring *Villages*, erewhile)
Had no such pleasingness as heretofore,
For ev'ry place, a mask of sorrow wore.                      (1180)
The walks are unfrequented, and the path,

Late trodden bare, a grassy Carpet hath.
I could not see (of all those Gallants) one
That visited *Hyde Park* and *Marybourne*.
None wandred through the pastures, up and down,
But as about some petty Country town,
Nor could I view in many Summer's days,
One man of note to ride upon our ways.
  Lord, what a diff'rence didst thou put between
That Summer and the rest that I have seen!     (1190)
How didst thou change our Fields and what a face
Of Sadness, didst thou set upon each place!
Yet oh! how few remember it or feel
The touches of it on their hearts of steel!
And when our banisht mirth thou didst renew,
Who did return to thee the praises due?
  What others apprehended, they know best,
But if it could be fully here exprest
What of that alteration I conceiv'd,
When of their pleasures, God our fields bereav'd,   (1200)
It would much more be minded, for they had
Naught in them but what moved to be sad.
Not many weeks before, it was not so,
But *Pleasures* had their passage to and fro.
Which way soever from our Gates I went,
I lately did behold with much content,
The fields bestrew'd with people all about,
Some pacing homeward and some passing out;
Some by the banks of *Thames* their pleasure taking;
Some Sullabubs among the Milk-maids, making   (1210)
With music; some upon the waters, rowing;
Some to the next adjoining *Hamlets* going;
And Hoxton, Islington, and Tethnam-Court,
For Cakes and Cream, had then no small resort.
Some sat and woo'd their Lovers in the shadows;
Some straggled to and fro athwart the meadows;
Some in discourse, their hours away did pass;
Some playd the toyish wantons on the grass;
Some of Religion, some of bus'ness talked;
Some coached were, some horsed, and some walked.  (1220)
Here Citizens, there Students, many a one;
Here two together and yon one alone.
Of *Nymphs* and *Ladies*, I have often ey'd,
A thousand walking at one Evening tide;
As many Gentleman, and young and old

Of meaner sort, as many ten times told.
　　And when I did from some high Tower survey
The Roads and Paths which round below me lay,
Observing how each passage thronged was
With men and Cattle, which both ways did pass;　　　　　(1230)
How many petty paths, both far and near,
With rows of people still supplied were;
What infinite provision still came in,
And what abundance hath exported bin.
Methought this populous *City* and the trade
Which we from ev'ry Coast about her had,
Was well resembled by an *Ant-hill*, which
(In some old Forest) is made large and rich
By those laborious creatures, who have thither
Brought all their wealth and *Colonies* together,　　　　(1240)
For as their peopled *Borough* hath resort
From ev'ry quarter, by a several Port,
And from each Gate thereof a great Road hath
That branches into many a little Path,
And as those *Negroes* do not only fill
Each great and lesser tract unto their hill,
But also spread themselves out of those ways,
Among the grass, the leaves, and bushy sprays—
Ev'n so, the people here did come and go
Through our large Roads, disperse themselves into　　　(1250)
A thousand passages, and often stray
O're neighboring Pastures in a pathless way.
　　This formerly I saw, and on that *Station*,
Where this I markt, I had this *Contemplation*:
How happy were this People; did they know
What rest our God upon them did bestow!
On us, what showers of blessings hath he rained,
Which he from other Cities hath restrained?
And from how many mischiefs hath he freed us,
Which fall on those that in good works exceed us?　　　(1260)
Here lurk no ravenous Beasts to make a prey
On those fat Cattle which these Fields o're-lay.
Within our Groves no cruel Outlaws hide,
That in the blood of passengers are dy'd.
Our Lambs, unworry'd, lye abroad, benighted;
By day, our Virgins walk the Fields unfrighted.
No neighboring Country doth our food forestall;
No Convoys need to come and go withal;
No foreign Prince can suddenly appall us,

For Seas do mote us, and huge Rocks do wall us.                    (1270)
No rotten Fens do make our air unsound;
No Foe doth with a trench enclose us round.
We neither tumults have by night or day,
Nor rude unruly Garrisons in pay.
No Taxes, yet our Land doth over-load;
Our Children are not prest for wars abroad.
From Spanish Inquisitions we are free
(God grant that we, forever, so may be)
We are compeld to no Idolatries;
Our people do not in rebellions rise;                             (1280)
No factious spirits much disturb the State;
No Plagues, our dwellings, yet depopulate.
No Rots or Murrains have our Cattle kild.
Our Barns and Storehouses with fruits are fild.
On ev'ry threshold, store of children play.
Our breeding Cattle fill both street and way.
And were we thankful unto him that gave them,
There are no blessings, but we here might have them.
    See, how like Bees upon a Summer-Eve,
(When their young Nymphs have over-fill'd the hive)               (1290)
They swarm about the City, sporting so,
As if a winter gale would never blow.
How little do they dream, how many times,
While they deserved ruin for their Crimes,
God, natheless, hath showed mercies on them,
And stopt those Plagues that coming were upon them!
How seldom is it thought, the pow'r of him,
Whose love they much forget (if not contemn)
Might heap upon them all those fearful things,
Which he upon our neighboring Nations brings.                    (1300)
For, in a moment, he could summon hither
His Judgments, and inflict them, all together,
Ev'n all, but one of these which he hath brought
On other Cities would enough be thought.
    If, in displeasure, he should call from thence
Where now it raves, the slaughtring Pestilence,
Or else the Famine, what a change were that
To them that are so healthy and so fat?
How desolate in less than half a year,
Might all our lodgings and our streets appear?                   (1310)
How unfrequented would that rendezvous
Be made in which we throng and jostle now?
How lonely would these walks and fields be found,

Wherein I see the people so abound?
    Or should he whistle for his armed Bands,
(Which now are wasting other Christian Lands)
To put in action on our Comic Stage
The Tragedies of War and brutish rage,
What lamentations then here would be made,
And calling unto mind what peace we had.                      (1320)
Should we in ev'ry house, at board and bed,
Have Soldiers and rude Captains billeted,
That would command and swagger as if they
Had all the Township (where they lodge) in pay,
To wait upon their pleasures and should see
Our own defenders, our devourers be?
Should we behold these Fields (now full of sport)
Cut out with Trenches: there, a warlike Fort;
Another here; A Sconce not far from that;
A new rais'd Mount or some fire-spitting Cat                  (1330)
From which the Foes our actions might survey
And make their Billets on our houses play?
Should we behold our Dwellings beaten down,
Our Temples batter'd, Turrets overthrown,
Our seats of pleasure burning from afar?
Hear, from without, the thundring voice of War?
Within, the shrieks of children or the cry
Of women struck with fears or famisht nigh?
Should we behold what painfully we got,
Possest by those that seek to cut our throat,                (1340)
Our children slain before us, on the ground,
Ourselves pierc't through with some deep mortal wound,
And see (ev'n there) where we have wantonni'd,
Our beauteous wives by some stern Troup surpriz'd,
And ravisht in our view? Or (which is worse)
When we have seen all this, be force't perforce
To live and live their slaves that shall possess
Our wives and all our outward happiness?
And then want also that pure Word of Grace
To comfort us, which yet adorns this place?                  (1350)
    Should such a Destiny (as, God defend)
This people and this place, thought I, attend?
(For this may be, and ev'ry day we hear
That other Nations do this burden bear.)
Should we who now for pleasure walk the field
Be fain to search what weeds the pastures yield
To feed us, and peek hungerly about,

Some Roots or Haws or Berries to find out
To keep from starving, and not gain a food
So mean without the hazard of our blood?                    (1360)
Should some contagious sickness, noisome make
This place, wherein, such pleasure now we take?
Should in these places, whither we repair
Our bodies to refresh with wholesome air,
Those blastings or Serenes upon us fall,
Which other places are annoy'd withal?
Should from the wife the husband be divorc'd,
Or from the parent should the child be forc'd,
While here they walkt, and perish by the sword,
Or should here be a famine of the Word,                     (1370)
On which would follow, to our grief and shame,
A thousand other Plagues which I could name?
Should these things be, then, what our blessings are,
It would by such a curse too soon appear.
      Then feel, we should, what comforts might arise
From those great mercies, which we now despise
Or think not on. Yea, so we might enjoy
But part of that which now we misemploy,
We think it would a greater happiness
Than yet we find in all we now possess.                     (1380)
We then should know how much we have been blest
In our long time of plenty, health, and rest.
How sweet it is that we may to and fro
Without restraint or fear or danger go.
How much we owe to him that hath so long
Our Granards filled and our Gates made strong,
Permitting us to walk for our delight
About our fields, whilst others march to fight,
And suffring us to feast, whilst others fast
Or of the bread of sour Affliction tast[e].                 (1390)
      As heretofore the peopled *Fields* I walked,
To this effect, my thoughts within me talked,
And though all present *Objects* gave content,
My heart did such *Ideas* represent
Of *Judgments* likely to be cast upon
So great a City and a sinful one,
That much I feared I should live to see,
Some such afflictions as here mention'd be.
And lo (though yet I hope, not in his wrath)
God, part of that I fear'd, inflicted hath:                 (1400)
A warning *War* he hath begun to wage

Against the crying sins of this our age,
And of this place, and in a gentle wise,
Pour'd out a taste of those Calamities
Which others feel at large, that we should mourn
For our transgressions and to him return.
Vouchsafe, oh! God, that soon return we may,
Lest thou, in anger, sweep us all away.
  If we observed well what God hath done,
And in what manner he with us begun, (1410)
How he forewarn'd us of those *Plagues,* which he
Vouchsafed *David* should a chooser be.[9]
(And how, ev'n he himself, in mercy choosed
To keep us from what *David* had refused)
We should perceive that our most loving God
At first did threaten with a *Father's* rod.
  A little while before this *Pestilence,*
Of this just wrath we had intelligence
By diverse tokens, which we did contemn,
Or, at the best, but little heeded them. (1420)
The *Spring* before this *Plague,* one jerk we had
By *WAR,* which made no little number sad,
By calling many from their ease, by taking
Some husbands from their wives, and childless making
Some *Parents,* which permitted was to show us,
In part, what sharp corrections God did owe us,
And make us mind that this unhallow'd place
Is thus long spared merely of his grace,
Else to awake us with some touch of that
Which he hath brought on many a foreign State. (1430)
  For that he might but touch us, he did call
No *Armies* hither to afflict us all,
But as a *General* in time of war,
When all his Troops of somewhat guilty are,
On them the fortune of the *lot* doth try,
That some as warnings to the rest may die—
Ev'n so, the *God of Armies,* in like case,
Pickt here and there a man, from ev'ry place,
To meet the sword, that ev'ry place might learn
His *Mercies* and his *Justice* to discern (1440)
And leave off sin, which, if we break not from,
His *Plagues* and terrors all will shortly come.

---

[9]  *David should a chooser be.* See King David's choice of plague over famine and war
(2 Samuel 24.13–15).

If any shall object, we lost in these
But some corrupted blood, which did disease
The common *Body*; let them understand,
That it portends hot *Fevers* in the Land,
When such *Phlebotomy* is needful thought,
And that good blood, as well as what is not,
Is lost at ev'ry op'ning of a vein.
The foot was prickt, and we did feel no pain;                    (1450)
The next blood letting may be in the *Arm*,
Where lies our strength. God shend us from the harm
Of such like *Surgery*, unless we see
The *Sign* be better than it seems to be.
God scar'd us lately also by a *Dearth*,
And for the people's faults did curse the Earth:
The *Winter* last before the *Pest* began,
Throughout some Northern *Shires* a Famine ran
That starved some, and other some were fain
Their hungry appetites to entertain                              (1460)
With swine and sheep and horses, which have dy'd
By chance, for better could they not provide.
Some others on boild nettles gladly fed,
Or else had oft gone supperless to bed.
And this was much, considering the soil
And ordinary plenties of this *Isle*.
Nay, since the *Sickness*, we small hopes possessed
Of that wherewith this Kingdom God hath blessed.
For when *Earth's* womb did big with plenty grow,
When her large bosom and full breasts did show                   (1470)
Such signs of fair increase, that hope of more
Was never in our lifetimes, heretofore,
A later frost, our early blossoms cropt;
The heav'ns, upon our labors, leanness dropt,
And such perpetual showers and floods we had,
That of a *Famine*, we were fearful made,
And fierce had any hope (in common reason)
Of harvest either in or out of season.
Yet he withheld that *Plague*, the Sky grew clear,
A kindly weather drove away our fear.                            (1480)
The Floods did sink, the Mildews were expell'd,
The bending ears of corn their heads upheld,
And *Harvest* came, which fild our Granards more
Than in the fruitful'st of sev'n years before.
And doubtless, had we gone to meet our God
With true repentance when this fearful Rod

Was raised first, it had away been flung
And not continued in this *Realm* so long,
For as a *Father*, when his dearest child
Grows disobedient, rude, and over-wild,                                (1490)
First warns, then threatens, then, the rod doth show,
Then frowns, and then doth fear him with a blow.
Then doubles and redoubles it until
He makes him grow more pliant to his will,
And leave those wanton tricks, which in conclusion
May prove the parents' grief and child's confusion—
Ev'n as this Father, so our God hath wrought
Us. By his *Word of Grace*, he first besought,
Then of his *Wrath* and *Justice* spake unto us.
Next, hanging over us, he plagues did show us.                          (1500)
Yea, diverse months before this Vengeance came,
The spotted *Fever* did forewarn the same,
Was made her *Harbinger*, and in one week
Sent hundreds in the Grave, their bed to seek,
Which naught prevailing, he did thereupon
(As being loath to strike) first strike but one,
Then, two, or three, then stayed a while, and then
To smite another number he began,
And then a greater. Neither did God show
This mercy only in the public blow,                                     (1510)
But deign'd it, also, in that chastisement,
Which he to ev'ry man in private sent
To hasten his repentance: first, he smote
Some one of those he knew in place remote;
Within a week, another better known;
Next week a friend; the next a dearer-one;
A little after that, perhaps, another;
And then a kinsman or an only brother,
Which, no amendment working, God did come
(To make him heedful) somewhat nearer home:                            (1520)
Knockt at his neighbor's house, and took out all
Or most who lodg'd on t'other side the wall;
Then called at his door, and seized on
A servant first; soon afterward, a son;
Next night was hazarded a daughter's life;
And e're that morning came, he lost his wife;
At last fell sick himself, and then repented
Or dy'd, or liveth to be worse tormented.
    Thus, as it were by steps, God came upon us,
That either Love or Terror might have won us,                           (1530)

To seek our peace, but yet so few were warned,
(And this long-suffring, so few souls discerned)
That some the nature of this *Plague* beli'd;
The number of the dead, some strove to hide.
On groundless hopes, God's Judgments some deferred.
Some scoffed others when they were deterred.
Some rais'd a profit from it. Yea, so few
Conceived what was likely to ensue,
That when we should like *Nineveh* have fared,
For sports and causeless *Triumphs* we prepared.                    (1540)
Of pleasure, in excessive wise, we tasted.
We *feasted*, when we rather should have *fasted*.
And when in sack-cloth we should loud have cry'd,
Ev'n then, we ruffled in our greatest pride.
Which God perceiving, and that we were grown
Regardless of his smiles and of his frown,
He did command his *Mercy* to let go
That hand which did restrain his *Justice* so.
Then, catching up a *Vial* of his wrath,
(Which he in store for such offenders hath)                         (1550)
He did on this our City pour it down.
And as strong poison shed upon the crown,
Descendeth to the members from the head,
And soon doth over all the body spread—
Ev'n so, this noisome plague of *Pestilence,*
On our head City falling, did from thence,
Disperse, and soak throughout this *Empery*,
In spite of all our carnal policy.
        Our want of penitency to allay
God's wrath and stop his anger in the way,                          (1560)
Enflamed and exasperated so
This *Fiend*, that he did thousands overthrow
In some few minutes, and the greedy *Grave*
Devour'd, as if it none alive would save.
*Death* lurkt at ev'ry angle of the street
And did arrest whomever he did meet.
There scarcely was that house or lodging found
In which he did not either slay or wound.
In ev'ry room his murders acted he.
Our Closets, nay, our Temples, were not free.                       (1570)
From his attemptings—no, not while men pray'd—
Could his unbridled fury be delay'd.
In sundry *Families* there was not one
Whom his rude hand did take compassion on,

Nay many times he did not spare the last,
Until the burial of the first was pass'd.
For e're the *Bearers* back again could come,
The rest were ready for their graves at home.
Nor bad nor good, nor rich nor poor did scape him;
Nor fool nor wise man, an excuse could shape him;				(1580)
He shunned not the young man in the saddle,
Nor him that lay and cried in the cradle.
So dreadful was his look, so stern and grim,
That many dy'd through very fear of him.
For to men's fancies he did oft appear
In shapes which so exceeding ghastly were,
That flesh and blood, unable was to brook,
The horror of his all affrighting look.

    Ev'n in that house whose roof did cover me,
Of this, a sad experiment had we.							(1590)
For there, a plague-sick man (at least conceived)
That Death, a shape assuming, he perceived,
Deform'd and ugly, whereat loud he cries,
"Oh! hide me, hide me, from his dreadful eyes.
Look, oh! look there he comes; now by the bed
He stands, now at the feet, now at the head.
Oh! draw, draw, draw the Curtain, Sirs I pray,
That his grim look no more behold I may."
To this effect, and such-like words he spake,
But that their hearers' hearts they more did shake.				(1600)
Then, rested he a while, and by and by
Up starting, with a lamentable cry,
Ran to a Couch, whereon his wife (who waking
Two nights before had been) some rest was taking,
There, kneeling down, and both his hands up rearing,
As if his eye had seen pale *Death* appearing
To strike his wife, "*Good Sir*," said he, "*forbear*
To kill or harm that poor young woman there.
For God's sake do not strike her, for you see
She's great with child. Lo, you have wounded me				(1610)
In twenty places, and I do not care
How me you mischief, so that her you spare."
Ev'n this, and more than I to mind can call,
He acted with a look so tragical,
That all bystanders might have thought his eyes
Saw real objects and no fantasies.

    To others, Death, no doubt, himself convey'd
In other forms, and other *Pageants* play'd.

Whilst in her arms the mother thought she kept
Her Infant safe, Death stole him when she slept.          (1620)
Sometimes he took the mother's life away,
And left the little babe to lie and play
With her cold paps and childish game to make
About those eyes that never more shall wake.
　　　Sometimes when friends were talking, he did force
The one to leave unfinish his discourse.
Sometimes their morning meetings he hath thwarted,
Who thought not they forever had been parted
The night before. And many a lovely *Bride*,
He hath deflow'red by the *Bridegroom's* side.          (1630)
At ev'ry hand, lay one or other dying.
On ev'ry part, were men and women crying:
One for a husband; for a friend another;
One for a sister, wife, or only brother.
Some children for their parents moan were making;
Some for the loss of servants care were taking;
Some parents for a child, and some again
For loss of all their children did complain.
　　　The mother dared not to close her eyes,
Through fear that while she sleeps, her baby dies.          (1640)
Wives trusted not their husbands out of door,
Lest they might back again return no more.
And in their absence if they did but hear
One knock or call in haste, they quak'd through fear,
That some unlucky messenger had brought
The news of those mischances they forethought,
And if (with care and grief o're-tyr'd) they slept,
They dream'd of *Ghosts* and *Graves*, and shriekt and wept.
　　　He that o're night went healthy to his bed,
Lookt e're the morning to be sick or dead.          (1650)
He that rose lusty at the rising Sun,
Grew faint and breathless e're the day was done.
And he that for his friend, this day did sorrow,
Lay close beside him in a grave the morrow.
Some men amidst their pleasures were diseased.
Some in the very act of sin were seized.
Some hence were taken laughing, and some singing,
Some as they others to their graves were bringing.
Yea, so impartial was this kind of *Death*,
And so extremely venomous his breath,          (1660)
That they who did not in this place expire,
Were saved, like the *Children in the fire*.

It may be that to some it will appear
My Muse hath only poetized here,
And that I fain'd expressions do rehearse,
As most of those that use[d] to write in verse,
But in this Poem I pursue the story
Of real Truth, without an Allegory,
And many yet surviving witness may,
That I come short of what I more might say. (1670)
But what I can, I utter, and I touch
This mournful string so often and so much
As in this Book I do that I might show
To them that of these griefs forgetful grow,
What sorrows and what dangers they have had,
That all of us more thankful may be made,
And if to any these things do appear
Or tedious, or impertinent, I fear
That most of them are they, who take no pleasure,
For good and useful things to be at leisure, (1680)
And more delight in Poems worded out,
Than those that are God's works employ'd about.
    Methinks I cannot speak enough of that
Which I have seen, nor full enough relate
What I declare, but still it seems to me
I leave out somewhat that should utt'red be.
For though in most the sense thereof be gone,
It was God's *Judgment*, and a fearful one.
    And *LONDON*, what availed then thy pride,
Thy pleasures, and thy wealth so multiply'd? (1690)
Or, then, oh! what advantage didst thou get
By those vain things, whereon thy heart is set?
How many sev'ral *Plagues* did God prevent,
Before this Judgment was upon thee sent?
How many loving favors had he done thee,
Before so roughly he did seize upon thee?
And that thou mightst his purposes discover,
How long together, did he send thee over
The weekly news of those great Desolations,
Which he inflicts on many other Nations? (1700)
How often did he send, e're this befell,
His *Prophets* of his *Judgments* to foretell?
How many thousand *Preachers* hath he sent,
With tears to pray and woo thee to repent
To tell thee that thy pride, and thy excess,
Thy lusts, thy surfeits, and thy drunkenness,

Thine idleness, thy great impieties,
Thy much prophaneness, thy hypocrisies,
And other vanities, would bring at last
Those plagues whereof thou now some feeling hast?    (1710)
  How did thy *Pastors* to repent conjure thee?
How strongly did God's Ministers assure thee
That all thy love, thy labor, and thy cost
Bestow'd on carnal pleasures would be lost?
That, thou hereafter shouldst become ashamed
Of that whereof thy comforts thou hadst framed,
And that those evils would at length befall
From which no mortal hand reprieve thee shall.
  Thou canst not but acknowledge these things were
Ev'n ev'ry moment rounded in thine care,    (1720)
And that thy *Sons of Thunder*[10] did presage
What for thy sins should be thine heritage.
Yet thou to hear their message didst refuse,
And as the stubborn unbelieving *Jews*
Despised all those *Prophets* who foreshew'd
The times of their approaching servitude,
Yea, punisht them, as troublers of the Land,
And such as weakned much the people's hand—
So, thou accountedst of thy Teachers then,
But as a crew of busy-headed men,    (1730)
Who causelessly, thy quietness disturbing,
Had for their sauciness deserved curbing.
But with amazement, now thou dost behold
That they have no uncertainties foretold.
For God in this one single *Plague* comprised
Those other *Judgments*, all, epitomized,
Which for thy ruin he at large will send,
If this be not enough to work his end.
Observe this *Pestilence*, and thou shalt see,
That as there may be some one *sin* in thee    (1740)
With other great *Transgressions* interlaced,
So, diverse Plagues in this great *Plague* were placed.
  It show'd thee (in some fashion) their distresses,
Whom *WAR*, in a besieged Fort oppresses.
For lo, thou wert deprived of all Trade,
As if thy Foes blockt up thy *River* had.

---

[10] *Sons of Thunder.* From Mark 3.17, referring to Christ's disciples: "And James the *son* of Zebedee, and John the brother of James; and he surnamed them Boanerges, which is, The sons of thunder."

And though no armed Host thy wall surrounded,
Yet (which was worse) thou by thy friends wert bounded,
For whatsoever person passed from
Thy Ports, upon an enemy did come.                              (1750)
And none more cruel to thy children proved,
Than some of thine, who from thy *Plagues* removed.
*Confusion* and *Disorder* threatned thee,
(On which attendeth all the *Plagues* that be)
For most of thy grave *Senate*, who did bear
Thy names of office, far departed were
To other places, leaving thee, nigh spent
And languishing for want of Government.
Yea, they that were thy *Trust* and thy *Delight*
In times of health did then forsake thee quite,                (1760)
To teach us that those men and vanities,
Which have our hearts in our prosperities,
Will in affliction be the first who leave us,
And when we most expect, then most deceive us.
    Oh! whither then; oh! whither were they gone,
Who thy admired Beauty doted on?
Where did thy *Lovers* in those days appear,
Who did so court thee, and so often swear
Affection to thee? Whither were they fled,
Whom thou hast oft with sweetest junkets fed                   (1770)
And they, whom thou so many years, at ease,
Didst lodge within thy fairest *Palaces*?
Where, *London*, were thy scarlet *Fathers* hous'd,
Who in thy glory, were to thee espous'd?
What were become of all thy children, which
Were nursed at thy breast, made great and rich
By thy *good-huswifry* and whom we see
In thy prosperity so hugg'd of thee?
    Where were thy rev'rend *Pastors* who had pay
To feed thy Flocks and for thy sin to pray?                    (1780)
(I must confess) the meanest, and some few
Of better sort, were in affection true,
And gave thee comfort. But oh! where were those,
Those greater ones, on whom thy hand bestows
The largest portions, those who have profest
A zealous care of thee above the rest,
Those, who (as I conceive) had undertaken
A charge that should not then have been forsaken,
Those many *silken-Doctors*, who did here
In shining satin Cassocks late appear,                         (1790)

They who (till now, a thing scarce heard of ever)
Do flaunt it in their Velvet, Plush, and Beaver,
And they, whom thou didst honor far above
Those mean ones? Who, then, showed thee most love?
    Where were they? And where were thy Lawyers too
That heretofore did make so much ado
Within thy Courts of *Justice*? Prithee, where
Were those *Physicians*, who so forward were
To give thee physic when thou neededst less
And wert but sick of ease and wantonness?        (1800)
Where did their foot-cloths wait? Where couldst thou call
For their assistance? What became of all
Their *Diets* and *Receipts,* and why did they
In that necessity depart away?
    Where lurkt those *Poetasters*, who were wont
To pen thy *Mummeries* and vainly hunt
For base reward by soothing up the Crimes
Of our Grand *Epicures* in lofty Rhymes,
And do before each other's *Poems* raise
The fruitless Trophies of a truthless praise?        (1810)
Dar'd none of all those matchless wits to tarry
This brunt, that his experienc'd Muse might carry
This News to after times and move compassion,
By his all moving strains of *Lamentation*?
What, none but me? Me only leave they to it,
To whom they shame to yield the Name of *Poet*?
Well, if they ever had a mind to wear
The *Laureate Wreath*, they might have got it here,
For though that my performance may be bad,
A braver Subject, *Muses* never had.        (1820)
    Where were thy troops of *Rovers*? Where were they
Who in thy Chambers did the wantons play,
Provoking God Almighty, down to cast
Those plagues from which they fled away so fast?
Yea, whither were those *Nothings*, all retir'd,
Of whom thou wert, of late, so much desir'd?
Alas! was there not any of all these
Who stayed to comfort thee in this Disease?
Did all depart away, and, being gone,
Leave thee to bear thy sorrows all alone?        (1830)
 Left they upon thy *Tally*[11] all that sin,
Which had by them and thee committed bin?

---

[11]   *Upon thy Tally* On the tab, on credit, running up a score.

Yes, yes, they left thee, ev'n all these, and they
So left thee, *London*, when they went away,
That thy afflictions they did aggravate,
And make more bitter thy deplored *Fate*.
A *Dearth* mixt also in this *Pest* was found,
For they who did in riches most abound,
(And should have holpen to relieve the poor)
Departing hence, diminished thy store.                              (1840)
To other *Boroughs* they themselves betook,
Their sick distressed brethren, they forsook,
And left on those that would be hospitable,
A burden which to bear they were unable.
Those few of worth who did in thee remain,
Had multitudes of beggars to sustain,
And from the Country (as before I said)
The sending of supply was long delay'd.

There was a *Famine* also, which exceeded
This other, though the same by few was heeded.                     (1850)
We had not so much scarcity of bread,
As of that food wherewith our souls are fed.
For of our *Pastors* (in the greatest dangers)
Some left us to the charity of Strangers.
And many souls, whom they were bound to cherish
Depriv'd of timely sustenance, did perish.

Who could have thought this *Vineyard* heretofore
So fruitful and wherein the savage *Boar*
Of *Turkey* rooted not, and whose thick fence
Hath long time kept the *Bulls* of *Bashan* thence,                (1860)
Should then (ev'n in the *Vintage* time) be found
So bare of what so lately did abound,
And, then (a thing worth note), when ev'ry Field
And meanest *Villages* did plenties yield?

Indeed, not long before, we surfeited,
And play'd the wantons with our heav'nly bread.
Our appetite was cloy'd, and we grew dainty,
And either loath'd or murmur'd at our plenty.
Yea, many of us, when at will we had it,
By private *Cookeries*, unwholesome made it.                       (1870)
For which, and for our base unthankfulness,
Our portion and allowance waxed less,
And we who (like fond children) would not eat,
Unless, this man, or that man carv'd our meat,
Then (like poor folks, that of mere alms do live)
Were glad to take of any that would give.

The *Laborers* were few, the *Harvest* large,
And of the best of those that had the charge
To spread God's *Table*, some grew faint and tired.
By their perpetual travail, some expired                                    (1880)
Their painful souls and freely sacrific'd
Themselves for us, that we might be suffic'd.
    Among which happy number I do bless
The memory of learned *Makerness*,
And zealous *Eton*, whose large congregations,
Bemoan'd their loss with hearty lamentations,
And worthily, for they did labor here
With cheerfulness and in their *Callings* were
So truly diligent whilst vigor lasted
That they then lifeblood, yea, their spirits wasted,                        (1890)
And ev'n unslackt the very nerves and powers
Of their own souls to help enable ours:
To *bury*, nigh a hundred in a day;
To church, to marry, study, preach and pray;
To make betimes at night late watch to keep;
To be disturb'd at midnight from their sleep;
To visit him that on his death-bed lies;
Oft to communicate; more oft baptize;
And daily (and all day) to be in action,
As were those two, to give due satisfaction                                 (1900)
To their great *Flocks*; more Laborers there needed;
And their consumed strengths, it much exceeded.
    But they are now at *rest*, their *work* is done,
Their *Fight* is finished, their *Goal* is won,
And though no *Trophy* I to them can raise—
Save this poor wither'd *Wreath* of mortal praise—
Their *Master* (to reward their faithfulness)
For them reserved Crowns of Happiness,
Because, unto his *household*, they the *Bread*
*Of Life*, in season, have distributed.                                     (1910)
Nor was the Food of life diminisht more
By such men's want alone, than heretofore,
But to our discontent, we also had
Our due allowances the shorter made
Ev'n by command, for some (I know not why)
Had falsely misinform'd *Authority*,
That our promiscuous meetings at the *Fast*
Increast the *Plague*, which was believ'd in hast[e].
And being urg'd, perhaps with such fame shews
Of *Reason* as *Conjecture* could infuse,                                   (1920)

(The matter being aggravated too,
With such untruths, as travel to and fro)
The public preaching on the *Fasting day*
Was, in an evil season, took away.
    For when the flesh was fed and soul deprived
Of two Repasts which weekly we received,
Prophaneness and hard-heartedness began
To get new rooting in the mind of man.
We missed those good helps and those examples
Which had been preached to us in our Temples.                    (1930)
The poor did want full quickly, to their grief,
Those Alms the *Fast* brought out for their relief.
And when with *Prayers*, *Preaching* did not go,
Our cold *Devotions* did far colder grow.
    What instrument of mischief might he be
Who caused that? And what a Fool, was he!
If *Wensday-Sermons* help infect, I pray,
What kept us safer on the *Sabbath day*,
Since most fast then till noon without refection?
Or what at *Funerals*, did stop infection?                      (1940)
    Good God! in thy affairs, how vain (to me)
Doth carnal *Policy* appear to be!
How apt is flesh and blood to run a course,
Which makes the soul's condition worse and worse!
To venture on eternal death, how toward!
And in a temporal danger what a coward!
    Sure, had not such a project, had a scope
Beyond the reaching of the *Devil's* hope,
And been too damnable for anyone
To be his *Procurator* thereupon.                               (1950)
Some would have made the motion that we might
Have liv'd excluded from our *Churches* quite,
And that till God his hand should please to stay,
None should in public, either preach, or pray.
    'Twas well the weekly number of the dead,
By God's mere mercy, was diminished,
Before the prohibition of the *Fast*;
The *Fiend* had else, for evermore, disgrac't
That *Discipline*, and carnal *Policy*
Had so insulted o're *Divinity*,                                (1960)
That, in succeeding Ages, men unholy,
Would thence have proved such Devotion Folly.
But God prevented it, that we should take
Good notice of it and good uses make,

And I have mention'd it, that here I may
God's *Wisdom* and Man's foolishness display.
    Oh! let us to our *Fasts* again return.
Let us for our omissions truly mourn,
And not capitulate with God, as though
He first his Rod out of his hand should throw          (1970)
Ere we would come unto him, for if thus
A son of ours should bear himself to us,
It would our ire exasperate the more
And make the fault seem greater than before.
    Why should we in an action that is just
The mercy of our gracious God distrust?
Or unto any place be loath to go,
Where God is to be heard or spoken to,
Through fear of that which may be caught at home
And in a thousand places where we come?          (1980)
Our sins and plagues were public, so should we
In *Pray'rs*, and *Tears*, and *Alms*, and *Fastings* be.
For that strong *Devil,* which hath tortur'd thus
Our general body, is not cast from us
By single *Exorcisms*; neither shall
Our privacies advantage us at all,
Except in what conduces to the health
Of private men or of their private wealth.
    If we in close retirements (by our fear),
At markets, or where worse Assemblies are,          (1990)
Infected grow, the *Devil* by and by
With us persuadeth either to belie
The *Church*, our constant *Fasting*, or some one
Good work or pious action we have done.
(As visiting the sick in time of need,
Or any other such like Christian deed)
For he those practices doth greatly spite,
And to disparage them hath much delight,
Because he sees that such as are inclin'd
To pious means will soon by trial find          (2000)
Good hopes to thrive beyond their expectations,
Their knowledge fool his cunning machinations,
Their faiths grow strong, temptations weak appear,
Their joy most perfect, where most sorrows are,
And know, that when the *Lord of Hosts* is armed
With all his *Judgments*, that he least is harmed,
Who, bold through *Love, self-trust* quite from him throws
And runs with confidence to meet his blows.

Let no man then be fearful to repair
Unto the house of *Preaching* or of *Pray'r*,                    (2010)
Or, any whither else, those works to do,
Which he by Conscience is obliged to.
No, though the Devil in the passage lay,
Or strew'd most fearful dangers in the way,
For if, in such a case, our death we take,
Our death shall for our best advantage make.
     Yet let none think I this opinion carry,
That ev'ry *Church* will be a *Sanctuary*
To all that come, for sure, if any dare
Without *Devotion* in God's house appear,                        (2020)
To them, that place more peril threatens than
A chamber thronged with infected men.
Some fainted in the *Church*, as others did
Within their houses (where themselves they hid),
Yet not so often, for though some did please
To blame the *Church* for spreading this disease,
No places were more harmless. None did we
Behold more healthy or to scape more free
From this *Infection* than those persons, whom
We saw most often to God's worship come.                        (2030)
Nor were there any houses more infected
Than theirs, who most the house of God neglected.
I speak not this by rumor, for ev'n thither
Resorted I, where thronged were together
The greatest multitudes, and day by day
I sat, where all the crowd I could survey.
Yet I nor man, nor child, nor woman saw,
To sink, look pale, or from their place withdraw.
And doubtless, if such faintings there had been,
As many prated of, I some had seen,                             (2040)
Which, since I did not see, I wish again,
None would at such a time God's house refrain,
Except in Congregations not their own,
And where infection feared is or known,
Or in their own Assembly, where disorder
Committed willfully, the Pest may further,
Or when their bodies' weakness, or the Air,
Their safeties may some other ways impair.
Excepting to (in times of *Visitation*),
When they are markt with marks of *Separation*,                 (2050)
As *Risings*, *Blains*, or *Sores*. Or newly from
The company of such like persons come,

Or whensoever they or do or may
Suppose themselves Infectious any way.
    These (as the *Lepers* did, by *Moses*['s] Law)
From public Congregations should withdraw,
For sure, if any such themselves intrude
To mix among a healthy Multitude,
(Though prayers or devotions they pretend,
Or whatsoever other pious end)                                    (2060)
Their foolish practice is Unwarrantable.
Yea, their condition so uncharitable,
That I abhor it and believe that for
So doing, God their *prayers* doth abhor.
    And here (although it may impertinent
By some be thought) I cannot choose but vent,
How I dislike our so much liked fashion
Of burial, where the public Congregation
Are bound to meet, and then, especially,
When of infectious griefs, great numbers die.                     (2070)
I know both Custom, and Opinion, have
So rooted this, that I my breath may save
In reprehending it. Yet when I must
Be taken hence, and turn again to dust,
Let naught but Earth and Heav'n my carcass cover,
And neither Church nor Chapel roof me over,
Nor any other Buildings, saving those
That only serve such relics to enclose.
    For though I do ingenuously confess,
We should, to show our Christian hopefulness                      (2080)
Of rising from the dead, lodge decently
Their flesh, who in Christ's Faith profess to die,
And that Churchyards or plots distinguisht from
The vulgar use do best of all become
That purpose, yet I know the common guise
Of bur'ing in the Church did first arise
From ancient Superstition and to gain
Some outward profit to the priestly train.
For many simple men were made conceive
That if (when they were dead) they might have leave               (2090)
To rest within those plots of hallowed ground,
Which either Church or Chapel did surround,
No wicked Spirit should permittance have,
To trouble or abuse them in the grave,
Whereas (which yet old fools believe they do)
They might else rise and walk at midnight too

About their streets, and houses, or cross ways,
Till some Mass-monger them,t quiet, lays.
And then it was suppos'd, how much the nigher
They lay unto their Altar or their Choir,                              (2100)
By so much more the safer they should rest,
Which brought no petty sums to Dagon's chest.[12]
    Thence was it, that our Churches, first of all,
Were glaz'd with Scutcheons like a Herald's hall,
And that this age in them depainted sees
So many vain and lying Pedigrees.
Thence comes it that we nowadays behold
Some Chancels filled up with rotten, old,
And foolish monuments, from hence we see
So many puppet Images to be                                           (2110)
On ev'ry wall within our Oratories,
So many Epitaphs and lying stories,
Of men deceast, and thence the guise was gotten,
To let so many Banners, dropping rotten,
Deform our pillars, and withdraw our eyes
From pious objects to those vanities.
If any man desirous be to lie
Within a Monument when he shall die,
Let ev'ry noble Family erect
Without their Cities some fair Architect,                             (2120)
Within the compass of whose roofed wall
There may be founded some good Hospital
Or buildings for the lawful recreation
Of youth and for the honor of the Nation.
And of that Name or kin, when any dies,
There lay their bones, or to their memories
Erect, there, Tables, and let them that had
Such minds, and fortunes, to the Structure add.
Yea, thither (if they please), let them translate
Their Ancestors. But I have spoke too late.                          (2130)
Those times are pass'd in which our noble ones
Were able to erect such piles of stones
As might be eminent. Our kingly race
Had by the seventh Henry such a place
Erected for them, so magnificent,

---

[12]   *Dagon's chest.* The national deity of the ancient Philistines; represented with the head, chest, and arms of a man, and the tail of a fish; here, a metonym for the Catholic church, which accounts for the reference to a "mass-monger" above.

That to this Land it is an ornament.[13]
Let them that cannot reach the cost of these,
Raise Cawsies, Bridges, and make Docks, and Keys
For public use, which with as little cost,
As now upon their peddling Tomb is lost                              (2140)
Should make them live far longer in their fames,
For we would those entitle by their Names.
    All they that love their Country, now they know
Which way they may their money best bestow,
(To memorize their Friends, with profiting
The public) will consider of this thing
And build them Tombs, where we may praise the work,
Not in a Church obscure, unseen to lurk,
Where few shall view them, and where most who shall
Behold them take no heed of them at all.                            (2150)
    If some good Patriot would begin the fashion,
It might allure, perhaps, to imitation.
And if it were not greediness of gain
Among Church-Officers, which did maintain
Such Customs, we should somewhat more forbear
To lay so many stinking bodies there,
Where God we seek (and him should seek to find,
With purity of body and of mind).
Indeed our sin alone pollutes, and yet,
An outward decency is also fit.                                     (2160)
Was't well, that in the Church (where throngs and heat
Did make us in the crowd to pant and sweat)
Ev'n in the midst of our Devotions too,
Men should, as oft it pleased them to do,
Thrust in (where we could hardly stand in ease)
With four or five strong smelling Carcasses?
Was't fit, so many Graves, at such a season
Should gape and breath upon us? Was it reason,
That heaps of rubbish, Coffin-boards, and stones,
Late bury'd bodies, and half rotten bones,                          (2170)
God's Temple should pollute and make it far
More loathsome than most Charnel houses are?
Was't fitting that to gain their griping fees,
They should endanger multitudes to lease
Their lives or healths or that they should fulfill
A foolish motion in a dead man's will

---

[13]  *such a place.* The special, elaborate chapel in Westminster Abbey that Henry VII
designated by will for his resting place with Elizabeth of York.

By wronging of the living? God forbid
It should be reason, and yet thus they did.
    Thus did they? Yea, far worse, for should I tell
At what high rates some Churchmen, here, did sell        (2180)
Their burying grounds; what fees they did exact;
How Readers, Clarks, and Sextons did compact,
To rack the dead; to what a goodly sum
Their large Church-duties (in some cases) come;
What must be paid for Bearers, though men have
Their friends to help convey them to the grave;
What for the Bells, though not a Bell be rung;
What, for their mourning clothes, though none be hung
Upon them but their own; what pay did pass
For Fun'ral Sermons, where no Sermon was;        (2190)
And what was oft extorted (without shame)
To give him leave to preach, who freely came.
If here (I say) I should discover what
I might of these things mentioned relate,
Those men who die (that charges they may save),
Would fear they might be beggar'd in the Grave,
For more to take that lodging had been spent,
Than would have bought a pretty tenement.
    Thus, as one matter drew another on,
My *Muse* hath divers things discourst upon        (2200)
To many sundry purposes, but what
I chiefly in this *Canto* aimed at
Was to preserve in mind an awful sense
Of what we suffred in this *Pestilence*,
What we deserved, and how variously,
God's *Justice*, this one *Corsive* did apply,
To eat out all Corruptions, which bespotted
Our souls, and had, ere this, our bodies rotted.
    I might as well have memorialized here,
How divers'ly God's *Mercies* did appear        (2210)
Amid his *Judgments*; how he comforted,
When outward comfort failed; how he fed,
When oil and meal were wasted; how he gave
Their lives to them, whose feet were in the grave;
What *Patience*, what high *Fortitude* he granted;
And how he still supplied what we wanted.
I might commemorate a world of Grace
Bestow'd in this affliction on this place,
Both common and in private. Many a vow
(Of theirs, who will, I fear, forget it now)        (2220)

Was daily heard. Ten thousand suits were deigned.
*Reprieves* for souls condemned were obtained.
Friends prayd for friends, the parents for the lives
Of their dear children, husbands for their wives,
Wives for their husbands beg'd with tears and passion,
And God with pity heard their lamentation.
    In friends, in servants, in the temporal wealth,
In life, in death, in sicknesses, and health,
God manifested *Mercy*. Some did find
A *Friend*, to whom till then, none had been kind.                    (2230)
Some had their servants better'd for them, there,
By God's correction. Some left wealthy were
By dying kindred, who the day before
Were like to beg their bread from door to door.
Some by their timely *deaths* were taken from
Such present pains or from such woes to come
That they are happy. Unto some, from heav'n,
The blessing of a longer life was giv'n,
That they might call to mind their youthful times
Repent omissions and committed crimes,                    (2240)
Amend their courses, and be warisome
That they displeas'd not God, in times to come.
    Again, some others by their sicknesses,
And by the tears they had in this *Disease*,
Grew aweful of God's Judgments, and within
Their hearts, good motions were, where none had bin,
Ev'n in their hearts who fear'd nor God nor Devil,
Nor guilt of sin, nor punishment for evil.
And some had health continu'd, that they might
God's praise extol and in his love delight.                    (2250)
Should I declare, in what unusual wise
God op'ned here their souls' dim-sighted eyes,
Who blinded were before; how nigh they reacht
To highest *Mysteries*; what things they preacht
Ev'n to their neighbors and their family,
Before their souls did from their bodies fly,
Or, should I tell but what young *Children* here
Did speak to take from elder folk their fear
Of Sicknesses and Death; what they exprest
Of heav'nly bliss, and of this world's unrest,                    (2260)
What faith they had, what strange illuminations,
What strong assurances of their salvations,
And with what proper terms and boldness they
Beyond their years, such things did open lay,

It would amaze our *Naturalists* and raise
A goodly *Trophy* to our Maker's praise.
But this for me were too too large a task,
And many years and volumes it would ask,
Should I in these particulars record
The never ending mercies of the *Lord*.                                    (2270)
For he that would his meanest act recite,
Attempts to measure what is infinite.
    That story therefore in particular
To meddle with I purpose to defer,
Till in the Kingdom of eternity
My soul in honor of his Majesty
Shall "*Hallelujah*" sing and overlook
With hallow'd eyes that great eternal Book,
Which in a moment to my view shall bring
Each past, present, and each future thing,                                    (2280)
And there my soul shall read and see revealed
What is not by the LAMB as yet unsealed.
    Meanwhile I'll cry "*Hosanna*," and for all
His love to me and mercies general,
His three times holy and thrice blessed Name
I praise and vow for aye to praise the same.

\*

# William Austin,
## *Epiloimia epē or The Anatomy*
## *of the Pestilence*

The British, Guildhall, Bodleian, and Huntington Libraries each hold one copy of the only edition of this three-part poem from 1666 (Wing 2nd ed., A4260). The full poem is represented here by its first part. Prefatory prose sections include "The *Printer* to the *Reader*" and "Errata"; the last page offers the advertisement, "Books Printed for *Nathaniel Brook*, and are to be sold at his Shop at the *Angel* in *Cornhill*."

Επιλοιμια επε[1]
OR
THE ANATOMY OF THE Pestilence
A POEM
In three Parts
Describing
the deplorable Condition of the City of London
under its *merciless* dominion, 1665,
What the *PLAGUE* is, together with the *Causes* of it,
As also The *Prognostics* and most *Effectual* Means
of Safety, both *Preservative* and *Curative*

---

By William Austin, of Grays-Inn, Esquire

---

*London*, Printed for *Nath. Brook*, at the Angel in *Cornhill*, 1666.

Part 1.

  Drawing a *Map* of this *sad* place, my quill
Seems in the *frightful* hand that writes a *Will*.
We can't abscond or show our *Tyrant-fears*,
But in black robe of *mourning characters*.
If you agrade such, *fitly,* then, the while
You'll with your *tears*, to grace them, mix a *smile,*
And no less *justly* look they should be made
To have, like day or emblem, *light* and *shade.*
Others to whom the thoughts of *Death* seem dull,
Like bits cram'd down the throat when belly's full,    (10)
May know they *spirit* or clear *eye-sight* lack,
Or *eyes have none*, who cannot look on *black.*
And he who now dares not be *cheerful*, hath
Great scruple, doubtless, but small heart or faith.
Then, whilst I write *Life's* hasty post, grim *Death,*
Hold not my pen, nor come to stop my breath.
One fully resolute nowhere to ramble,
Now life so doubtful is, needs no preamble.
  Fancy --- *But stay*, lest this offence may give,
We should ask leave to *write*, as well as *live.*    (20)
Some Politicians "*silence*" charge, when grief,
Backt with our health's chief foes, hath play'd the thief

---

[1]  *Επιλοιμια επε Epiloimia epē.*   The most literal translation is "a crying out" (epe) "against the plague" (epi loimia), but the title suggests Austin takes it to mean "anatomy of the pestilence."

(From *Physic* prove their rule, that *those fare best*,
Who, very sick, lie still and speak the least);
*Wisely*, sure, treat on *roast meat*, when they find
*Butcher* and *Cook* have blandished their mind;
If faring *ill* differs from *well*, their skill,
Judging of *other* flesh, will thwart their will.
That *Royal Sir*, who had for happy lot,
*God's* heart, and *King of politics* begot,                     (30)
When his great breast within was orb of fire,
The breath his silence kept in, flam'd it higher.[2]
And he who by afflictions did commence,
The *Oracle* of tacit *patience*,
Saw his contrasted victory o're death,
Lay in the vocal virtue of his breath.
His tyrannous *malignant* dolors gave
No other choice to him but *speech* or *grave*.[3]
When nothing else will do, *complaint* prevails,
While pain with vapor from the mouth exhales.                     (40)
*Confession oft saves life*; when we endure
The smartest sores, our *crying* turns the *cure*.
Deep wound, to *hide* and *lock* [it] *up closely* will[4]
Such safety be as to *preserve* it still.
In dang'rous sickness *then* to hold one's peace,
Is like mute sleep to nourish the disease.
Your *septum lucidum* a while yet keep[5]
Lockt to our woe; don't grudge us time to weep,
Who think our *setting sun* most fitly seems
So painted as to cast his *longest* beams;                     (50)
That *Plague* with *Cause* and *Cure* most modey goes,
When in a *large* grave cloak of *mourning* prose.
Such, on the subject, will refuse to hear
*Meter*; Apollo twitches by the ear.
He, who with smiling cheer on *music's hill*
*Plays* to the sick his *therapeutic* Skill,
Invigors flaccid body, drooping soul

---

2    [marginal note] Psalm 30.2. ["O LORD my God, I cried unto thee, and thou hast healed me."] *That* Royal Sir. King David; see 1 Chronicles 7–14 and 2 Samuel 24.13–15.

3    [marginal note] Job 13.19; John 1.9. [respectively, "Who is he that will plead with me? for now, if I hold my tongue, I shall give up the ghost"; "If we confess our sins, he is faithful and just to forgive us our sins, and to cleanse us from all unrighteousness."]

4    [marginal note] Κρύπτειν την νόσον λυγρήν. [In Latin, this is a proverb, *occultare morbum funestum* meaning to conceal disease is fatal].

5    [marginal note] Seat of fancy. [*Septum lucidem* means seat of fancy]

With his illustrious rays and *chants* them whole—
He, license gives, who, *Poet* and *Musician,*
The pleasant is all-curing God *Physician.*                    (60)

τέχνη δ' αμφιλαφής ούτις τόσον όσσον Απόλλων⁶

*Inventum medicina suum est, opisexque per orbem*
*Dicitur: herbarum and subjecta potentia vati.*
*--- Ex illo didicerunt funera primum,*
*Differre and gelidae vitare pericula mortis.*⁷

    Fancy when blub-cheek't *Boreas* does strain
To make a dreadful tempest on the *Main,*
When the *Sea Arms* in mutiny require
Oceans to quench their element of fire,
Waters on waters horridly are laid,
As first they lay before the *World* was made,                 (70)
Pretending ne're to be suffic'd with *men,*
They gape as if they'd gorge the *world* again.
Their *gulfy* mouths *rocks* open and provoke,
Opposing Rocks with deaf'ning noise and smoke.
Wave *murders* wave, then suddenly does *burn*
With *briny* thirst to be its neighbor's *urn.*
This drinks that's blood, dies, then anew does roll,
As if it had imbib'd the other's soul.
Jupiter, Neptune, Mercury together
Join, as of old, to wander *God knows whither.*                (80)
*Neptune* with all his forces does arise,
To take *Auxiliaries* from the *Skies.*
The bottom of the Sea confusedly thrown
Upward, contemns the *mountains in the Moon.*
Deep answers deep; the waters there and here,
Above and under heaven compose one sphere,
When rabid *winds,* like *Furies* wak't from sleep,

---

⁶ *τέχνη δ'αμφιλαφής ούτις τόσον όσσον Απόλλων.* There is no art so abundant as that of Apollo's (from the hymn of Callimachus For Apollo, translated by Evdoxia Kolydaki..

⁷ *Inventum ...vati.* "I am called Help-Bringer throughout the world; and all the potency of herbs is given unto me. Alas, that love is curable by no herbs, and the arts which heal all others cannot heal their lord" (Ovid, *Metamorphosis,* trans. Frank Justus Miller. The Loeb Classical Library (London, W. Heinemann; New York, Putnam, 1922–25], 1.521–24; 39); *Ex illo ... mortis* "From Phoebus do leeches know the deferring of death" (Callimachus, "Hymn to Apollo," trans. A. W. Mair, *Callimachus, Hymns and Epigrams. Lycophron. Aratus,* trans A. W. Mair and G. W. Mair, The Loeb Classical Library (London: William Heinemann, 1921), 53.

Design the ruin of poor floating ship;
O're *Hell* the billows boiling, how the wrack
Inebriates the mates with toil and tack!                              (90)
Some torn from mast, a while with sail's proud top
They fly, and then like *Icarus* they drop;
Others reel from the bark on either hand,
And sink where faithless *Peter* could not stand.[8]
Here one with fear *freely resigns* his breath;
Another there, tir'd out, *is forc't* to death.
*Ralph* hastily following *Clem's* call and beck,
Jostles 'gainst *Sam*, and thumps him over deck,
Like the known sport on *Venice* bridge or boat,
A *Castellane* against a *Nicholote*,[9]                             (100)
Or in a formal *combat*, as if he,
Killing before he dy'd, should *victor* be.
Some past all hopes of life, grown desperate,
Quickly to b'out of pain, conspire with *Fate*;
The ship *falls* as she *rides* and faintly speaks
Her inward bleeding wounds by sundry leaks.
The *sail* first tears, and then the stately *mast*,
Like some great tumbling house, exclaims its last.
Now vessel, cast at *Boreas*, his foot,
Bursts, as a fir'd *Granado*, all about.                             (110)
One then on th'other takes fast hold, and neither
Scapes, but like *oak and Ivy*, die together.
To buoy them up a while, each broken piece
They fasten on, and stick like *Solon Geese*;
Sporting there, with their limbs at stake, they're soon
Lost to some *Shark* that tears them one from one.
If no such greedy cozening gamester come,
They drop into the *mare mortuum*,
Like blossoms in the spring, that some sharp cold
Hath sorely nipt; they quickly lose their hold.                      (120)
      Thus 'tis with us: our dearest darling breath,
The air we take, is not our life but death;
That by which we should nimbly *kick up heels*,
Spread sails to post along, inverts our keels.

---

[8]   *faithless Peter.* See Matthew 26; Mark 14; Luke 22; John 13, 18. In Luke, this is
rendered, "And the Lord turned, and looked upon Peter. And Peter remembered the word of
the Lord, how he had said unto him, Before the cock crow, thou shalt deny me thrice. And
Peter went out, and wept bitterly" Luke 22:61–62.

[9]   [marginal note] Two Factions in *Venice*, that at a set time in the year contend for the
mastery upon a bridge; whence they tumble one another into the water.

In ev'ry moment of swift *time*, we have
*Surges* and *ravening fishes* for our grave.
*Destiny* has the learn'd *Physician's* trick,
And by consent of most, *lives by the sick*,
Lies as an *infant* swaddled up in bands,
Who for her help uses her *parents'* hands— (130)
Thousands kills daily, yet as if her powers
Were too too weak alone, makes use of ours.
Such, are luxuriant cluster'd grapes, and such
Fruit hoarded up rots others by the touch.
As readily as *flint and steel*, we make
Fire—are as spark and tinder, *touch and take.*
    As did of old, those *fought with heaven*, so we;[10]
Each is his fellow's murdering enemy.
See when in fight, *Mars* ragingly does ride
Through armed ranks to triumph on each side, (140)
When ev'ry noise being voic'd with fire and smoke,
Sounds dismally, as when the heart is broke.
Soldier on soldier in distracted ire
Tumbles, like unbound faggots on the fire.
One deeply wounded, *dead friend* does bemoan,
Till he fall on him for his *burying stone.*
Like *Partridge, chicken-tail'd,* that you retri[e]ve,
Here and there drop those can no longer live.
Here stands a straddling *Hector*, that hath lost
As many collops as old pissing post;[11] (150)
At last with others he's compell'd to yield
His body to be pavement to the field.
Some nimbly rifle others; then, as those
Who took the golden treasure at Talouse,[12]
Another wounds them, so they fall down where
They spoil, as under load too big to bear.
They see their friends expire, but must not have

---

[10]   [marginal note] 1 Samuel 14.10; Judges 7.22 [respectively, "But if they say thus, Come up unto us; then we will go up: for the LORD hath delivered them into our hand: and this shall be a sign unto us"; "And the three hundred blew the trumpets, and the LORD set every man's sword against his fellow, even throughout all the host: and the host fled to Beth-shittah in Zererath, and to the border of Abel-meholah, unto Tabbath."]

[11]   *collops ...pissing post.* A collop is a thick fold of flesh on the body as evidence of a well-fed condition; this usage suggesting with humor some serious weight loss.

[12]   *golden treasure at Talouse.* The hoard of treasure Celtic warriors allegedly stole from the temple of Delphi in the third century B.C.E, as they exited the Balkans in defeat; it vanished and was thought hidden in the French city of Toulouse. Although the silver was found, the gold never was.

Life so long to be witness to their grave.
Who glory most in valor or in strength,
Cannot inch time out longer than their length.                    (160)
One's sent t'*eternal silence*, while his jaws
Stretch wide in his victorious friend's *applause*.
Another, *heartning* of his neighbor, feels
His own *faint wounded soul* run down his heels.
Thus we (God help us) our sick warfare find,
Being *fruit* that hang but till the first brisk wind.
We're *standing-corn* today; then by and by
With sickle cut, we do but *live to die*.

    Where the *judicious* make but a *retreat*,
*Timorous* vulgar crowds have their *defeat*.                     (170)
One, seeing how they tremble as they stand,
Would think they were on *Gabian's* quaking land.[13]
They goods imprison in each chest and hutch,
As if they were made guilty by their touch.
As tim'rously they talk, look pale and stare,
As if they had been frighted by the air.
E're they do firmly stablish their intents,
First shuttlecock and stoolball arguments,
They're bid to *fly*, and then they're bid to *stay*,
And so are hail'd and tortur'd ev'ry way.                         (180)
Some strive to *change*, at least their vote *Prorogue*,
But the far greater number bears the vogue:
"Should pelf," *say they*, "so far with us prevail,
As to outweigh our *lives* in th'other scale?
Linger we here like *Archimede*, till we
*Circle* ourselves out of all *Geometry?*
No. *Balak* bids, where *God* shows angry face,
To build him altar in another place.
Let's therefore lock up all and hasten out." [14]

    And so they turn the sail and talk about.            (190)
Both of them and their goods we are bereft,
While their *fear* seems concomitant to *theft*.
They run to *hide their heads* in ev'ry hole,
As if their *bag and baggage* they had *stole*.
Have y' ever seen a routed army, how
They mount up *head and tail* like cap'ring cow,
Bound as *Tre-ding-te-do*,[15] or as when shot

---

[13]    [marginal note] *Pliny.*

[14]    *Balak ... altar.* Reference to the biblical king Moab at Numbers 23.1–30.

[15]    *Tre-ding-te-do* Obsolete term.

Falls in the rear, and rouses lazy *Wat?*[16]
Leap hedge, then fall in ditch, scape ditch, and then
Flounce into bog, then out, and in again?                    (200)
Think us as light of heel, as wild and mad,
As new hatcht Partridge of the *Tribe of Gad*.[17]
But as *unlucky birds*, it is our lot,
That scarce one of a flock escapes the shot.
Haply we're safe the first day of our flight,
But go into our *winding-sheet* at night.
So have I seen poor panting hunted deer,
Wounded by fatal arrows here and there,
*Sigh, fly, wind, turn*, but does as vainly fret,
As rambling Coney struggles in a net,                        (210)
Heightens her dole, and after all her course,
The *life* she'd save is *torn* from her by *force*.
From her own self she posts away apace,
And makes the greater speed to lose the race.
By those infectious fires that she flies,
Like squib i'th' air quickly consumes, she dies.
    *Physic*'s suspended now; you'll soon see why,
As herbs, their season come, hung up to dry.
No man that *sells his wisdom* here will be,
Where *Patient* dies e're he can come for *fee*.             (220)
You must allow that they who *Judges* sit
On life and death *should* go the circuit.
What would a man chides the *Physician* have?
What should he do where he wants skill to save?
It cannot be *honest* or *wise* man's part,
To meddle with a thing beyond his art.
The Plague, being out of human power, doth prove
That there's infallibly *a God* above.
To see men die and never make complaint,
More than by Purge or Pill, would fright a Saint.            (230)
Pity with fear would move an heathen's sense,
And bring his frailty to his conscience.
'Twould make him as a Christian Physician,
Try well the Simples of his Composition.
Simpling's a part of Physic; and you know,

---

[16]  *lazy Wat.* The meaning is any typical lazy soldier; we might now use the name Jack or Joe or some other common name instead of Wat, which is an abbreviation of Walter.

[17]  *As a new hatcht Partridge.* See 1 Sam 26:20: "Now therefore, let not my blood fall to the earth away from the presence of Yahweh: for the king of Israel is come out to seek a flea, as when one doth hunt a partridge in the mountains."

Solomon said, "take simples where they grow."
Doctors must needs be wanted where they're gone,
For all the Country's strangely liver-grown.
The sorrow that to us does intervene,
Makes us extremely troubled with the *Spleen.*          (240)
Much honesty and kindness they do show,
Telling us all their mind before they go.
They say *mox, longè, tardè,*[18] and thus put,
As wise men should, their *Iliads in a nut.*[19]
Who is not satisfi'd with this may fret,
Till *Passion* prove his antidote by *Sweat*—
A medicine that is taken e're 'tis given,
Good to drive out their *old* (and druggy) *leaven.*[20]
If any with their *Lord have mercy's* blest,
He may get *Parish-Priest* to do the rest.          (250)
*Physicians,* so, into *Divines* will run
And then exhale as *Spirits* in the Sun.[21]
They'd reprehended be to go away,
Like those who would not heal on *Sabbath day;*
Withdraw from the disease their helpful skill,
When it hath got the greatest force to kill;
Claim so great *fame* of us, and when they come
To merit, leave their *titles* in their room.
Like *distant* spreading trees, some sinking wretch
Reaching out to, does only *shadow* catch,          (260)
But none can be dishonor'd, sham'd, or shent,
For wanting[22] his *full* power they represent.
They never were intended such renown,
To have, with Doctor's style, great Nature's crown.
They're still but Mortals, who our crazy harms
Are not to help by miracles or charms.
Their *absence* intimates they do endure

---

[18]  *mox, longè, tardè.* Plague-time saying: Fly quickly from the place infected, abide far off, and stay away long; also known as *"cede, recede, redi."*

[19]  *Iliads in a nut.* An epic in brief; a lot conveyed in little space. This may also refer to George Wharton's *England's Iliads in a nut-shell. Or, A brief chronology of the battles, sieges, conflicts, and other most remarkable passages from the beginning of this rebellion to the 25. of March, 1645* (1645).

[20]  *old* (and druggy) *leaven.* Combining usages of leaven as an additive to simples ("druggy") and as the residue of sin ("old leaven").

[21]  *Exhale ... sun.* Evaporate, this particular process based on early meteorological principles governing sublunary elements.

[22]  *wanting* lacking.

Hardship with detriment for Patient's cure,
And for the good of *Nature* are design'd
To help her work that way she's most inclin'd.[23]                    (270)
Their Patients their co-partners they make;
The prescripts they give them, themselves they take.
What though the air common as water be,
*Jordan* could serve to cure the *Leprosy.*
Those that have *care of souls* have *bodies*
And *these* must be provided for, *you know*,
Therefore that honest neighbor don't esteem
One next himself, the farther off from him.
They tell him what no *Heathen* is so strict,
Learned, or wise to have wit to contradict:                          (280)
"That virtuous man can ne're offend or sin,
Who makes his Charity at home begin."
So, having pleasur'd those that would complain,
As with thick cloak against a shower of rain,
That *blessing* want not, which the *sick* require,
Make us as happy as we can desire.
E're they depart, bid us *adieu*, and thus
Leave God, the best Physician, with us.
They leave us, and we well do know the matter,
That shepherds, when the sheep are smitten, scatter.                 (290)
Who t' Aaron, now, or Moses make address,
As of old, seek them in the Wilderness,
Where no more Grove-Idolatry we'll fear,
Since Levites, who God's judgments dread, are there.
We wonder not they leave us thus alone,
That Prophets fail us, since the Law is gone.
We would reprove them well to leave us here,
Like Priest and Levite vulned passenger.
If they, should people teach, could not abide
In town or life to have the *text apply'd*;                          (300)
If where they cannot *save*, they should employ
Their breath and lucubrations to *destroy*;
If they with *fear* should have so little *grace*,
To think themselves *less* sinners for their *place*,
Were not the *bodies* of the *Saints* as dear
In *life* as are their *Relics* anywhere?
Did *Pastor* not for *Sheep,* in such mishaps,
To show them way of safety, *break the gaps*?

---

[23]   [marginal note] *Hippocrates, section* 1, *Aphorisms* 21. [Those things which require
to be evacuated should be evacuated, wherever they most tend, by the proper outlets.]

And was that *Patriarch* conquer'd *God*[24] *so brave*
T' *orecome Death* and not halt into his grave?                    (310)
    The *Law*, dispersed sundry ways, invites—
As did the Infant *Gospel*, Proselytes.
Each *Inns of Court*, shut fast up, seems to you
Mysterious as Synagogue of Jew.
Conveyancer is at Surveyor's hand,
As both in field design'd to measure land.
If any quarrels betwixt neighbors breed,
*Lawyer* no more than *Conjurer* he'll need,
For in a short time, he may lay his life;
One or both parties die, so end the strife.                        (320)
We'd blame these *Dons* to leave us in a State,
O're-power'd by th'*uncivil laws* of Fate;
To *back* the bench and bar, relax and thaw
This bitter biting weather from the Law.
Many would shrewdly chide them for their pains,
Condition'd, they'd but left them so much brains.
Who serv'd the *Tabernacle* did not fail,
They say, to keep it with *veil over veil*.
The *Court* disbands, as if the *rule of state*
Were like some long worn fashion, *out of date*.                   (330)
Each Officer, like a *Diagoras*,
Studies the difference 'twixt place and place:
How he with safety farthest may recule,
From those relate the nearest to his rule.
They fly, as if our judgment were the same
With *Sodom* and *Gomorrah's* sulfur flame.
These fain we'd blame, *I know not why*, unless
We thought our Plague, on them, would make it less
(As if by our ill husbandry w' had found,
That their deep channels well might drain our ground.)             (340)
Like such would all things, with one measure meet,
*Stand* on our *head* or have our *hands,* our *feet*:
When finding we're exceeding *ill*, we wo'd
Find fault with those could never *do* us *good*.
After we have *rebel'd*, we angry are,
That in our *punishment* they take no share.
When, for our stubbornness, we're scourged thus,
We'd cry, "Our Rulers won't be rul'd by us."
But, we see *Nature* kindly takes our part,
To keep untainted *liver*, *brain*, and *heart*;                   (350)

---

[24]   *that Patriarch conquer'd God.* Jacob.

When Hurricanes blow us away, heaven *shrouds*
The heads of *lofty mountains* in the clouds;
We see in gloomy tempests each fair light
Adorns those Orbs above, withdraws from sight,
And when to Earth, Heaven's Parliament did vote
*Plague-grave* of rain, the *Ark* did safely float.
    *Bacchus* and *Ceres'* worthies, such who shine
By th'agile, jovial rays of Ale and Wine,
Haunt Tippling-booths, and serve, *as many think,*
To talk up vap'ring spirits in the drink,                                      (360)
Or, as most modern authors phrase it, stand
To gauge the Liquor-casks with *sword in hand,*
Till in their *foil* they fall, as not being fickle[25]
To quit their service, though they sleep in pickle.
Of these (whom one listing affirm'd it truly,
They were as numerous as Flies in *July*)
Some *few* are left, but *most* are gone, we see,
To teach *rurigene* Bumkins, *Cocks* can *neigh.*
He's but a *Craven-cock* who cannot brave,
Unless he may his own known Dunghill have.                                      (370)
    So great a tempest beating on our *Shore,*
No wonder if the *fields* and *meadows* roar.
What place can you suppose fitter to yield
Such fruit as *Wildings* be than *hedge* or *field?*
Transplant them, or if you do them innest,
Much sweetness they acquire and prove the best.
None can courageous spirit qualify,
Better than with the Country honesty.
*Augeas' Stable* still had been unclean,
Had *Hercules* ne're from his City been.                                        (380)
These should be blam'd, for now when *Night* is drest,
They fail to tell the *spangles* in her vest,
Leave us the sad reversion of their wars,
(And in their stead) to combat with the stars.
They should be blam'd, for being now so scar'd
As to leave City without welt or guard.[26]
Did not their flight, their *ramage* prowess, meet
Friendly, and by their care prove it discreet,
Show by their *retrospection* that they've sense
Of *after world,* as men of Conscience,                                        (390)

---

[25]  *in their foil they fall.* From wrestling: the fact of being almost thrown.

[26]  *without welt or guard.* Phrase from shoemaking: without ornamentation or trimming.

And to our charity commend their *fear*,
As such have not *courage* enough to hear?
They'd be in fault, if, with their *souls,* they do
Trust *God* and do not with their *bodies* too.
Did not they signify, each of them strives
For future justice to preserve their lives?
    The *Trades* are in their *Hieroglyphics* now,
Their *Shops, Halls, Signs,* left only for a show.
Their progress they are gone to sundry parts,
T'instruct rude country towns and sow their arts.          (400)
They swarm in great ones and are fixed there,
As if our sad, *foul* weather made their[s] *fair*.
The only thriving trade that one can tell here
*Lives* by the *dead* (as Hangman), *Coffin-seller*.
You, judging of this mystery must know,
That sturdy Smith, who lives by thump and blow,
Shoemaker, Chandler, Glover, Baker, Grocer,
And she makes shirts and lives by "*Yes*" and "*No Sir*"—
All these, with almost ev'ry money-taker,
Are *summ'd* and *tomb'd* up in a *Coffin-maker*.          (410)
As each Disease, when the Plague rages, is
Turn'd to the Plague, so all trades turn to this.
At ev'ry door stand marshall'd in array
Biers, as green boughs are planted there in *May*.
Trades would be blam'd for going out of town;
They take our *City's* glorious Standard down–
That Standard *Fame,* for news shows *foreign Kings*
Each new day and relies upon for wings,
Enchants *Erinyes'* Snakes with rage to greet
Each other till their *Cadmus* teeth[27] do meet.          (420)
Can e're they *London's* interest repay,
Though they should *work* on ev'ry *Holy-day?*
Do they want *tools* or make they *tail of bricks*,[28]
That to the *woods* they go to pick up *sticks?*
Do they now, for the want of *Prentices*,
To Country go to be supply'd with these?
To their new streets inhabitants to win,

---

[27] *Erinyes' Snakes.* Mythological goddesses who seek justice against criminals; associated with rage; depicted by Aeschylus with snakes for hair. *Cadmus teeth* Mythological teeth of a slain dragon which, after being sown by Cadmus Prince of Tyre, produced soldiers.

[28] *tail of bricks.* A pattern in bricklaying, here adding to the humor in asking what people might lack that they should flee to the country.

Fly they as *Coy-ducks* to bring others in?
As *tir'd* and *heartless* must they take their *ease,*
And like *poor land* lie fallow to increase?                          (430)
Or should the grass in ev'ry street be seen
Florid and verdant as in *Bedlam-green?*[29]
With vacive houses do they lay a wile,
For *wandring Jews,* usurp them may the while?
Or *says some Prophet* [of] that great Turkish race
They may beget by changing of their place?
*No, no*; who'll neither *pity* nor *excuse*
Other's great loss, deserves himself to lose.
You'd scarce count such an *Artisan* discreet,
Knows how to use his *hands* and not his *feet.*                     (440)
When ev'ry one into the *Country* flies,
*Trades* here are wheels without their *axle-trees.*
Th' imbellic and meticulous, they were
By th' ancient laws exempted from the WAR.
It is not always *fear* makes men retire,
Nor always *cold* that drives them to the fire.
Muff upon glove and gate with door to house
Speak pleasure, mode, convenience, grace and use.
Who hath good words, will spare some to his neighbor
And bless as well those *rest,* as those that *labor.*               (450)
Who by his *birth* and *calling* too is *free,*
Hath double right to *lawful liberty.*
Well bak't bread hath good crust as well as crumb ·
And he writes best that hath his elbow room.
They get by their departure no disgrace:
The place did not make them; they made the place.
*Men* honor have, not *places,* unless those
Where we bare head or pull off hose and shoes.
His place must *out of measure* him bewitch,
Makes altar that does daily kiss his breech.                         (460)
When any at *death's point* their dear lives crave
What power ha's that *idol* then to save?
*City* should such *preserve* who give it fame,
Which from those't would *destroy* it cannot claim.
If they be *rich*, long service ushers *gain*
That bows low to their *hand* and thanks their *brain.*
If they have *honor*, 'tis not their *renown*
More than their *labors*, crops and *virtues* crown.

---

[29]  *Bedlam-green.* Likely referring to Bedlam-green, Herefordshire. A green is an areas
covered with a growth of herbage or foliage; verdant; (of trees) in leaf.

When calm bright day, with beauty to express
The most resplendent robe in glory's dress,                              (470)
Varying her look and tire, with *lightning, thunder,*
*Hail, wind and clouds*, changes admirers' wonder,
What fault have those, whose luckless dwellings lie
For quarter to such plundring enemy?
      Yet *all* forsake not home, but *thousands* stay,
Who ne're go out of Parish bounds to pray.
Haply (as who'd not wish?) when plague is o're,
May most be blest to multiply a score.
London's not in Cimmerian darkness then,
But robb'd of light to be return'd again.                               (480)
Its richly furnisht buildings seem to th' eye,
Like ships that in safe port *at anchor lie.*
*Principle* 'bides secure from all abuse;
Only a while it wants a little *use.*
Who with *malignant* sickness is at strife,
Ha's hardest task can be in human life.
None learns to *tutor Fate*, nor can be said
*Lord* of his *life* with *master* of his *trade.*
Who *needs* will *cavil*, when the sea apace
Posts o're the bank he sits, should keep his place.                     (490)
Or when he sees some fire-drake does assail
His face, neither hide that nor turn his tail.
Abroad we see huge *Pinduses* of men spite[30]
As if the deluge were to fall again.
While (*prais'd be God*) he from *Fates'* rage and
Tenderly keeps (*unquencht*) our *Israel's light*,
We're like *that people*, when the vulgar throng
Took the dimensions of right and wrong.[31]
We'd clamor at *those mounts*, but that we know
The *vales* would loudly echo back our woe.                             (500)
And e're we can with words our envious *pride*
Advance, our stolid *vanity* deride.
They should be blam'd, did not our reasons seem
To call them back in a sophistic dream.
Can aught within art's verge be found or made
To whet our wit or judgment to persuade?

---

[30]   *Pinduses of Men.* The Pindus Mountain in northern Greece and southern Albania, called "the spine of Greece," here referring to a massive migration spurred on by threat of plague.

[31]   [marginal note] Deuteronomy 12.8. ["Ye shall not do after all the things that we do here this day, every man whatsoever is right in his own eyes."]

We should be blam'd, and we ourselves should blame,
Did not *confession aggravate* our shame,
And make our own insimulating breath,
Sub'tly ally us to a double death.                                    (510)
'Tis not our stay but our disorder'd pranks
Betray our lives, like troops have broke their ranks.
Such are our frantic fits, they cry to have
For whip and scourge no *Bedlam* but the grave.
    We who remain, seeing each *attinent*
Deaf to our kindest words, remove his tent.
*Friends* were as dear as *flesh* can be to bone—
Or *heart* to *bosom*—leave us all alone,
That when we have the greatest need to use
Their friendship, then the *love-knot* should unloose.                (520)
In bitter winds, when't hails and rains and snows,
Then to be rob'd and stript of all our clothes,
That *men* and *money* temper'd are alike,
As cold to help as hard to move or strike,
That we should find our richest heaps so scant,
That they but serve to mind us of our want,
As one to *Westminster* some stranger brings,
To view the wealthy Sepulcher of *Kings*.[32]
The beauteous bulk and countenance of wealth,
*Personless* and without the *soul of health*,                       (530)
That our bags, when most *heavy*, should be found
*Only* of weight to *weigh* our hearts to ground.
Since th' *eye* assures us now, we must not think
'Twill *look* on us unless in *paint* or *ink*,
And th' *ear* no other *words* from us will hear,
But such as may be *current* with its *fear*,
Takes from our mouths only such gales as may
Carry its rocking vessel forth our bay—
    T' expect succor from *son*, as well one might
Day's *sun* expect at deadest time of night.                         (540)
Who seeks one for his blessing, as his son,
For blessing comes to Church, when Church is done.
No *mother's* tender hand nor piteous smile
Over her own *dear bowels* while they broil,
No *wise* to comfort. With the body, *heart*
First dies, as senseless; then *head* dies apart.
Sister, brother, husband, not more disclaim
Their kindred than the hearing of their name.

---

[32]  *Sepulcher of Kings.* Tombs in Westminster Abbey.

In their assistance all no better are,
Than th' empty echo answers from afar. (550)
In neighbor's house we think to give our moan;
That ease and scope it finds not in our own.
With open mouth we run forth, but the door
Answers our mouth as it was *shut* before.
Then haste we to *acquaintance*, who—the worst
Fearing—had took th' *alarum* to be horst.[33]
To send them gifts would seem such flattery
As theirs, who court old men with gifts to die.
*Carriers* too are in like cross *restive* mood,
Neither with *words* nor *presents* to be woo'd. (560)
As if they should be prest here, did they come,
To carry biers to grave, they stay at home.
Finding ourselves each one as left *perdu*,
In labyrinth without Ariadne's clue,
And having for our bitter sole relief,
Musings, suspicions, malady, and grief,
All things *without* and *in* us full of woe,
We'd succor beg, but *from whom* do not know.
          Then, like such totally subjected are
To th'effrene, maniac manage of despair, (570)
With ev'ry rule we are at mortal strife,
Would draw us from th' anomaly of life.
Orders confound, and morals send to beg
In fields and woods, with neither arm nor leg.
As if *reason* were *stupid sloth* to feel;
Aculeate *spur*, we place it at our *heel*.
Justice and dignity we only put
Before, to take the first place of our foot.
In harming *others*, that we harm not less
*Ourselves*, we murder our own consciences. (580)
Then when our souls' tell-clocks are husht, that we
Without remorse may *sleep* in villainy,
We *dream* of nothing but such freaks as they
Usually act, who with the *Fairies* play.
What may unriddled *folly* be? Else what
On other's name or body leaves a spot?
To scape the Plague we see lascivious Dame,
Who gives it us but by another name.
We surfeit and luxuriate till the Pest,
Though not invited, boldly shares the feast. (590)

---

[33] *Horst*. Unidentified. Implies silence, an alarm one will not answer.

This *pledges us our healths* that freely spare
Liquor of life to the infected air.
We give ourselves to each enormity
Will let us have the least ado to die.
Our valor, since we'd try what would come on't,
So favor as to place us in the front;
We [en]list under such vices seldom fail
But speedily do with the Plague prevail.
They such be nothing have to do with it,
*As we suppose*, no more than flies with meat.                    (600)
Such as no more will let us feel our bane,
Than did *Vitellius* his boozing vain—
No more with plague confederates are than Cloister
With Market, Sword with Quaker, Lark with Oyster.
The Captain *Zephyrus* his project hath
Like Precedent to school our cheated faith.
As *he*, so *they* lead us with friendly word,
But yet, at last, consign us to their *Lord.*
        By *Searchers* we are govern'd, such as feel
Whether a man be made of *wood* or *steel*.                      (610)
They're pilgrim-*weemen-seers*[34] who can tell,
Not whether one be bound for *heaven* or *hell*,
But what's of more importance, *many think*,
To know the ill and welfare of his chink.[35]
They prate not much of health, as others, but
Are of the *Gentle-craft* to fit his foot:
Speedily they prepare him for the grave,
And then take measure of whate're he have,
Confess and then absolve him all alone,
With power as much as ever had *Pope Joan*.                      (620)
Better that you may know with theirs our state,
They may be term'd *the middle magistrate*,
Not for their *sex* but *ways*, for they'll be sure
To come between *heir* and *executor*,
Just in the *center* fall, where's understood
Whatever can be valued as *good*.
They fear no rebel forces may them brave,
For none will strive with them for what they have
They're Captains of th' *Amazonian* shades,
Whose dismal territories none invades.                          (630)

---

[34]  *pilgrim-weeman-seers.* This is meant sarcastically, that the searchers are itinerant
women who are "seers" only after their own increase in money, not of futures or of health.

[35]  *chink* A humorous colloquial term for money in the form of coin; ready cash.

For all their *age*, they're left us for a *breed*,
Serving us always at our *greatest need*,
Serve dying man to *multiply* his store,
*Increasing* with what he can use no more,
Engender with the dead, *as on a tomb*
The *Spaniard* did with the *Pope's* niece in *Rome*.[36]
Whom shall we spend our breath more to commend,
Than one [who] is left our last and only friend?
They are our friends beyond what can be said,
For they do not forsake us when we're dead.                    (640)
Our *spirits* awe and keep our *ghosts* in fear,
As you may see by the small *wand* they bear.[37]
    With *Searcher*, *Nurse* and *Quack* to rule our state,
To make completely a *Triumvirate*.
Her *Politics* are not from *Aristotle*,
But from the *grave*, the *purse*, the *bag* and *bottle*.
Her task is hard; therefore one must allow
Her food as much as if *he* were her plough.
Her danger being great, he cannot think
Her analeptic worse than *Spanish* drink.                    (650)
Though she take many a *preservative*,
*Quicksilver*'s that which keeps her best alive.
Her daily pay as commonly is known,
As hers that *lover* serves for *half a crown*.
Her *hands*, to take, are nut hooks, and her *feet*,
As ready are to run for *winding-sheet*.
She keeps the sick from *want*, which she does ward
Off so, it can't touch her who is his *guard*.
*Narcotics* are the best things he can keep
By him, for she thrives best when he's asleep.                    (660)
He never *chides* her, nor indeed is't *reason*
He should, for well he knows 'tis out of *season*.
*Passion* uncurb'd by *fear* is mastiff dog
To raging fury left and freed from clog.
The Pestilence like Frigate then will ride,
Hard-goaded in the poop with w*ind* and *tide*.
And soon his life's dear longing he may loose,

---

[36] [marginal note] A marble Figure upon a tomb in St. *Peter's* Church of a very beautiful Lady, with which a Spaniard was so enamored that he expiated his lust upon it, as if it had been alive.

[37] *wand.* Those caring for plague-sick associated with carrying of a rod or other sign of warning to others to remain at a safe distance, in this case "wand" related humorously to the "spirits" and "ghosts" of superstition.

Who for his *Nurse* is nice to pick and choose.
Suppose such are as scarce as may be tare
In corn that's weeded well: one here, one there.                    (670)
Discarded *nurse* may do him as much harm,
As *Devil* sent away without a *charm.*
For want of *Nurses* think as many shoals
Of sick have died, as hops without their poles.[38]
For her *neglect* or *absence* his content
Is *patience*, as best fitting *patient.*
He'll ne're give out she kill'd him, for 'tis said,
He's to be always silent when he's dead.
And while he lives, *Nurses* he'll never curse,
Knowing few *good*, most *bad*, and many *worse.*                    (680)
Quietly he'll conclude she's such a thing
About his person, as is *plague-sore ring.*
       You, now to know the mystery of *Quack*,
May jumble *walnuts* in a *musty* Sack.
As many knick-knacks, *many will avouch it*,
Lurk in his brain, as in a *Tinker's budget.*
Now be'nt in wrath to see *Quack* hindmost here,
*Greatness* and *office* put him in the *rear.*
Knowing not to lead, he is not *first* nor *middle,*
Having no soul of *harmony* to fiddle.                    (690)
Therefore, as best of all to please your taste,
Like sugar after physic, comes at last.
*He*, or *some* for him, setting out a throat,
The patches speak in *Tom of Bedlam's* coat.
As variously his pedigree he brings,
As flies from sorts of reptiles take their wings.
He never broke his brains to know or bear
A *Doctor's trouble*, who runs here and there,
But his *first principles*, that you may think
He's *knowing* man to deal with *pen and ink*,                    (700)
He was bred up to *keep accounts*, or know
The subtlety of *weaver's art* or so,
But since *counts* fail, and *ends* are broke, he lays
A new design, and falls to *vary phrase.*
By *Physic* he thinks best he may prevail:
So "What d'ye lack," he turns to "What d'ye ail?"
Finding his state sink, and almost past hope,
His spirits like brave soldier, musters up,
Resolves to *save* himself, or by some limb

---

[38]    *hops without their poles.* A climbing perennial plant that needs a pole for its ascent.

Catch others, and so make them *fall* with him. (710)
Then without further thought, or needlessly
Hackny'ng his breech to th' *University*,[39]
As rebel Cobblers in the Pulpit where,
He from the *shop* steps into *Doctor's chair*,
So when some course, old *Holland* napkin rots,
'Tis dishcloth turn'd, and serves to scour the pots.
What hurt do *many* medicines, well is known;
Therefore to mend this fault, he hath but *one*,
Somewhat that on diseases *foul will fall*,
And like the fire consume and conquer all; (720)
Some *water*, *pill,* or *powder* can give birth
To wonders, bring out all things like the earth;
Somewhat can mollify the *hardest corn*,
And straight the windings of a *crumpl'd horn*.
With his *rule*[r] he can take *Paul's* height, or use
To lay foundation to a winking house.
The *guts* that do but learn his skill in part,
Are thought the *close Meanders* of his art.
The body's ev'ry limb and bowel greet
With as much pride his worth as gouty feet. (730)
His instrument's a saw, nail, scourer, rammer,
Wedge, chisel, plane, cord, bellows, forge and hammer.
Oft 'tis but one, but hath as many joints,
As *merchant*'s shop with rattles, pins and points.
Expect his ware not new and in the fashion,
But what as old is as dissimulation,
Under a new name vampt, as strange appears,
As when the *Farrier* cuts off *horses'* ears;
As when for your convenience you do
Turn heel down and make *slipper* of a *shoe*. (740)
To ev'ry form and thing change this he can;
As *Jesuit*, they say, is *ev'ry man*.[40]
Like serpent with its old skin off, it is
Just as some new-born issue, christened his,
Lest barren he by others be revil'd,
For heir of arts, fathers another's child.
He's very *humble*, you must understand,
Taking his fees by others, *underhand*.

---

[39]  *Hackny'ng his ... University* Associating himself dishonestly and quickly with the university physicians.

[40]  *Jesuit ... every-man.* The anti-Catholic saying closes with the idea of the Jesuit as a chameleon—a phony, not to be trusted.

Whether his *calling lawful* be'nt or be,

H' ha's luck to find a *lawful deputy*.                                    (750)

     Some *Bookseller* or *Pothecary*, these

Till he fare better, find him bread and cheese.

These two, while he at *tick-tack, passage, ruff*,[41]

Is diligent, make money of his stuff,

While he consults to make his *golden calves*,

As *Jeroboam* did, they go his halves.

You've seen an *highway gelding* turn to *jade*,

So does his *doctor's science* turn to *trade*.

Of these he learns to set himself out bigger,

And bind his phrase in *form*, if not in *figure*.                        (760)

They for his credit will not let him lack

Hard words would break a plowman's teeth to crack.

To trim him up, they are his *looking-glass*,

Or serve as *scouring sand* to bright his *brass*.

If he outlive the times, he'll never blush

In meaner habit than of *rival plush*.

A Doctor's fellow he for wealth will be,

In judgment only of a low degree.

Meanwhile his prescript and his physic form,

As *Hymenaeus'* speech, proves canker-worm,[42]                           (770)

Mangies our purse, eludes our life, and hath

Authority to stigmatize our faith.

And he, himself, as his great acts may tell,

Like *Jambres* is monkey of miracle.[43]

These are the times in which he must commence,

Being to the *Plague* a very *pestilence*.

     This is our tott'ring *three-leg'd* stool we've found

For fine device to tumble on the ground.

Upon *these three* we lean our painful heads,

As in a *Jesuit's* chamber with three beds?                               (780)

Here *young and handsome maids* fearless to fall,

Keeping the street great distance from the wall

---

[41]   *tick-tack.* A variety of backgammon, played on a board with holes along the edge, in which pegs were placed for scoring; *passage.* A gambling game for two people played with three dice; *ruff* A card-game.

[42]   [marginal note] 2 Timothy 2.17. ["And their word will eat as doth a canker: of whom is Hymenaeus and Philetus."]

[43]   [marginal note] Exodus 7.11, 2 Timothy 3.8 [Respectively, "Then Pharaoh also called the wise men and the sorcerers: now the magicians of Egypt, they also did in like manner with their enchantments"; "Now as Jannes and Jambres withstood Moses, so do these also resist the truth: men of corrupt minds, reprobate concerning the faith."]

Walk in the midst the way alone, as though
They might *conceive* if any *near* them go,
As if they in great danger were to get
For plague, great belly by the men they met.
Along street's length *blind man* may walk in dream,
And not a louse give any touches him.
    Each *Change*, now chang'd, fast barricado'd is,
As *Janus Temple* in the times of peace. (790)
Their flaunting gallantry hide all their heads,
As when gay flowers sink into their beds.
As when an old man's feet in frosty weather,
To make nest warm, lie crumpled up together.
Where we had *"Pater noster"* in our way,
We sighing now, *"Ora pro nobis"* say.[44]
Many not broke by trade, but breaking that
For change of life in far more honor'd state,
Knowing the great advantage by't, before
They die, desire their *Will* hang out at door: (800)
Gift door with *prophesy*, how it may teach
Others the *dying discipline* they preach;
Persuade more after them, that they may find
They've little reason long to stay behind;
Invite them there to dwell, and so become
The *first* door to their *sempiternal* home.
When *one* dies in an house, the *rest* they get
Abroad, and then the *grave* is to be *let*.
None count it strange that money should be given
For *passage* makes the nearest way to *heaven*. (810)
Those *well* have liv'd, and so are fit to die,
*Atropos* there can teach her mystery.
They help and do her service in the place.
For many hands make work go on apace,
But patch and paint don't always join, nor are
All faces in *disgrace* for mark of *scar*.
House, neither goods nor master wants, for he
Secures his *venture* by a policy,
Rules it by *poliza* script; *twine* or *clue*,
Can easily his *labyrinth* undo. (820)
It only serves as ticket to the master,
To go to raise his faith in change of pasture,

---

[44]   *Pater noster.* Beginning of the Lord's Prayer, "Our Father"; *Ora pro nobis* Pray for us, part of the Hail Mary prayer, "Holy Mary, Mother of God, pray for us sinners now and a the hour of our death."

Entreats house may not be by any thought
Upon account of *chance* or *time* in fault.
'Tis ornamental-frieze, that, by its place,
Insinuates the *prayer's* turn'd to *grace,*
Emboldens fear, and none the Tenant will
Blame; house secures t' himself by bond or bill.
'Tis to be let, as *Isabella* is,
When wife to *Tristram,*[45] by *antiphrasis.*                    (830)
'Tis to be let, i.e. be let *alone*
To tenant, ha's ear-markt it for his own.
       A *Soldier* stands at many doors with spear,
As if black *Pluto* had his palace there,
Or that the soldier must his weapons carry,
Being death's *life-guard* and *stipendiary,*
As though with our *profession* we would vaunt
We members are of the Church militant.
Halberds and spears stand watching there alone,
While *guard,* as fear'd, with their own *arms* are gone.        (840)
They seem *Dodona's grove,* to speak a law,
Like *Oracle* to force one to withdraw,
Not that any design'd with him to fight,
But as if *master* of those arms were *spright[ly].*
Think of the watchman's service, and he shows
But as a *man of clouts*[46] to fright the *crows,*
Like gazing person in the market, who
Sits kicking heels and nothing has to do.
What cares he if his *porch* and *fort* you take,
When plaguey *victor champion*s at his back?                     (850)
But he—say we suppose him strong and stout—
Keeps not the sick within, though others out.
As if sick persons swell'd t'a *mighty* state,
To let them out, he's *porter* at the gate,
Thinks it hard nature to withhold those, who
Would of the world but *take leave* e're they go.
So up and down among the rest they crowd,
Now in, then out, as sun that's under cloud,
To earth; persuade us with touch, sigh, and groan,
As if't were *mortal sin* to die alone;                          (860)
Swarming like bees on ev'ry herb they fall,

---

[45]    *Isabella and Tristram.* Mythological mother and son; perhaps Austin confuses their
relationship or this is his twist the notion of antiphrasis: a figure of speech by which words
are used in a sense opposite to their proper meaning.

[46]    *Man of clouts.* Man of patches; scarecrow; fool.

Not to get *honey*, but disperse their *gall*,
Esteem it light, wherever they resort,
If they revive *Joab* and *Abner's* sport,[47]
As in a dance where many go *the round*,
One falling pulls down others to the ground.[48]
    Coaches and Carts (our plague in health) we are
Free from, as if the stones they must not wear,
And these as clean from use are kept, as though
Ev'ry day were to be the *Lord Mayor's show*.                    (870)
The coaches left, scare us to see them come
In *mourning* towards us like gaping tomb.
So sorrowful a spectacle to one
They seem, as *body* when the *soul* is gone.
They look as if they penitently mourn'd,
Because they had their *masters* overturn'd:
For sake of business, pastime, friend or wife,
*Carried* him quite beyond the *stage of life*.
As if not *ghost,* as is the common talk,
But when a man is dead, his *house* must walk.                   (880)
So sadly do they look and mope about,
As if *pleasure* were turn'd the *inside out*.
    Those open shops sell any ware or stuff
In *Cheapside*, now do make it *dear* enough.
They're very few, and that there may be made
Good bargain, you'll scarce find two of a trade;
Most nail'd and lockt up are, and seem to you
Like picture buildings, can't be lookt into,
Presents seal'd up and ready to be sent,
Where e're their *Landlords* are to take the rent,               (890)
One gazing on them easily believes,
Whose e're they be, they're very fit for thieves.
Stranger might think all the week long we keep
Some solemn feast, as *Holy-day of sleep*,
That all the *day* we lockt up *night* and lackt,
Nothing to know, 'twas *noon* but to be waked.
Did *Cesar* now enter our City gate,
His prize would make him think h'had found a cheat;
Doubtless he'd lose it all, and in derision
Go out again for want of opposition.                             (900)
    Our *Cash-bank*'s dry, so little is there in 't,

---

47   *Joab and Abner's sport* From 2 Samuel 2, a lesson in the bitterness and danger of
warlike sport used for military practice; such sport may turn deadly.
48   *One falling ...ground.* Related to the children's game-song Ring Around the Rosie.

That parts abroad bring *money* to our *mint*.
Our *treasury* and glutted soul's delight
Devour'd such wealth, now craves the *Widow's mite*.
As if like *corn sacks* of the *fathers*, so we [49]
Had, fast when dead, in our mouths all our *money*.
As if t'appease the *manes* with the dead,
All his whole substance too were buried.
Or for the last abuse of worldly store,
As if the *rich* did *die* to *starve* the *poor*.                    (910)
So fast we die, so poor live, that what's sent
To feed us, on our burials is spent.
Our gaudy robes can make no better brags,
Than from each shire to be supply'd with rags.
*Nature's* inverted, for this place the heart
Should feed is fed by ev'ry other part,
Unless you'll say the waters from the *Main*
To *rivers* run do but refund again.
But so our *Ocean* does the rivers need,
That most of us seem of true beggar's breed.                    (920)
*Strangers* for alms we thankfully do greet
Abroad, and here beg of the next we meet.
*Beggar* hunts *benefactor*, yet no worse
He'd handle him than merely take his purse:
"I have been sick these thirteen days," *says one*,
"And now, like *bird* from *nest* am newly flown."
"Good Sir," *another cries*, "have pity on me,
For I, *God wot*, have five *plague-sores* upon me."
Thus *benefactor,* fear'd, dares make no stay;
So *Charity* with *Justice* flies away.                    (930)
     *Two* days and nights fires in our streets did burn,
To light th' *infectious spirits* to their urn.
*Three* days by order they should have been there,
But to be out of pain of life and fear,
Like niggards, who to their last end arrive,
We would not be at so much charge to live.
The fires were, after, precedent of such,
Old grandsires knew what fire was by the touch,
But the Plague being in our flagitious lives,
And as the creature that in fire survives,                    (940)
*God* with our sacrifice would not be pleas'd

---

[49]  [marginal note] Genesis 42.35. ["And it came to pass as they emptied their sacks, that, behold, every man's bundle of money was in his sack: and when both they and their father saw the bundles of money, they were afraid."]

The *physic* e're should touch the *part diseas'd.*
　　By night and day the dead walk ev'ry where
As if the *day of doom* drew very near.
*Dis* shows us his *black princes* in the dead,
Being more tall than others by the head.
As they are softly carried on their way,
*Death* seems to make triumphant *holy-day.*
Many [who] attend them to the graves are taught
How to come there next day, so then are brought,　　　　　　(950)
As if *sin's punishment* with *sin* did meet,
To be alike infectious and sweet.
Thus, as such in their duty are well read,
We do but *let the dead bury the dead.* [50]
The doleful Parish-bell all night and day
Beating, as *pulse*, its sickness does *betray.*
*"Mortality"* all sermons does contain,
As ev'ry silver *fountain* courts the *Main.*
All divine rays are center'd in this text,
As amply round us spreads as heaven's convex.　　　　　　　(960)
T' illustrate *holy Scripture* well, his breath
Best does it to the life, best sets forth death.
The *Gospels* full sum and epitome:
To prove life's warfare is *"Prepare to die."*
　　In this the grave's great jubilee, we choose
No place but *Churchyard* for our rendezvous.
We need not, when our life begins to fail,
Fall straight to dig our graves *with tooth and nail*;
Nor stay till we are by some long disease
Consum'd; we may in *grave* walk when we please.　　　　　　(970)
Who goes from street to street in *City* roams,
Like the possessed man among the tombs.
No subtle wit th' *infernal God* betrays,
Whose palace gate lies open nights and days.
His meskite's porch opens to all that come,
To stay and be prepar'd to hear their doom.
There we receive the vapor and the steam
Of those we lost before, so follow them.
Graves' mouths gape wide along our way to force—
At least, invite—us to our lives' *last course.*　　　　　　　(980)
And that a *lonely* place may not displease,
They've room to welcome many *families.*

---

[50]　[marginal note] *Non est vivere sed valere vita.* [Latin proverb: Life is not just to live but life is to be strong.]

Though we before our *exit* from the womb
Lay there *alone*, we're *crowded* in the tomb.
Wisely they leave graves open to the dead,
'Cause some too early there are *brought to bed.*
Those there we thought bid us their *last adieu*,
Before they can *repent*, are *born anew.*
They waking speak, thinking they may be bold
Wanting their clothes, to say *they are a cold.*                    (990)
One out of trance return'd, after much strife
Among a troop of *dead*, exclaims for *life.*
One finding himself, as some *maid*, hard lace't
Or as a *Watch* for pocket, straightly case't,
Equally terrifi'd with *pain* and *fear*,
Complains to those can neither speak nor hear.
One having broke his elbows, heels and toes
Continues on the *alarum* with his nose.
Another, he, instead of lice and fleas,
Feeling himself worse pincht in *little ease*,                     (1000)
Dejected with arms hanging, whines a ditty,
Like pris'ner goes to suffer, *Psalm of pity*,
Having with cold and speaking lost his throat,
Makes noise as bird that sings his *rural note.*
One too too weak to raise his aching head,
Throws off the *sheet* when friends have sold his *bed.*
Another, not being us'd to *silent life*,
Calls daughter *Doll*, maid *Sue*, and *Kate* his wife.
At last they come and gape to what is said,
Like unlearn'd clowns that hear a letter read.                     (1010)
They cry for help, as if they had disgrace
By lying there or did not like their place.
They seem as favors to the world again
Sent to convert their sinful brethren.[51]
     We fear no *grave* (if we may, *dying*), for though
Buried *today*, we may arise *tomorrow.*
The *day of judgment* can be no surprise,
For graves gape wide, and the sepulchr'd rise.
By grinning heads that are before us hurl'd
From thence, we're scorn'd and flouted from the world.            (1020)
*Death* shows us not his teeth to scare, but kill,
As morglays beared to execute his Will.
These when our plotting heads would work our pride

---

[51]    [marginal note] Luke 16.28. ["For I have five brethren; that he may testify unto
them, lest they also come into this place of torment."] *Favors.* Favorites; people favored.

To great designs, our policy deride.
When we laugh much, our fellow *skeleton*
Shows us our sides we hold, from bone to bone.
When the world makes us sigh, lament, and cry,
*Memento mori*'s always in our eye.
The *Stygian lake* receives again new birth,
And makes profound eruptions from the earth.                     (1030)
Brimstone *Vesuvius* and *Aetna* have
Vast *Gaetanean* channels in each grave.[52]
*Heaven* rains down scorpions, while the *earth* presumes
To stifle us with deletory fumes.
We cannot quench or cool that flaming breath
The air swells up our lungs with, but by death.
In our choice drink we do the *Lethe* taste,
And our dear bread is made of arsenic paste.
The flesh we eat gives us with strength but power
To feed those greedy wolves, our hearts devour.                     (1040)
We're as *Aegisthus'* sons[53] or such cross guest,
Found in the *wilderness* a dying feast.
We stew, bake, boil, with such success to follow
To those that eat, as when there's *mors in olls.*[54]
Warm vest, like robe of *Hercules,* was wet
In *Nessus'* blood,[55] procures death's icy sweat.
Each thing *Paul* said was lawful though not fit,[56]
Now's so forbid: we die by touching it.
Letter of friend "*long life*" and "*perfect health*"
Gives us in wish, takes both away by stealth.                     (1050)
Though't bring us gold as *Palamede's*, each groat
Is for the carriage paid to *Charon's* boat.
It treason shows, and pays us our *last meed,*
While sadly we our *condemnation* read.

---

[52]   [marginal note] *Gaeta.* A great gaping mountain between *Rome* and *Naples*, supposed to be cleft asunder by an earthquake.

[53]   *Aegisthus's sons.* Austin may confuse Aegisthus with his father Thyestes, whose enemies killed and fed his children to him; he then slept with his daughter to create a son, Aegisthus, to help him avenge their deaths.

[54]   [marginal note] 2 Kings 4.40. [ "So they poured out for the men to eat. And it came to pass, as they were eating of the pottage, that they cried out, and said, 'O thou man of God, there is death in the pot.' And they could not eat thereof." *Mors in olls* literally means "death in the pot," as per the biblical passage.]

[55]   *robe of ...Nessus' blood.* Nessus was a famous centaur who was killed by Hercules, and whose tainted blood in turn killed him.

[56]   [marginal note] 1 Corinthians 10.23. ["All things are lawful for me, but all things are not expedient: all things are lawful for me, but all things edify not."]

We find by this exitial surprise,
The *whole Creation's* turn'd our enemies.
And to speak our condition at the best,
Our *City's* merely but great *house of Pest.*
To seem, though foes to all, t'ourselves good friends,
(Holding all day our noses by the ends)                    (1060)
Some mixed drugs or herbs together bound
We smell, as if we stank above the ground.
Our rooms with sulfur fumes are smoke't and air'd,
As if for *Purgatory* we prepar'd.
Our life, of which we can be sure of nowhere,
So *passive* is, we do not *act* but *suffer.*
We who are not permitted yet to die,
Seem left as *dregs* merely to *putrefy*:
As *broken hose* one by misfortune rends,
At ev'ry touch ready to run to *ends*;                     (1070)
As *tainted eggs* the parent birds will not
*Brood* longer on, so *addle* we and *rot.*
We who of late prais'd *heaven* for victories,
Now beg our lives to conquer *that* with cries;
After our joy, tears, sighs, and prayers, these
Make us concern'd to write upon our knees.
Forlorn and wretched, we who now remain,
Suddenly are as exuls, caught and slain,
Our lethal curse making our friends afear'd,
Like wounded deer we're horn'd off from the herd.         (1080)
*God* leaves us too. *Hell* falls from *heaven*, while thus
The *Devil* rains his *kingdom* upon us.
*Sad case*, could any fitly make appear,
No human *judge* were great enough to hear.
And ten to one who thus employ their breath,
Like swans they do but sing before their death.

## Epigraph
*Tali spiramine Nesis*
*Emittit stygium nebulosis aëra saxis*
*Antraque letiferi rabiem Typhonis anhelant.*
Lucan. l.6.[57]

---

[57]  *Tali ... anhelant.* With such an exhalation Nesis sends forth a deathly atmosphere
from her misty rocks, while the caverns of Typhon breath forth death and madness (Lucan's
*Pharsalia*, trans. J.D. Duff, The Loeb Classical Library [London: William Neiemann; New
York: G. P. Putnam's Sons, 1928] 6.91–93, pages 310–311).

\*

# Thomas Clark,
## *Meditations in my Confinement*

The British Library owns the single copy of the only edition of this poem from 1666 (Wing CD-ROM, 1996, C4562), which begins with a verse dedication to the author's "much Honored Friends" and ends with a postscript, both transcribed below.

MEDITATIONS
In my CONFINEMENT
When my House was Visited with the
SICKNESS
In April, May and June, 1666
*In which time I buried two Children
and had three more of my Family Sick.*

———

London,
Printed by W. G. for the use of the Author. 1666. [1]

**To my much Honored Friends, whose Kindness and Affection hath been
expressed to me in my late Affliction, to whom I render hearty *Thanks*, and
wish *Health* and *Prosperity*.**

    *Give ear* (my courteous friends) *and lend your vote,*
*To this my doleful and* Swan-like *note*;
*Though not so sweet (as that is said), more true,*
*Which causeth me my cheeks with tears bedew:*
That, *is a* Poet's fiction *of the* Swan;
This, *sobs and groans of an* afflicted man,
*One that with* sorrows God *doth* castigate,
*That he may fit him for a better* state.
    *Expect not now in these lines* Melody,
*Nor shall I promise any* Harmony.                (10)
*Where grief predominates, it is a rein,*
*To check the* Fancy *and* Invention's *strain.*
*This* Piece *at best is rough and impolite,*
*Not burnish'd o're with* art *to make it bright.*
*No* elegancy *here is interlac'd,*
*Which might the Reader* Court *to be embrac'd.*
Courtship *with me was then quite out of* fashion,
*When whole months pass'd and scarce a* salutation.
Sighs *here* are Accents, Periods *end with* tears,
*And for the* Burden, *'tis a mass of* fears.       (20)
*I have no argument that may incline*
*You for to read this Tract, but that* 'tis mine.
*Nor do I Judge it worth your pains, yet take*
*It, and peruse it, for the* Author's *sake.*
*Accept of my* endeavors; *where they're short,*
*I beg your patience and your pardon for't.*
Thomas Clark

---

[1]   *W.G.* This is most likely William Godbid; for more, see the Index of Names in the Appendices.

## Meditations in my Confinement, etc.

When mercies lose their *end* and cannot *draw*,
And *Sins* are froze so *hard* they will not *thaw*
By gentle means, then is *Correction's rod*
Sent, by *Afflictions*, to *drive* men to God.                    (30)
And may he grant that I so understand
The voice of his severe chastising hand,
That making the right *use* for which 'twas sent,
I may from *Sin* turn, God from's *Punishment*.
My house, the house of *mourning's* made; then how
Can *Mirth* or *Music* relish with me now?
Or if I should dare to compose a *Verse*,
What fitter subject than of *Grave* or *Hearse*,
Or *Winding-sheet?* These only be my *Theme*,
On which my thoughts are and whereof I dream,                    (40)
And waking find myself alive, and wonder,
That *Soul* is not from *Body* wrest asunder.
Then do I rouse and pluck my Spirits up,
And *hope* gets ground, that yet that *bitter cup*
May be prorogu'd and sweetened, so that I
Prepar'd may better be and fit to die.
And then again, my Sins start up and stare
Me in the face and ask me how I dare
Presume on mercy, since demerit's such,
That what's inflicted yet is but a touch                    (50)
Or taste of that Divine and most just *wrath*
The number of my Sins deserved hath;
Which thing (so true, my Conscience can't deny)
Doth heighten much my present misery.
But oh, besides this, how doth the *World* frown
Upon one by his *Maker* thus cast down,
Who (as *Job's* friends did, these) stand in amaze,
And at a distance too (as they) to gaze!
Again, as they did, so do these do here,
Rashly prejudge, and condemn too, I fear;                    (60)
And well it were, if pity these so-take
As (doubtless) was in them for good *Job's* sake;
Yet (to a Proverb) are they on record
Mis'rable Comforters, to be abhorr'd.
But now (alas) if I should speak my mind,
How justly may I call this Age unkind?
Who is it that remembers *Joseph's* smart?
Or his afflictions ever takes to heart?

Nay, rather, is not shame, reproach, and scorn,
The portion here of most that lie forlorn?                              (70)
And chiefly, such whom God, to evidence
His mighty pow'r by his wise providence,
Hath humbled by severest *dispensation*
Of the Distemper, or the Visitation;
The *Pestilence* (I mean), or now as 'tis
Called "the Sickness" with an Emphasis;
A name peculiar for it, and most fit,
Denoting and comprising *"all"* in it.
And if the *name* do carry too much *dread*,
What wonder if the *thing* itself strikes *dead?*                       (80)
Of those three Judgments, supereminent,
So often threatned by th'Omnipotent,
This of them all doth seem unto a Land,
The most immediate stroke from his own hand.[2]
This God's *Artill'ry* is, and Himself like;
Who's he that can defend, when it doth strike?
An *arrow* (call'd for swiftness) from a *Bow*,
Pointed to rich and poor, to high and low:
It *Sex*, nor *Age*, nor *Person* doth respect,
Nor can exemption be. Who may expect                                    (90)
Favor? The force of Youth's no Privilege;
No strength of Constitution blunts its edge;
*The* Sovereignty *of* Drugs *cannot* resist;
It wounds and kills ev'n where and whom it list.
This *arrow* flies by *day*, yet who can see it?
A terror 'tis by *night*, and none can flee it.
It walks in *darkness*, and who then can shun it?[3]
And vain it is to think they may outrun it.
What shield can guard the angry *Angel's* blow,
Who hath so many by his stroke laid low?                                (100)
What Rhetoric either can persuade or charm
This furious *Messenger* to slack his *Arm?*
The rich man's *Coffer* nor his Bags can bribe it,
Neither the skillful *Artist* can prescribe it;
The valiant *Soldier* dareth not alarm it,
Nor can the *black Magician's* philters charm it.

---

[2]    A reference generally to plague, famine, and war. See also David's choice at 1 Chronicles 7–14 and 2 Samuel 24.13–15.

[3]    *walks ... shuns it.* A reference to the popular plague Psalm 91: "Thou shalt not be afraid for the terror by night; nor for the arrow that flieth by day; / Nor for the pestilence that walketh in darkness; nor for the destruction that wasteth at noonday" (verses 5–6).

The *Lord* and *Beggar* equally do stand,
And both alike accounted in *Death's* hand.
Death is the King of Terrors, and a man
At very thoughts thereof grows pale and wan.        (110)
And though whats'ever sickness causing *Death*
Pays Mortals *debt* to *Nature*, stops our *breath*—
Yet this of all *Diseases* mark'd doth lye,
(As I may say) dip'd to a *double-dye*
And which is like the Serpent's deadly *sting*,
Poisons all o're; *that*, whence all *woes* do spring
To Body, State, Relations, Liberty,
To Friends, Acquaintance, and Society,
And all discomforts else to humankind,
'Tis couch'd here in the *Abstract*, we may find.        (120)
Some *Characters* whereof, I here shall give,
To show it is, in kind, *superlative*
Unto all other, for *disconsolation*
Which take in this epitomiz'd *Relation*.

### The Extremity of this Distemper to the Body and Person

In Body, see what tumors ulcerating,
Tearing the flesh, ev'n unto macerating,
With Biles and Botches, Carbuncles and Blains,
All which do torture with excessive pains,
Or if not so, it worse in bowels lies,
Unspeakably tormenting till it dies,        (130)
Complexed always and in high extremes
Of Ague's chillness, mix'd with Fever's flames.
And if (in ought, unto the Patient sick)
It favor shows, 'tis in dispatching quick;
Or else in this, unto the party showing
By its Death-marks where suddenly he's going.
But oft not so, for many long do lie
In extreme languishing, sad misery
With Entrail-racking-laxes vehement,
And retching vomitings most violent.        (140)
Oft times the mind too's held with stupefaction,
And is bereft of reason by distraction;
Which thing enough is to bring desperation,
At least a hind'rance 'tis to preparation.
    Next unto life itself, health's preservation
And lawful means for *Body's* restoration
By men esteem'd is much, both to prevent,

And when there's need to cure the Patient.
All count Physicians useful, commendable,
Their calling noble, practice laudable,                                    (150)
In wisdom, learning, known experience, grave,
And carriage suitable to all they have.
These persons of such honor are and worth,
As some almost for Demi-Gods set forth,
Believing they have pow'r to rescue Death,
At least to lengthen out the lease of Breath.
But here, the Doctors' scruple, are not free
In anything except in taking fee;
And as to that, they're ready men, and quick,
But slack enough in visiting the Sick,                                     (160)
And chiefly then, the time when there's most need,
Their height of Art and Skill to show indeed.
This is to very many much addition,
Unto their sad deplorable condition,
Because on these men they did much depend,
From Sickness' rage their *Bodies* to defend;
At least, expecting, if it should them seize,
These would within call be, to give them ease.
But they are fled (perhaps); if not, how e're,
To see such Patients, they will give no ear.                               (170)
Here I must leave them too, and if they die,
Let their great Doctors answer't, and not I.
        Such are the *Body's* sufferings, whilst there's breath,
And some there are (I'll show) that survive Death.
For Death's not all in this Distemper: here
The mere Concomitants thereof (which fear
And terror works upon the Patient so)
Makes Death (as 'twere) to strike a double blow,
And its Attendants are so represented,
As if Death's stroke by horror were prevented.                            (180)
The bitterness is multiply'd by th'quality,
Which swells the product of Calamity
Into so vast a sum, figures can't do't
Nor number or proportion can reach to't.
'Tis sudden, solit'ry, incurable,
And what so comfortless? So terrible?
This Sickness also, after Death, doth seem
To trample o're the dead with disesteem,
And (Victor-like, o're Captives) with despite,
Denies such Obsequies and fun'ral rite,                                    (190)
Which in a solemn manner is most due,

As we have seen in this late time, not few.
How hath some posted been to Graves before
They were quite cold and scarce found cov'ring o're?
And 'stead of Friends and Mourners following there,
How did all shun them, that they did come near?
'Twas well if Bearers could be got for money,
Men's hearts through fear were grown so hard and stony.
How were some thrown in Carts and drawn in pace
Much like Offenders, t' Execution place?                    (200)
And as for Burial, one in many score
Had not a word of any Pray'r said o're.
And (in the Country) some were ty'd to poles,
Dragg'd by the Neck with ropes, and pok'd in holds;
Whilst other Carcasses were left in field,
To see what Burial Beasts and Fowls would yield.
This, like a second death, here did appear,
Which did cost many a heart-piercing tear,
Of such as did survive, fearing that they
Themselves, if seized, might go the same way.             (210)
    And thus much of the Dying, or the Sick
Of this Distemper; something of the quick
May here be said: the healthy and the sound
That ne're have touch by't yet receive a wound.
This seems a Paradox, but it is true,
As Instances I could give, not a few,
For (others being dead) this doth bereave,
These of the comforts which they should receive.
Alas! how fares it with whole Families,
Whereout (perhaps) one only thereof dies?                 (220)
Whenas the rest (pent up and all in tears
In hourly expectation of their fears)
Transported are, with grief and terror made,
As if that all their Necks o'th block were laid.
And we well know such spectacles have been,
That this (God's Besom) hath swept houses clean.
These thoughts, amazements, and suprisals strange,
(Acted by fear alone) such sudden change
Hath wrought in some (it hath so dear been rated,
Their lives at state) Death hath been ante-dated.        (230)
    suff'rings more to *Body* or the *Mind*,
Are usher'd in, when thus a man's confin'd,
Must here in this place waved be, lest I
Be justly taxed with prolixity.
I could here tell ye, how the Neighbors keep

Their distance, as not daring scarce to peep
Out of their doors or on that side to look,
Lest that Infection may be thereby took,
And how all Passengers that go that way,
Will o're the Kennel skip as from a fray;                    (240)
How few of many that go by, and know,
Will ask, "How do ye?" or like kindness show.
These things dismay a *Body* very much,
(But here, I'll leave, I meant only a touch)
And though this is the course us'd constantly,
Yet I confess I've found much courtesy,
For neighbors have been very kind to me
In this my long and sad extremity.

### The extraordinary Expense and damage to *Estate* that this Distemper brings

   Next, for *Estate*, how can there a worse foil
Befall a man than this or greater spoil                    (250)
Unto his fortunes: 'specially, if low,
And weak i'the world, for then down he must go.
A two-fold sting 'tis, 'gainst both which, no fence:
One points to loss, the other to expense.
It stops *Gain's* current, causeth that ebb low,
And set ope *Charge's* sluice to Overflow.
As first, it blocks up Commerce, bars all Trade,
For of a Shop no use at all is made,
Nor other Craft, the only means whereby
A man maintains himself and Family.                    (260)
So thus, no *gain* is got; that's known full well,
For none with such will either buy or sell.
And for *Expenses* daily running out,
I need say little, for that's out of doubt.
'Twixt Doctors, Surgeons, Physic, pay of Nurse,
(As in the Proverb) "hand ne're out of purse."
   Upon this Subject, I might more enlarge,
Having had sad experience of the charge,
Not only of *expense*, but damage-cost
Th'account whereof's not yet made up what lost;                    (270)
All which in Characters are written so,
That still lies legible in Folio.
Should I speak pain, sure there could not be worse:
Sickness of *Body to* make sick the *purse.*

**The Uncomfortableness of this Distemper**
**In Debarring the Visits of Relations and Kindred**

Touching *Relations*, Bonds of strongest tie,
By *Nature* seal'd, do almost Cancell'd lie
As out of date, during this time of danger,
One to another being as a stranger.
Whenas to other times, this near Connection
Mounted upon the Wing of dear Affection, (280)
Such pow'r hath in't that nothing should have hindred
The swift and frequent Visits of their *Kindred.*
Like as a burning Beacon at *invasions*
Calls quick assistance, so 'tis with *Relations*:
If any be assaulted in their health,
How soon the rest in that small *Commonwealth*
Haste to th'afflicted Member for to yield
All succor to it, him from Death to shield,
By Counsel, Care, and what else may conduce
Both to the outward means and Comfort's use. (290)
But this hath such malevolent Aspect,
As if that *Nature* did herself neglect,
And unto admiration works this wonder:
Nearest of *Kin* are oft farthest asunder.
The *Daughter* dareth not approach the *Mother*;
Nor dares one *Brother to come at* another.
The *Father* may not his own *Child* come near,
Nor may the *Child* the *Parents* see for fear.
The *Mother* doth bewail her *Child* at distance;
The *Child* oft wants the *Mother's* kind assistance. (300)
Yet may we not these judge unnatural,
Nor in the least for this "unkind" them call.
Nor do I mean as if their love, good will,
Or sweet affections stifled are: these still
May in their vigor flourish, be as green,
As firm, and strong as ever they have been.
The fire hid in the Embers is not out;
The seeming-dead Tree in the Spring doth sprout.
*Relations*' care and kindness doth not quite
Consist in outward visits and in sight (310)
Of their Allies, nor doth it argue lack
Of Love in them, whom danger thus keeps back.
This showeth only Fear's predomination,
The strongest passion in his operation,
And boundless in th'extreme, for (out of doubt)

By this are strange effects past finding out.
And now assuredly 'twill be confess'd,
Greatest Discomforts must lie in the Breast
Of such who are afflicted with this sore
And saddest punishment (spoke of before),                    (320)
Which doth reciprocally add much grief
Either to other, even past belief,
When solemnly they may not at last breath,
Take leave of one another before Death.
These piercing Aggravations are indeed
To sink the spirits, make the heart to bleed.

### The Abridgment of Liberty, by Confinement in this Distemper

    And now I come to treat of *Liberty*,
Or how that is abridg'd (by this) to see:
That which opposeth *Liberty withal*
As is a *Rise* the opposite to *Fall*,                       (330)
So contraries compar'd with one another,
Doth Illustration bring each to the other.
In this case (sure) it's verify'd what's said:
A man's own *house* is then his *prison* made,
For either he's therein most strictly *lock'd*
By Law's constraint upon him or else *yok'd*
By *self-confinement* (which is little less)
On his Parol (not daring to transgress
Lest he offence in any kind should give
Unto his Neighbors, who about him live).                     (340)
This then enough is and a proof sufficient
That herein lies *restraint* and detriment;
For Liberty's privation (in extent)
Differs but little from *Imprisonment*,
Except herein, and then the diff'rence much,
That these God's *Pris'ners* are (others not such),
And He alone, and none but he, can ease
Their smart and pain and seal them a *Release.*
'Tis He offended is, enters the *Action*,
Orders th'Arrest, requireth satisfaction.                    (350)
He will withdraw his *suit* and set such *free*,
Who on him do depend for *Liberty*,
And though provok'd, yet prone to mercy still,
To them that humble are and wait his will.
And since they cannot *satisfy*, 'tis done
If but believe their Bail is his own Son.

Oh! that men would take pattern here and see
That they as merciful to *Pris'ners* be,
That patiently they would forbear and stay,
With them that have it not, till they can pay.                    (360)
    But for my own part, I must here confess,
Much Privilege I had in my distress.
I was not padlock'd in, nor by a *guard*
Of Watchmen by constraint of freedom barr'd,
But wholly left unto my own discretion,
Which kindness show'd in me too much Impression.
This I acknowledge was my Neighbors' love,
Which (prais'd be God) did them no damage prove;
No further use did I of that here make
Than lawfully I might with good leave take.                    (370)

**The Uncomfortableness of this Distemper,**
**Dissolving for the present the bands of**
**Friendship.**

    The next thing is to show how palpable
This is to *Friends*, and indemonstrable,
For herein such a high discomfort lies,
That greater cannot amongst *friends* arise.
Twixt real Friends, indeed, a *True-love-knot*
Is ty'd, not to be loos'ned or forgot,
So long as life doth last in this our station,
Which without doubt surpasses all relation.
The wise man saith, "A *friend* is more than brother.
*Affection* is so grafted each in other,"                    (380)
And sure *this* is the strongest tie that can
Here in this world be to link man to man.
For how, by Counsels sweet and Courtesy,
Doth one *Friend* strive another to outvie?
And search the heart, if grief do lie hid there,
To vent it thence, that each their share may bear?
And through thick and thin, mount high, low dive,
That they each other's spirits may revive.
When good news is, these do congratulate.
When sorrowful, or bad, commiserate.                    (390)
In health and happiness, they harmonize.
In sickness and discomforts, sympathize.
*Friendship's* a ray of the Diviner love,
Which sets the wheels awork, and pity move
In *friends* towards th'afflicted. But alas!

Pity can't be exerted in this Case
As it should be, for it will not amount
To one bare visit, upon this account:
*These* cannot more than *others* quit their fear.
They love *friends* well, but their own life is dear,　　　　(400)
Or should they dare, 'twould charg'd be in effect,
As foolhardy fam'ly disrespect;
Therefore *friends, friends* must pardon, when 'tis so.
*That way* fear turns the beam, the Scale will go,
As when the Huntsman's Bow hath mark'd a Deer,
The Herd the chafed one will not come near,
And though for help or shelter it may run,
Sometimes amongst them, yet they still it shun—
So 'tis with those whom this Disease doth take,
All *Comforts* and *Associates* straight forsake.　　　　(410)
Though ne'r so intimate perhaps before,
No converse now can be on any score.
*Friends* stand at distance; all do such men fly,
Nor dare for fear to keep them Company.
Yet though fear doth thus *friendship's* bands dissolve,
'Tis but for present; 'twill again revolve.
Now since fast *friends* thus bounded are in dangers,
Why think we much, or expect more, from strangers?
　　But let not me complain 'tis dark, when light
Shined on me ev'n in the gloomy'st night:　　　　(420)
I mean, favor's bright beams on *friendship's* score,
Which were not merely "*how d'yees*" at the door
But *real visits*, and so influential,
Yielding refreshings to me, most essential
'Twas a *supply*, for kind, most answerable
To all things, and a *support* suitable,
A healing *Plaster* made for any sore,
And a *key* fitted unto ev'ry door.
What shall I more say? I'll not Counsel keep:
This bounty did me make for joy to weep.　　　　(430)
Which love of theirs, I shall acknowledge ever,
And to my slender power will endeavor
To quit myself from base Ingratitude,
By a self-Off'ring of such servitude
As either I can study, they Command,
Or may expected be from such a hand.
In the meantime, this shall not wanting be,
My thanks to them for their good will to me.
And as a foretaste of that due respect

I owe unto them, let me here direct (440)
This fervent *Option*, which as an *Oblation*
I tender, winged with my heart's *Oration:*
    May health and happiness always attend ye.
    A *Prosp'rous gale* in all things may *befriend* ye.
    Wisdom in all your actions may direct ye.
    The Pow'rs-Divine from dangers may protect ye.
    No *Violent Distemper* may e're seize ye.
    Nor ought that's hurtful may I'th least disease ye.
    May *friends* increased be, and *foes* that hate ye,
    With shame convinc'd, may strive to imitate ye. (450)
    May *Virtues* flourish in and so improve ye
    That others may both *Emulate* and love ye.
    Your *persons* honor'd so, may none dare slight ye.
    Your *Wives* and *Children* such may most delight ye.
    May your *good names* be still preserved by ye.
    May sland'ring *Tongue-detractors* not come nigh ye.
    In '*States* and *Families*, may *Angels* guard ye.
    And at the last, may *Heaven's King* reward ye.

## The Uncomfortableness of this Distemper in reference to breaking of all Acquaintance and Society

    As for Acquaintance and Society
(For these may well together joined be) (460)
It is a large theme to discuss, but how
By this 'tis interrupted, I may show
In few particulars, as well as many;
The rest are eas'ly understood by any.
The life of man's much sweet'ned by Discourse,
Communication having such a force,
And virtue (like a Load-stone) drawing to't,
That comforts manifold spring from this root.
Without Society, how would men mourn?
And live like Anchorites and Monks forlorn? (470)
Man when in Paradise (that blessed state)
At first, while yet alone without a mate,
That happiness itself, seem'd not complete,
Until a *help* was found out for him *mete*,
Which (as recorded is in holy-Write)
Almighty God himself did count most fit,
And *join'd* one to him for *Society*,
Which argues plainly that *good Company*

May lawfully be kept, which may improve
*Virtues* and *graces* in us, and our love                                (480)
Increase in one another and invite
Each to good works and thereunto incite.
That man who hath no *friend* must needs be *sad*,
And his Condition miserable bad.
*Friendship* (that sweet and necessary tie)
At first is got by *familiarity*,
And that doth through *Acquaintance* rise, but he
That is debarr'd of all *Society*,
How anxious must his life be to him, when
He wants so chief a happiness of men?                                    (490)
To such as have been us'd unto a *Cell*,
And so accustomed themselves to dwell,
It is not irksome, no discouragement,
'Twas their own choice, and they are best content,
But those that have frequented *Company*,
And place'd there in a great *felicity*,
When unexpected *Sickness* checks delight,
And banishes *Associates* from their sight,
By a sequest'ring each from other, so,
Those dare not come to them, nor can these go—                           (500)
Oh what an ecstasy and surprise strange
This interposal causeth and what change!
How do they then like solitary doves
Bemoan their Widow'd state and dear lost loves.
So hard it is for custom to dispense
And yield to that, for which there's no defense;
Thus 'tis with many whom this *Visitation*
 Ties and Confines unto their habitation.
     And now in this my long and sharp Confinement,
By which I was depriv'd of all Employment                                (510)
That in the least might any way amount
Or turn unto a livelyhood-account,
(Which thing, next to my Children's loss, was chief
And greatest of my smart and worldly grief)
If it should here demanded be of me,
How I did brook want of *Society*,
I must confess, that loss, I found hard trial,
(And most unsav'ry 'tis without denial)
For (if I should speak freely and the truth)
*Society* I've lov'd ev'n from my youth,                                 (520)
And *Conversation* amongst *friends*, hath bin
Oft-times to me a thing delighted in,

My business also that I have, when any,
Leads me thereto, which doth depend on many.
But being thus constrain'd to house-abode,
And so withheld from following work abroad,
Also of all things else almost bereft,
This yet some solace was and comfort left,
That though debarr'd *Society* with me,
I still might have *converse* with *Book* and *Pen:*                    (530)
These (though small refuge for to fly to be)
Yet were means yielding much content to me.
(For idleness I always hate, and fly it,
Knowing no goodness ever can come by it.)
With *Pen* and *Ink* I kept my hand in ure,
Hoping this Exile would not long endure,
And such good *Books* I had (though read before)
I now found time enough to re-read o're,
With profit too (I hope) for *Information*,
Which may conduce to practice[al] *Conversation.*                    (540)
This studious course, to which I was inclin'd,
Diverted many sad thoughts from my mind
And thereby did that saying versify,
"When most alone, then least alone was I."

**The Conclusion**

   I Fear if it should now here be inquir'd
The Answer should be that my Reader's tir'd.
My Discourse, therefore, on this sad *occasion*
I'll break off and conclude with *exhortation.*
(For here I would a word or two wedge in
In season, which upon my friends might win)                    (550)
To such, whom God hath *hid* and heads did *cover*,
Whilst the destroying *Angel* did pass over,
Who, like the *Israelites* in *Goshen* dwelt,
In midst of *Judgments*, and yet nothing felt,
Or like to *brands*, which from the *fire* were snatch'd
When thousands round about I'th *flame* were catch'd
Who, with *distinguish'd mercy* to this day,
Have had their *lives* giv'n to them for a *prey:*[4]
How are these bound, by special *Obligation*
To pray God for this signal *preservation?*                    (560)
And thankfully record his mercies high,

---

4    *For a prey.* As a reward for righteousness .

Living up to them in sincerity?
Let these take heed not fearless be secure,
Since there can none of one day's life be sure.
God's scourge is not thrown quite out of this hand,
His *Judgments* still doth hover o're the *Land*,
And whoso marched not I'th *Van* last year,
May be press'd this, and made to bring up the Rear.[5]
What, though the *Death-bill's* now but low amount,
Who knows whose lot may fall in *next week's Count?*          (570)
    Let therefore none presume here to deprive
Almighty God of his *Prerogative*;
I mean, by *censuring*, let that remain
To him, to whom it only doth pertain,
Nor let them dare into his *Counsels* pry—
These secrets be (*Arcana Imperii*).[6]
All *actings* here have not their *reasons* given,
And he'll fall short that fetches them from *Heaven*.
Think not that where *affliction's* rod is sent,
There always is deserv'd most *punishment*.          (580)
(This was *Job's* friends' fault, and it is related
To be avoided, and not imitated)
God hath his sev'ral *ends*, past finding out,
In all his *Dispensations*, without doubt;
As for *trials*, some *examples* made
That others may look on and be afraid,
And when a public *Judgment's* on a Land,
His precious ones do feel his angry *hand*
As well as others, and recorded lies
In *Sacred Writ* by *Solomon* the wise,          (590)
That as *to bad* so doth *to good* befall,
And all things here happen alike to *all*;
As *Common mercy* unto all is sent,
So *gen'ral Judgments* have the like extent.
Yet God as a free *Agent* worketh still:
He spares, or strikes, according to his will.
If he says, "Strike," *Death* must and will come in,
For *Death* we know is the reward of *Sin*.
Whoso hath no *Sin*, then only *he*
From *Sickness* is exempt and from *Death free*,          (600)
but if none such, let all be then concluded,

---

   [5]   *Van ... press'd this.* Who was not enlisted in Death's Vanguard last year may be pressed into Death's service this year.

   [6]   *Arcana Imperii.* State secrets of the empire.

As under *Sin*, so not from *wrath* excluded.
What now remains? But that we all submit
Unto his *providence*, as is most fit,
Waiting his *will*, and let us moderate
Our *fears*, which often are inordinate.
    Oh whereby may I, or who is't that can
Fully describe the Plague-affrighted man!
'Twere well we could the *Pest* o'th *Soul* so shun,
As we do from the *Body's sickness* run,         (610)
And regulate our *lives*, so that we may
Stand in the *breach*, and turn God's *wrath* away.
Thus we by true *repentance* might prevent
His high displeasure and our punishment,
Then needed not our *fears* so to possess us,
Having God's *promise* in his *Word* to bless us.
Shall *passing-bells* for dying men afflict us?
And not the *Judgments* of our God affright us?
Shall Weekly Bills of Parish-Clerks more move us
Than *Oracles* of Ministers improve us?         (620)
Would we then *fly*, because we fear *Infection*?
Let's *fly* under the *wings* of God's *protection*;
Let us our hearty *pray'rs* to him direct,
Avoid the *Cause*, and so prevent *th'Effect*.

**POSTSCRIPT**

This ne'r intended was t'have seen the light
Had not some friends importun'd me, it might,
But since 'tis so, a further boon I crave,
Under your wings it may protection have.
FINIS

\*

# Christopher Pitt,
## *The Plague of Marseilles*

At least nineteen copies of this poem from 1721 (The Eighteenth Century; reel 7446, no.02) exist in British Isles and North American libraries. Preceding the poem is a prose preface "To the Reader," and following it is an advertisement for books "Just Published, and Sold by J. BATEMAN at the *Hat* and *Star*, and J. NICKS, at the *Dolphin* and *Crown*, both in St. Paul's Churchyard."

THE PLAGUE
of
MARSEILLES
A
POEM
By a Person of Quality

*Tristius haud illo Monstrum, nec saevior ulla*
*Pestis and ira Deum Stygiis sese extulit undis.*[1]
Virgil
LONDON
Printed for J. BATEMAN, at the *Hat* and *Star*,
And J. NICKS, at the *Dolphin* and *Crown*,
Both in *St. Paul's Churchyard*. 1721.
(Price Six Pence)

Why with such Care will poor deluded Man
His Moment shorten and contract his Span—
The Sport of ev'ry treach'rous Passion made,
By all caress'd and yet by all betray'd?
He blindly hugs the faithless Guests within,
Lost in the mazy Labyrinths of sin,
His God, by Earth-born Insolence, defy'd.
The Puny Mortal swells with Giant Pride,
And Scales the sky, by fond Ambition driv'n
To tempt the sacred Majesty of Heav'n,                    (10)
Assaults the Almighty's everlasting Throne,
Nor lets him lay th'uplifted Thunder down.
    Awake at length, thou drowsy World, awake.
Hear, O ye Realms and Kingdoms! Hear and shake,
To see that Vengeance which you never felt!
Rouse from this stupid Lethargy of Guilt.
Rouse and attend to Heav'n's Decrees in haste,
Or else this Sleep of Sin will be your last.
    For lo! the Great JEHOVAH, from the skies,
Bears his red Arm and bids his Vengeance rise,            (20)
Over all the Nations shakes his Iron Rod;
The World shall groan beneath the Hands of God.
    Lo! the Destroying Angel by Command,
(The Heav'nly Sword all flaming in his Hand)
Leads out his Host of Judgments to their Prey,
In dreadful Pomp and terrible Array.

---

[1] *Pestis .... undis.* No monster more baneful than these, no fiercer plague or wrath of
the gods ever rose from the Stygian waves. Virgil, *Aeneid,* in Fairclough, 3.214–215, pages
362–63.

I see, I see, the Sword of God display'd,
In horrid Circles waves the brandish'd Blade.
From far the formidable Glory streams,
And shoots a baleful Length of dismal Beams. (30)
I see the purple Glutton gorg'd with Food,
Pamper'd with Death and surfeited with Blood.
Grim Fate with Famine in the Front appear;
Behind, the sweeping Pestilence and War.
    Unhappy *Gallia*! for what tow'ring Crimes,
Unmatched in Guilt, unparallel'd by Times,
Are thy wide Realms to this Destruction giv'n?
Thy sons thrown out into the Wrath of Heav'n?
That first thy Kingdoms are by Fate ordained
To feel the Weight of the Almighty's Hand, (40)
Curst with the sad Preeminence of Woe,
That swept away whole Nations at a Blow.
    The dreadful Pest from *Sidon's* guilty Shores,
With fatal Course, reach'd fair *Massilia's* Tow'rs.
On Her she lavish'd her infectious Breath,
Her Funds of Poison and her Stores of Death.
With a resistless Rage the Fury came,
Nor could the Length of Oceans quench the Flame.
Wrapped on the gloomy Pinions of the Wind,
She flew and left her native Realms behind. (50)
The loaded Winds were heard to groan and roar,
As if they mourn'd the Ruin which they bore.
    And now to aid the Pestilential Flame,
From Angry Heav'n a mortal Influence came.
From sullen Stars the mingled Poisons flow,
Who gleam Destruction on the World below,
Like Comets shoot malignant Beams from Far,
Like them with livid Plagues they taint the Air.
High o'er the Walls the tow'ring Fury soars,
Marks out the Realm and measures round the Shores. (60)
O'er the devoted land extends her Bound,
And draws the Line of Desolation round.
    But oh! what Numbers can be found to show
In all its Forms th'Extravagance of Woe!
In the soft Impotence of Tears to grieve,
Is all the sad Variety can give.
The Scene's vast; the Images so strong,
They leave behind the Energy of Song.
    The Pestilential Pow'rs the Haven seize,
And blow in Death at once and the disease. (70)
From thence divided, the grim Terrors pass'd

Thro' ev'ry Street and laid the city wast[e].
What is this Victor whose unbounded force,
O'er Bulwarks breaks, with unresisted Course?
Scorns to attack like other Foes in Form,
And takes, without a Siege, the town by Storm.
While Nations feel his unrelenting ire,
And a whole People in one Groan expire.
    The Foe first storm'd with his tremendous Train
The Head, the fair Metropolis of Man,                                    (80)
And seiz'd of that, the Purple Monster knew
It could with Ease th' inferior Pow'rs subdue.
In dizzy Rounds and Whirls, the tortur'd Brain
Confest th'Extremities of mortal Pain;
That Seat of Reason, where the Soul of late
Reigned o'er the rest in Intellectual State,
Lies now dismantled by the barbarous Foe,
Who lays the towring Height of Reason low,
And tears (insulting o'er the gaudy Prey)
The painted Scenes of Memory away.                                       (90)
O'er the distracted Fancy wildly roam,
Ten Thousand Images of Things to come.
In all her Shapes, Confusion seems to rise,
Eternal Horrors swim before their Eyes.
As o'er their Minds the horrid Phantoms go;
Ev'n now they feel th'imaginary Woe,
But dread no greater Pains, no heavier Doom,
Than what they suffer Here, before they come
To the last cold Retirement of Tomb.
    Next to the Heart the swift Contagion came,                      (100)
And brought new Heats unto the nat'ral Flame.
From thence the propagated Monster ran,
Fir'd ev'ry Part, and boil'd in ev'ry Vein:
Thro' all the Streams of Life its Course pursu'd,
And follow'd round the circulating Blood.
    The Lungs, whose vital Airs once fann'd the Heart,
Forget their Office now, and kindle ev'ry Part.
No more the Fibers with soft Breath inspire,
But blow the Flames and aggravate the Fire.
Still the Contagious Pow'rs their Conquest stretched,                    (110)
And bar up all the Avenues of Speech.
The wild Infection grown more bold and strong,
Untunes th' harmonious Organs of the Tongue.
The Sap of Life in ev'ry Vessel dries
And drinks the vital Juices as it flies.
Gasping in Death, the Wretches strive in vain,

With streaming Tears to calm the glowing Pain.
For ev'n their Tears are lost, the sad Relief,
To soothe the last Extremities of Grief.
The spreading Flame exhausts the closing Eye,                    (120)
Drinks up, and leaves the Crystal Sluices dry.
Insatiate Tyrant! whose unbounded Will,
Not yet contented with the Pow'r to kill,
Bids the poor dying Wretch, his Groans forego—
His Groans, the common Charter of his Woe—
Deny'd to mourn the Miseries he bears,
And barr'd th'unhappy Privilege of Tears.
　　　Stay, dreadful Plague, thy rapid Fury stay.
Lie down a while, and slumber o'er thy Prey.
Allow thy busy Pestilence at least                              (130)
Some gentle Pause, some Interval for Rest.
Dream of past Conquests o'er Destruction spread;
Brood o'er thy Heaps and Mountains of thy Dead.
Ah no! the raging Monster scorns to hear
The Force of Sighs or Eloquence of Pray'r.
What Arms, what Methods can withstand this Foe,
Who gathers Strength from ev'ry fatal Blow?
　　　Unblest *Massilia*! how wer't thou before
The lawful Pride of *Gallia's* Southern Shore?
From all his Bounds the Tributary Sea                           (140)
Paid then the Homage of his Waves to Thee.
Thy floating Tow'rs adorn'd thy guarded Side,
And *Asia's* Wealth flowed in with ev'ry Tide.
Such once was *Athens*, such her prosperous State,
Till such as Thine the Measures of her Fate.
Oh! could my Bosom with such Raptures glow
As His, who sung her memorable Woe?[2]
So just my Fire, so regular my Rage,
Thy bleeding Wounds should stream thro' ev'ry Age.
With Thine Posterity should mix their Tears;                     (150)
Thy Groans should echo through the length of Years.
Yet those loud Groans, and these low Strains confess,
Thy Woes are greater, as my Skill is less.
　　　How does the City mourn her dreadful Fate,
That pour'd forth Thousands once at ev'ry Gate?
How is the Queen of Nations fall'n from high?
How does she see her Tribes confus'dly die?
She that o'er Kingdoms rear'd her tow'ry Head,
And aw'd old *Ocean* in his inmost Bed,

---

[2]　[marginal note] Dr. Sprat.

Her wealthy Merchants then like Kings in Pow'r,                                        (160)
Her active Traffic stretched from Shore to Shore,
But now the solitary Mother moans,
In all the Rage of Grief, her slaughter'd Sons.
    So wept proud *Memphis* when by Fury driv'n,
Her Tyrant dar'd th' Omnipotence of Heav'n.
When the destroying Angel from on High.
Flew charg'd with all the Terrors of the Sky,
On a proud pointed Pyramid he stood,
Let loose the Plague, and pointed out its Road,
And breathed out all the Vengeance of his God.                                        (170)
    But yet when *Egypt* felt the mighty Woe,
The Chosen Race escap'd the gen'ral Blow.
The Angel read the Character Divine,
Passed by with Rev'rence and ador'd the Sign;
Of God's own Foes, the First-born only slew.
O'er all the rest, he innocently flew.
Is such *Massilia* thy distinguish'd Fate!
Condemn'd to drink the Dregs of heav'nly Hate?
When the Commission'd Angel went abroad,
On thy sad Doors he found no Pledge from God,                                          (180)
No kind Divine Protection writ in Blood.
'Twas hence the delegated Vengeance ran,
And slew thy Sons by Nations, not by Men.
    Oh! with what Pangs I tremble to relate,
The horrid Scenes and Mysteries of Fate!
The dreadful Spectacles of Death to view,
And trace the vast Variety of Woe!
Old Age feels here th'inexorable Doom;
There sinks the sprightly Youth in all his Bloom.
In vain the Tim'rous would Protection find;                                            (190)
The winged Fate arrests him from behind.
Soon as the Wretch resigns his tainted Breath,
His last sad Gasp communicates his Death.
The Fury now, her boundless Pow'rs to spread,
Calls out again her Poisons from the Dead.
From all th'envenom'd Mass of putrid blood,
She darts the pointed Pestilence abroad.
So, some brave HERO, when his foe is slain,
Tugs out his spear and launches it again.
    Now ev'ry Street, a Pile of Death had crown'd,                         (200)
And one promiscuous Carnage heap'd the Ground.
What fatal Vapors from the Dead arise
In livid Streams and float along the Skies!
What Clouds of Poison stain the Heav'ns purer Ray,

Taint the clear Air and violate the Day!
A thousand Ways the swift Contagion takes,
Flows with the Streams or stagnates with the Lakes,
O'er the wide Sea in fatal Triumph rides,
Born high, and wafted by the bounding Tides.
The Winds infected with the fatal Breath,                          (210)
Bear on their sooty Wings the Scents of Death.
And each confed'rate Element ally'd
Declares for Heav'n and scourges Human Pride.
　　　Here, ov'r her tender Babe, a Mother smil'd,
And gaz'd with eager Fondness on the Child,
The clinging infant to her Bosom prest,
And strain'd the pleasing Burden to her Breast.
The little lovely Innocent as yet
Hung at the breast, unconscious of his Fate,
Nor thought he drew his Death in that sad Hour,                   (220)
From whence he drew the Means of Life before.
　　　There lay the faithful Husband and his Wife,
A while both hover'd o'er the Verge of Life.
Now Hand in Hand through Death's dark Paths they move,
Nor the last Moment can divide their Love.
Still join'd they share the universal Doom
And mix their last Embraces in the Tomb.
　　　Here dying Fathers to their Sons bequeath
At once their Riches and at once their Death.
To the same Fate th'unhappy Sons resign'd                          (230)
Soon leave the same sad Legacy behind.
There too, the Merchant's closing Eyes behold,
His Heaps of Wealth and Pyramids of Gold,
Though from the rifled East his Vessels come,
And in proud Triumph bring all *Asia* Home.
Yet what avail his Ships with Riches stor'd
To calm the Pains and Tortures of their Lord?
Not his vast Treasures can extend his Date,
Nor buy one Moment from the Hands of Fate.
　　　Others, who catch their Friends' departing Breath,            (240)
Join in the dark Society of Death.
In vain each breaths his tributary Groan,
For while they mourn his Fate, they meet their own.
They take one melancholy last Embrace,
Then sleep together in the Arms of Peace.
　　　The Earth no more a kind Reception gave:
The Dead crowd up the Chambers of the Grave,
In num'rous Sholes the swarming Specters go,
And fleeting Crowds fill all the Realms below.

Hell throws in vain her gloomy Portals wide, (250)
And stretches out her Bounds on ev'ry Side,
Tho' yet too narrow for the mighty Tide.
 With joy the vultures scent the distant Prey,
And call in haste their feathered Tribes away.
Bent on the Banquet, flies the gath'ring Crowd,
And ov'r the Dead descends the living Cloud.
Lur'd by the Feast, the hungry Savage roves,
Leaves his wild Mountains and his native Groves,
With sullen Pride and with a stern Disdain
To gorge so largely on his Sovereign, Man, (260)
But e'er he tasted, from his Prey he fled,
And fears his ancient Terror, now he's dead.
From the dire Banquet hastes the greedy Guest,
And finds a Famine in too full a Feast.
 And now each gloomy Ghost, each wand'ring Sprite,
Who sport and wanton in the Mask of Night,
Who roam malignant thro' this World below,
And triumph in th' Excess of Human Woe,
O'er the tall Piles of Carcasses advance,
And o'er the Waste of Desolation dance. (280)
In Consort mixt, their midnight Revels ply
Nor see one solitary Face go by.
The stars alone their hideous Forms affright,
And the sick moon grows paler at the Sight.
 Genius of *Britain*, with Indulgence hear,
The sighs of *Albion* and the Poet's Prayer:
Exert thy utmost tutelary care,
To curb this purple Tyrant's lawless Pow'r.
Stretch thy auspicious Wings from Shore to Shore.
To guard her Natives from the dire Disease, (290)
Oppose the watery Bulwark of her Seas.
Screen all her Kingdoms from the fierce Attack.
Bid the kind Tempests blow her Poisons back.
Bid the devouring Plague this Island spare,
Nor stretch her Circle of Destruction here.
Or if thy delegated Pow'r is gone,
Fall low before Heav'n's everlasting Throne,
And make the Cause of *Britain's* Realm thy own.
To stay the Vengeance of thy God, appear
Armed with the sacred Violence of Pray'r (300)
Present the Incense of thy Britain's Vows.
Weigh down eternal Justice with her Woes,
Till her Repentance wrests away the Rod,
And sheath the Sword of an offended God.
FINIS

# General Glossary

*abstruse.* Concealed, hidden, secret.

*accite.* To arouse, to excite.

*aculeate.* Furnished with a sting.

*affrappeth.* To strike against.

*against.* Facing, in front of, in full view of.

*agrade.* From Italian *gradire* to be pleased with.

*ague.* An acute or violent fever.

*amain.* In or with full force.

*amort.* In the state or act of death; lifeless, inanimate.

*analeptic.* Restorative medicine.

*anchorite.* A person who has withdrawn or secluded himself or herself from the world, usually for religious reasons.

*angelica. Angelica archangelica*: a common perennial herb with large compound umbels of white or greenish-white flowers.

*apoplexy.* A malady, very sudden in its attack, which arrests more or less completely the powers of sense and motion; it is usually caused by an effusion of blood or serum in the brain, and preceded by giddiness, partial loss of muscular power, etc.

*apostrophe.* A figure of speech, by which a speaker or writer suddenly stops discourse and turns to address pointedly some person or thing, often in an exclamatory address, common in epic poetry.

*arrant.* Errand; short journey; referring to the arrant journey of a knight, for example.

*artificer.* Artisan.

*askant.* Askance; to turn aside.

*attinent.* Related, belonging to.

*axle-trees.* The fixed bar or beam of wood on the rounded ends of which the opposite wheels of a carriage revolve.

*augurist.* Augur; a soothsayer, diviner, or prophet, generally; one that foretells the future.

*auxiliary.* Helpful, assistant, affording aid, rendering assistance, giving support or succor.

*aye.* Ever, always, eternally; yes, even so.

*bale.* Evil, especially considered in its active operation, as destroying, blasting, injuring, etc.

*balm.* A healing, soothing agent or agency, also called a balsam.

*bane.* That which causes death, or destroys life.

*baron.* The lowest rank in the nobility, just below *viscount.*

*basilisk.* A fabulous reptile, also called a *cockatrice*, alleged to be hatched by a serpent from a cock's egg; ancient authors stated that its hissing drove away all other serpents, and that its breath, and even its look, was fatal.

*bearer.* One who helps to carry a corpse to the grave, or who holds the pall in a funeral procession.

*behest.* Vow or promise.

*beldame.* An aged woman, especially with depreciative sense: a loathsome old woman, a hag; a witch; a furious raging woman.

*besom.* A bundle of rods or twigs used for sweeping or as an instrument of punishment.

*besought.* Sought after.

*bewray.* Expose by divulging secrets.

*bezoar stone.* Various substances formerly held as antidotes: specifically, a calculus or concretion found in the stomach or intestines of some animals, chiefly those that chew cud.

*bier.* Movable stand on which a corpse, whether in a coffin or not, is placed before burial; that on which it is carried to the grave.

*bile.* The bitter fluid secreted by the liver, of a brownish yellow color, passing sometimes into green; one of the 'four humors' of early physiology, also called yellow bile or *choler*, supposed to cause irascibility of temper.

*billet.* A short written document; a small paper, notice, or note.

*billeted.* Quartered by billet (official order), the addressee to provide board and lodging for the soldier bearing it.

*bill-man.* A soldier armed with a bill; see *brownbill.*

*blain.* An inflammatory swelling or sore on the surface of the body, often accompanied by ulceration; a blister, botch, pustule.

*blastings.* The production of blasts of wind or breath; sometimes also flatulence.

*blithe.* Compassionate.

*botch.* A hump; a swelling; a tumor, wen, or goiter.

*bourd.* Make a jest or game of.

*brake.* A clump of bushes, brushwood, or briers.

*brawler.* A quarrelsome, wrangling fellow; a breaker of the peace.

*broker.* Pawnbroker.

*brownbill.* A kind of halberd painted brown, formerly used by foot-soldiers and watchmen.

*brown-paper merchants.* Tradesmen who wrap their goods in cheap, course brown paper.

*bruising.* To crush, pound, or grind down; a process used to prepare food and medicine.

*bulwarks.* A substantial defensive work of earth, or other material; a rampart, a fortification.

*busse.* Kiss.

*caitiff.* A base, mean, despicable 'wretch', a villain.

*canicular.* Of or pertaining to the dog-days; see dog-days.

*cans.* Vessels for holding liquids.

*capon.* Castrated cock.

*carbuncle.* Any of various inflammatory or infective lesions of the skin, so named after the fiery red precious stone of that name.

*carle.* See *churl.*

*carnal policy.* Secular policy.

*carrier.* Any person undertaking, for payment, the transport of goods by land or water.

*carter.* A person of low birth.

*cassock.* A kind of long loose coat or gown.

*cater.* A buyer of provisions or 'cates'; in large households the officer who made the necessary purchases of provisions; caterer.

*cat.* A lofty work used in fortifications and sieges.

*cavil.* To object, dispute.

*cawsy.* A mound, embankment or dam, to retain the water of a river or pond.

*chamber.* A room in a house.

*chancel.* The eastern part of a church, appropriated to the use of those who officiate in the performance of the services, separated from the other parts by a screen or railing.

*chapman.* A person whose business is buying and selling; a merchant, trader, dealer.

*chastment.* Chastisement, punishment.

*charet.* A wheeled vehicle or conveyance.

*cherubin.* In certain biblical expressions describing the seat or dwelling of the Deity; angelic.

*choler.* See *bile.*

*chuff.* Any disliked person; specifically, a miser or close avaricious man.

*churl.* Used as a term of disparagement or contempt; base fellow, villain.

*cinque port.* Applied to the five senses; originally a group of sea-ports (originally five, whence the name) situated on the south-east coast of England.

*clacking.* The making of a sharp, hard noise.

*clark.* Clerk. After the Reformation, the lay officer of a parish church.

*clog.* A block or heavy piece of wood, or the like, attached to the leg or neck of a person or a beast, to impede motion or prevent escape.

*coact.* Coerce.

*coarse.* Corpse.

*cock-high.* Mounted aloft, perched up; cock-horse.

*cockatrice.* A serpent, identified with the basilisk. See *basilisk.*

*colic.* See *wind colic.*

*collops.* An egg fried on bacon; fried ham and eggs.

*common-weal.* The welfare of a country or community; the general good. See *weal.*

*concomitant.* An attendant state, quality, circumstance, or thing; an accompaniment.

*conveyancer.* A lawyer who prepares documents for the conveyance of property and investigates titles to property; also used to denote a thief.

*cope.* The over-arching canopy or vault of heaven.

*copse.* A thicket of small trees or underwood periodically cut for economic purposes.

*cordial.* A medicine to comfort or invigorate the heart.

*corsive.* Corrosive.

*cormorant.* Insatiably greedy.

*cowherd.* One whose occupation is to tend cows at pasture.

*craven-cock.* Self-acknowledged weakling or coward in a match.

*cruciate.* To afflict with grievous pain or distress.

*damps.* Exhalations, of vapor or gas, of a noxious kind.

*dankish.* Somewhat dank, humid.

*diapason.* Complete concord, harmony, or agreement.

*discommend.* To find fault with, express disapprobation of: the opposite of recommend.

*disgest.* To distribute.

*dog days.* The days about the time of the rising of the Dog Star, Sirius, the hottest time of the year linked with the visitation of the plague.

*dolor.* Physical suffering, pain. In the plural, *dolors* means diseases.

*doughty.* Virtuous; valiant, brave.

*dragon water.* A medicinal preparation, possibly consisting of water infused with dragons (*Dracunculus vulgaris*), a perennial plant with a distinctive purple-black spike enfolded in a similarly colored sheathing leaf.

*drench.* A medicinal, soporific, or poisonous draught, often forcibly given.

*dross.* Dreggy, impure, or foreign matter, mixed with any substance, and detracting from its purity.

*effrene.* Unbridled.

*eftsoons.* A second time again.

*eke.* Also; in addition.

*embulked.* Made bulky.

*entrail-racking-laxes.* Entrail torturing diarrhea.

*erst.* First in time or serial order.

*esquire.* A man belonging to the higher order of English gentry, ranking immediately below a knight.

*estates.* Groups in a community.

*exequies.* Funeral rites or ceremony.

*exitial.* Hurtful; destructive to life, deadly, fatal.

*exul.* Exile.

*eyne.* Eyes.

*fain.* Glad, rejoiced, well-pleased.

*falling-ill.* Epilepsy.

*farrier.* One who shoes horses; a shoeing-smith; also one who treats the diseases of horses.

*farthing.* The quarter of a penny; the coin representing this value.

*fell.* Fierce, ruthless; dreadful; destructive; enraged.

*fen.* Low land covered wholly or partially with shallow water; a marsh.

*film.* Membrane.

*fire-drake.* A fiery meteor or kind of firework.

*fire-spitting cat.* See cat.

*flux.* A morbid bodily discharge; an early name for dysentery.

*foins.* Thrusts with a pointed weapon.

*forsooth.* In truth; truly.

*foisting.* Practicing roguery, cheating.

*foot-cloth.* A large richly-ornamented cloth laid over the back of a horse and hanging down to the ground on each side, considered a mark of dignity.

*fondling.* A 'fond' or foolish person.

*foretimes.* Former times.

*freedom.* See *liberties*.

*frenzy.* Mental derangement.

*furlong.* The length of the furrow in the common field, theoretically regarded as a square containing ten acres.

*galping.* Gaping; yawing; vomiting.

*gentle-craft.* Shoemaker.

*glozing.* Flattering; deceitful blandishment.

*God wot.* God knows: used to emphasize the truth of a statement.

*gormandizing.* Excessively and voraciously eating; eating like a glutton.

*granado.* Grenade.

*granard.* Granary.

*griping.* Spasms of pain, pangs of grief or affliction. Also, the covetous actions of a miser or usurer.

*groat.* A coin equal to four pence in value and in weight, or one-eighth of an ounce of silver. *grove-idolatry.* Heathen worship in groves of trees in honor of deities, the groves often planted for that purpose.

*grutch.* To complain.

*halberd.* A military weapon: combination of spear and battle-axe, consisting of a sharp-edged blade ending in a point, and a spear-head, mounted on a handle five to seven feet long.

*halcyon.* Calm, quietude, halcyon days.

*hamlet.* A group of houses or small village in the country; *esp.* a village without a church, included in the parish belonging to another village or a town.

*haven.* Port.

*haw.* The fruit of the hawthorn.

*haycock.* A conical heap of hay in a field.

*herb of grace.* See *rue.*

*hests.* Biddings, commands.

*hie.* To hasten, speed, go quickly.

*hight.* To call, to name.

*hild.* To flay or strip the skin off.

*hind.* Female deer.

*holp.* Help.

*holpen.* Helped.

*imbellic.* Unwarlike.

*imp.* To engraft feathers in the wing of a bird, so as to make good losses or deficiencies, and thus restore or improve the powers of flight.

*impostume.* A purulent swelling or cyst in any part of the body; an abscess.

*incontinently.* Straightway, at once.

*Indianist.* User of tobacco.

*indite.* To utter, suggest, or inspire a form of words which is to be repeated or written down.

*ingenuously.* Honorably straightforward.

*inned.* Taken in, gathered in (as a crop).

*innest.* To age or mature as in a nest, to in-nest.

*insimulating.* Accusing.

*interposal.* Interposition.

*jars.* Quarrels.

*jerk.* A stroke with a whip or wand, a stripe, a lash.

*jerffe.* Giraffe.

**junkets.** Confections, sweets.

**kindles.** Without natural power, affection, feeling, etc.; unnatural.

**landship.** A vehicle serving the same purpose on land as a ship on the sea; a ship erected and kept on land for training purposes.

**lax.** Looseness of the bowels; diarrhea.

**leathern.** Made of leather; leather-like.

**liberties.** Areas of local administration distinct from neighboring territory and possessing a degree of independence.

**liver-grown.** Suffering from an enlarged liver, the liver also associated with cowardliness and   courage: lily-livered versus hot livered.

**lowne.** Person of low birth.

**lucubrations.** Nocturnal studies or meditations.

**manes.** The spirit or shade of a dead person, considered as an object of homage or reverence.

**mare mortuum.** The Dead Sea; figuratively sea of death.

**mass-monger.** A Roman Catholic, especially a priest.

**mattock.** A tool similar to a pick but with a point or chisel edge at one end of the head and an axe-like blade at the other, used for breaking up hard ground.

**maugre.** Notwithstanding; in spite of everything.

**maul.** Sledgehammer.

**meanders.** Patterns.

**meed.** Recompense.

**megrim.** Headache; migraine.

**mell.** Mingle; mix.

**meridian.** Of or relating to midday or noon.

**mess.** A serving of food.

**meskite.** Mesquite, mosque.

**mickle.** Much; great.

**minster.** A monastery or religious house.

**mishrump.** Upstart, deriving from the concept of the mushroom.

**mite.** Money or coin of a small or insignificant amount, as *not worth a mite.*

**mithridate.** Mithridatum, any of various medicinal preparations, usually electuaries compounded of many ingredients.

*mittimus.* A warrant issued by a justice of the peace, etc., committing a person to custody. To "make a mittimus" often means "to arrest."

*modey.* A version of moody: brave, bold, high-spirited, passionate; angry, wrathful.

*mold.* The ground considered as a place of burial; the earth of a grave; a grave.

*mole.* A person who works underground; a person who works in darkness or in secrecy.

*mollify.* To make soft or supple.

*moorish.* Boggy, marshy.

*morglay.* Sword.

*mould.* The top or dome of the head.

*mountainet.* A small mountain; a hillock, mound.

*mountebank.* An itinerant charlatan who sold supposed medicines and remedies.

*muckhill.* Muck-heap, manure heap.

*mummeries.* Ridiculous ceremonies, named for Mummer's (mimed) play.

*murrain.* Infectious disease, especially that striking animals.

*muster.* To assemble (v.); an assembly (n.).

*narcotic.* A drug which when swallowed, inhaled, or injected into the system induces drowsiness, stupor, or insensibility, according to its strength and the amount taken; *esp.* an opiate.

*ne.* A simple negative.

*negro.* In extended use: a dark or black type of animal or plant.

*niggard.* A mean, stingy, or parsimonious person.

*obit.* An office or service, usually a mass, held to pray for the soul of or otherwise commemorate a deceased person.

*oblation.* The presentation of money, goods, property, etc., to the Church for use in God's service.

*onsets.* Attacks; onslaughts.

*oraculous.* Oracular; of or relating to an oracle.

*ostent.* A portent or sign; a wonder, a prodigy.

*outparish.* A parish lying outside the walls or municipal boundaries of a city or town, but often associated with it.

*outroads.* An act of riding out; *esp.* a warlike excursion or raid.

*outwork.* Any part of the fortifications of a place lying outside the parapet, erected for defense.

*palsy.* Paralysis or paresis (weakness) of all or part of the body, sometimes with tremor.

*panders.* People who assists the immoral urges or evil designs of others.

*pare.* Cut; prune.

*partisan.* A type of spear with a long, triangular, double-edged blade.

*pash.* To hurl or throw violently.

*pate.* Head.

*paunch.* The stomach of a person or of an animal.

*peers.* Peerage; members of the upper class; nobility.

*pelf.* Stolen goods.

*penmen.* A clerk, notary, scrivener.

*pence.* Plural for *penny.*

*penny.* The smallest form of British coin used also as a weight in recipes and abbreviated *d.* for *denarius*, the Greek coin considered to be roughly of the same weight both of the penny and of the drachma, the basis for the dram.

*perdu.* Designating a sentinel's position which is so dangerous that death is almost inevitable; desperate; lost.

*petty.* Of secondary or lesser importance, rank, or scale; minor; subordinate.

*poetaster.* An inferior poet; a mere versifier.

*philter.* Love potion.

*phlegm.* One of the four cardinal humors, described as cold and moist, and supposed when predominant to cause constitutional indolence or apathy.

*pike.* A weapon consisting of a long wooden shaft with a pointed steel head.

*pied.* Dappled, speckled; metaphorically variable, inconstant, flawed.

*plaint.* Audible expression of sorrow.

*plaster.* A solid medicinal or emollient substance spread on a bandage or dressing and applied to the skin, often becoming adhesive at body temperature.

*plight.* To give in pledge.

*ploughswain.* Ploughman.

*plush.* A rich fabric of silk, cotton, wool, or other material.

*poetaster.* An inferior poet; a writer of poor or trashy verse; a mere versifier.

*poliza.* Policy.

*polling.* Cheating.

*postern.* A back or side entrance; any door, gate, etc.

*posthume.* A posthumous work.

*potsherd.* A fragment of pottery, a shard.

*prolixity.* Tedious lengthiness of spoken or written matter.

*proselytes.* Converts.

*prospectious.* Forward looking vision.

*puling.* Whining, plaintive piping or crying; a complaint.

*purples.* Any dark red or purplish lesion of the skin.

*puttock.* Bird of prey.

*quacksalver.* Quack; a person who dishonestly claims knowledge of or skill in medicine.

*quail.* To be suppressed, crushed, vanquished.

*qualm.* Death, esp. of a violent nature; (also) an instance of this.

*ramage.* Wild; untamed.

*rank.* Affected by or resulting from putrefaction; festering, rotten; contaminated.

*rape.* To take or seize (something) by force.

*raught.* To reach *after*, grasp.

*rave.* Rake, drag.

*reave.* Plunder; deprive; raid.

*recule.* Recoil.

*refection.* Refreshment with food or drink after hunger or fatigue.

*relive.* Resuscitate.

*remoted.* Remote, distant.

*restive.* Characterized by erratic or adverse behavior arising from discontent, disquiet.

*rheum.* Watery or mucous secretions, esp. as collecting in or dripping from the eyes, nose, or mouth.

*rife.* Widespread.

*rill.* Rivulet.

*rising.* A Swelling or tumor.

*roundelay.* A short simple song with a refrain.

*rout.* A company, assemblage, band, or troop of persons.

*rover.* Pirate; marauder, robber.

*rue.* *Ruta graveolens*: a perennial evergreen shrub having bitter, strong-scented leaves; also called *herb of grace.*

*ruffle.* To behave proudly or arrogantly.

*rurigene.* Rural.

*russet.* Rustic, homely, simple.

*ruth.* Pity, compassion.

*sallate.* Salad; a dish of cold herbs or vegetables.

*sconce.* A small fort or earthwork; especially one built to defend a ford, pass, castle-gate, etc.

*score.* A group or set of twenty.

*scutcheon.* Escutcheon; the shield or shield-shaped surface on which a coat of arms is depicted.

*sempiternal.* Enduring constantly and continually; everlasting, eternal.

*septum lucidum.* *Pellucidum*, a thin double layer of tissue forming a partition between the two lateral ventricles of the brain.

*serene.* A light fall of moisture or fine rain after sunset in hot countries, regarded as a noxious dew or mist.

*sexton.* A church officer with oversight of material affairs: ringing the bells, digging graves.

*shags.* A garment, rug, or mat of shaggy material.

*shamefast.* Ashamed.

*shark.* Applied to persons, with allusion to the predatory habits and voracity of the shark; one who enriches himself or herself by taking advantage of the necessities of others; a rapacious usurer, an extortionate landlord or letter of lodgings, etc.

*shend.* Defend, shield.

*shent.* Disgraced.

*shilling.* A silver coin the equivalent in value and weight of 12 pence.

*shoal.* A large number of persons thronging together or classed together.

*shuttlecock.* A small piece of cork, or similar light material, fitted with a crown or circle of feathers, used in games of "battledore and shuttlecock" and badminton.

*silly.* Deserving compassion; innocent.

*simony.* The act or practice of buying or selling ecclesiastical preferments, benefices, or emoluments; traffic in sacred things.

*simples.* Medical preparation consisting or composed of one substance, ingredient, or element; uncompounded, unmixed.

*sith.* Then, thereupon; afterwards, subsequently, since.

*slight.* Display of disregard; or, small matter, trifles.

*smitten.* Beaten, struck.

*sooth.* True.

*sooth up.* To render less objectionable.

*sophistic.* Given to the use or exercise of sophistry or speculation.

*spangle.* A small round thin piece of glittering metal with a hole in the center to pass a thread through, used for the decoration of fabrics; figuratively, a star.

*spleen.* Excessive dejection or depression of spirits; gloominess and irritability; moroseness; melancholia; referred to as "the spleen."

*spotted fever.* A fever characterized by the appearance of spots on the skin.

*sprite.* Spirit, in generalized sense: a being essentially incorporeal or immaterial.

*squib.* A common species of firework, in which the burning of the composition is usually terminated by a slight explosion.

*standish.* An inkpot.

*stead.* Served; stood for.

*stew.* Brothel.

*stipendiary.* Serving for pay, mercenary.

*stone.* Kidney stones, referred to as "the stone."

*stoolball.* An old country game somewhat resembling cricket, played chiefly by young women or, as an Easter game, between young men and women.

*strappado.* Torture to extort confession, in which the victim's hands were tied from behind to a pulley, the body hoisted from the ground and let down half way with a jerk.

*strew.* To scatter, spread loosely.

*sullabubs.* A drink or dish made of milk or cream, curdled by the admixture of wine, cider, or other acid, and often sweetened and flavored.

*swan-like.* In reference to the fabled singing of the swan just before its death.

*succor.* Aid, help, assistance.

*suckling.* An infant that is at the breast or is unweaned.

*swage.* Assuage.

*swain.* Serving-man, attendant, follower.

*sweepstake.* One who 'sweeps', or takes the whole of, the stakes in a game.

*sweeting.* A 'sweet' or beloved person.

*swerve.* Shift off of course.

*tabret.* A small tabor or drum.

*teen.* Vexation.

*tell-clock.* One who tells the clock, calls the time aloud.

*tett.* Teat; nipple; dug.

*text-bill.* A short printed advertisement.

*three score.* Three times twenty; sixty.

*tippling-booth.* A temporary dwelling erected for selling ale and other strong drink.

*token.* A spot on the body indicating disease, esp. the plague.

*tradefaln.* Trade-fallen, fallen or broken in trade, bankrupt.

*travail.* Bodily or mental labor or toil, especially of a painful or oppressive nature.

*treacle.* A medicinal salve composed of many ingredients, formerly in repute as an antidote to poisons. Also called *theriac.*

*tromp.* Trumpet.

*troth.* Faithfulness, good faith, loyalty; honesty; truth.

*truss.* To strike, strike against.

*tush.* An exclamation of impatient contempt or disparagement.

*turtle mate.* Turtle dove, noted for its affection for its mate; figuratively a name denoting conjugal affection and constancy.

*untoothsome.* Unpalatable, disagreeable.

*ure.* Used as "in ure": in or into use, practice, or performance.

*urinal.* A glass vessel or phial employed to receive urine for medical examination or inspection.

*vacive.* Empty, void.

*vail.* To take off or lower, as in a hat or weapon.

*vamp.* To furnish, supply; alter.

*van.* Vanguard; the foremost portion of, or the foremost position in.

*vaunt.* Boast or brag.

*venger.* Avenger.

*vent.* To sell or vend.

*verge.* The bounds, limits, or precincts *of* a particular place. Chiefly after the preps. *within, in, out of.*

*vild.* Vile.

*virid.* Vigorously blooming, verdant, green.

*viscount.* One acting as the deputy or representative of a count or earl in the administration of a district; high sheriff.

*visement.* Consideration, deliberation, reflection, thought.

*viz.* Abbreviated form of *videlicet*; namely, that is to say.

*vulned.* Wounded.

*warisome.* Cautious or careful.

*wain.* Carry.

*weal.* Wealth; welfare. See *common-weal.*

*weare.* Worn down.

*welt*

*weltering.* Tossed about by waves.

*whenas.* At the, or a, time at which; in a case in which; when.

*whereout.* Out of which, out from which.

*whilom.* At times; at some past time.

*wicket.* A small door or gate made in or beside a large one, for ingress and egress.

*wilding.* Any wild plant or animal, often used to denote the apple or crab-apple.

*wile.* A crafty, cunning, or deceitful trick.

*wight.* Person.

*winking house.* A place where one can sleep; a place where one "winks" at the activities taking place within.

*wormwood.* The plant *Artemisia Absinthium*, proverbial for its bitter taste. The leaves and tops are used in medicine as a tonic.

*wot.* To know.

*winks.* Sleeps.

*yelping.* Boasting.

# Index of Names

*Agamemnon.* Greek mythological hero of the Trojan war.

*Aesculapius.* Classical god of medicine, son of Apollo.

*Alsop, Bernard* (d. after 1653). Printer in London often in partnership with Thomas Creed, at the sign of the Eagle and Child; after Creed's death, he partnered with Thomas Fawcett and is here identified with Fawcett as a printer for editions of Abraham Holland's poems.

*Anabaptists.* Radical Reformation Christians who, beginning in 1521 in Germany, rejected conventional Christian practices such as wearing wedding rings, taking oaths, and participating in civil government while adhering to a literal interpretation of the Sermon on the Mount and Believer's baptism.

*Appelles* (fl. 4th c. B.C.E). Renowned painter of ancient Greece.

*Aratine.* Pietro Aretino (1492–1556) Italian painter and writer known for his pornographic literature, although his works were known in early modern England primarily through reputation rather than through translation.

*Aratus* (c. 271–213 B.C.E.). Greek didactic poety, best known for *Phenomena,* on astronomy and meteorology.

*Ariadne.* In Greek mythology, daughter of King Minos of Crete, who helped Theseus overcome the Minotaur by giving Theseus a thread to help him find his way out of a labyrinth.

*Archer, Thomas.* London bookseller who flourished 1603–1634, here identified as the bookseller for Thomas Dekker and Thomas Middleton's poem.

*Archimede.* Archimedes of Syracuse (c. 287–212 B.C.E.) Legendary Greek mathematician.

*Asteria.* The Titan goddess of prophetic dreams, astrology and necromancy pursued unsuccessfully by Zeus; in the process of escape she ultimately became the island of Delos.

*Atropos.* In Greek mythology, one of the three Fates who cuts each mortal's thread of life.

*Augeas.* In Greek mythology, king of Elis known for his stables that had never been cleaned until Hercules did so as his famous fifth labor.

*Avernus.* A lake in Italy, associated by Virgil and others with the mouth of Hell. .

*Bacon, Francis* (1561–1626). 1st Viscount Saint Alban, Lord Chancellor, lawyer, and philosopher, credited as the father of the scientific method; here Wither sees Bacon in his dream vision.

**Bashan, bulls of.** Psalm 22.12: "Many bulls have surrounded me; Strong bulls of Bashan have encircled me."

**Baskerville, Sir Humphrey** (1586–1648). Of Eardisley Castle in Hereford County; here offered a dedicatory poem by John Davies.

**Bateman, J.** London bookseller at the *Hat* and *Star* in St. Paul's Churchyard, here identified along with J. Nicks as one of the sellers of William Pitt's poem.

**Bedlam** The Hospital of St. Mary of Bethlehem, used as an asylum for the reception and treatment of the mentally ill; originally situated in Bishopsgate, in 1676 rebuilt near London Wall.

**Berkshire** An English county forty miles west of London, home to Windsor Castle and to the city of *Reading*, an alternative location for the English courts when prohibited in London due to plague.

**Blower, Ralph.** Printer in London 1595–1618, here identified as the printer for William Muggins.

**Boar of Turkey.** Noted for ferocity; boars generally represented as aggressively bestial versus civilized.

**Bodenham, Thomas, esquire.** Unidentified but by John Davies, who offers a prefatory verse dedication to him.

**Boreas.** The north-wind; the god of the north-wind.

**Brook, Nathaniel.** London bookseller 1646–77, identified here as such for William Austin's poem.

**Cary, Sir Philip.** (1572–1631) of Hertfordshire, brother of Elizabeth Cary (1585–1639), the first woman to write a full-length play and a political history in English, and here identified by Davies in dedicatory verse.

**Charon.** Ferryman of souls to Hades who in Greek mythology.

**Charybdis.** Whirlpool; of Greek mythology, the daughter of Poseidon and Gaia turned into the whirlpool by Zeus.

**Cheltenham.** Town in Gloucestershire, on the edge of the Cotswolds in the South-West region of England, abbreviated by Richard Milton as Cheltnam, to suite the pentameter.

**Chichester, Earl of.** Francis Leigh (d. 1653), later Baron Dunsmore, noted in Wither's dream vision.

**Chryses.** Apollonian priest of Greek mythology who figures in Homer's *Iliad*, praying to Apollo when Agamemnon takes his daughter as a war prize; in answer, Apollo sends a plague on the Greek troops.

**Cimmerian.** One of a people fabled by the ancients to live in perpetual darkness.

**Cox, Robert.** Author of commendatory verses "To my entirely beloved, Master, John Davies" and possibly author of *Actaeon and Diana* (1656).

**Creed, Thomas.** Printer in London 1593–1617, here identified as printer for Thomas Dekker and Thomas Middleton's poem.

**Crisp.** Ellis Crisp (*d.* 1625) of Hammersmith (but descended from a Gloucestershire landed family), a prominent merchant, alderman, and sheriff of London in 1625, here noted for the latter role by George Wither.

**Croft, Herbert** (*c.*1565–1629). Administrator and landowner cited in a marginal note by John Davies.

**Delphic.** Referring to the mythological birth place of Apollo.

**Diagoras.** Greek poet and sophist of the 5th century B.C.E.

**Dis.** Fictional city in Dante's *Inferno* that contains the lower circles of hell; an alternate name for Satan.

**Dodona.** Dodona is a mythological Greek oracle. *Dodona's Grove* (1640) is an historical allegory by James Howell, making extensive use of tree lore.

**Don.** A Spanish title, prefixed to a man's Christian name, often used for humorous emphasis.

**Dunkirks.** Dunkirkers; during the Dutch Revolt (1568–1648) the Dunkirkers or Dunkirk Privateers, were commerce raiders in the service of the Spanish Monarchy.

**Dutton, Elizabeth** (n.d.). Daughter of Thomas Egerton, Lord Chancellor of England and here subject with her sisters Mary and Vere Dutton of dedicatory verse by John Davies.

**Egerton, Thomas** (1540–1617). First Viscount Brackley, Lord Chancellor of England from 1603–1617, here the subject of dedicatory verses by John Davies.

**Egerton, Mary and Vere.** Daughters of Thomas Egerton, Lord Chancellor of England and here the subject with their sister Elizabeth Dutton of dedicatory verse by John Davies.

**Ephraim.** In the book of Genesis, the second son of Joseph and Asenath.

**Eton.** Called by Wither "zealous Eton" and noted for tending with care to his congregation during a plague visitation. This may be Martin Heton (1554–1609), the popular bishop of Ely who eschewed pomp and circumstance, as Wither did; or William Heton, vicar in East Marden, West Sussex, from 1607–1626.

**Fawcet, Thomas Holland** (*fl* 1621–43). Printer in London often in partnership with Thomas Creed, at the sign of the Eagle and Child; after Creed's death, he partnered with Bernard Alsop and is here identified with him as a printer for editions of Abraham Holland's poems.

**Gad, Tribe of.** One of the twelve tribes of Israel.

**Galen** (c. 130–200). Prominent Roman physician who codified classical medicine.

**Gallia.** France.

***Godbid, William.*** London printer from 1656–77, here perhaps the W.G. who printed Thomas Clark's poem.

***Gordian knot.*** An intricate knot tied by Gordius, king of Gordium in Phrygia. The oracle declared that whoever should loosen it should rule Asia.

***Gosson, Henry*** (*fl.* 1601–30). London bookseller admitted to the Stationers' Company on 3 August 1601.

***Gough, Richard.*** City of Hereford, gentleman, unidentified otherwise than as "Uncle" by Richard Milton.

***Greys, Anthony.*** Otherwise anonymous writer of commendatory verses, "To the Reader in praise of the Author," for John Davies of Hereford.

***Grismond, John.*** London printer in Ivy Lane c. 1639–66, here identified as the bookseller for George Wither's poem.

***Hamilton.*** Likely James Hamilton, second marquess of Hamilton (1589–1625), courtier, commissioner to the Scottish Parliament under King James; here Wither seems him in a vision.

***Harvey, Gabriel*** (1552/3–1631). Controversial scholar, writer, and Cambridge friend of Edmund Spenser.

***Hector.*** Mythological hero of the Trojan War.

***Hesiod*** (*fl.* 700 B.C.E.). Ancient Greek didactic oral poet, thought to be the earliest to produce the form and best known for *Days and Works*.

***Hippocrates*** (c. 460–370 B.C.E.). Greek father of medicine.

***Holderness, Earl of.*** John Ramsay, 1st Earl of Holderness (*c.* 1580–1626), Scottish aristocrat; here seen in George Wither's dream vision.

***Hoxton.*** Near Graves-end, Kent, frequented for its taverns and gambling-houses.

***Hubbard.*** Likely Sir Henry Hobart, first baronet (*c.* 1554–1625), lawyer and judge; here appearing in Wither's dream vision.

***Hyde Park.*** A park in central London, initially opened to the public under Charles I.

***Hymenaeus*** (*fl.* 50–65). was an early Christian from Ephesus, an opponent of the apostle Paul, who associates him with Alexander and Philetus. Hymenaeus and Philetus are included among persons whose profane and vain babblings will increase unto more ungodliness.

***Inns of Court.*** The four sets of buildings in London (the Inner Temple, the Middle Temple, Lincoln's Inn, and Gray's Inn) belonging to the four legal societies which have the exclusive right of admitting persons to practice at the bar, and hold a course of instruction and examination for that purpose; hence, these four societies themselves.

***Islington.*** In Middlesex County, England, sought out by Londoners for wholesome air and recreation.

*Islip, Adam.* Printer in London 1591–1640, printer for Davies.

*Jambres.* One of two men who opposed Moses and in Rabbinic tradition considered magicians (2 Timothy 3.8).

*Janus Temple.* The doors of the temple to Janus in the Roman Forum were always open in time of war, and shut in time of peace, as Janus was regarded as the doorkeeper of heaven.

*Jeroboam.* The first biblical king of the northern Israelite Kingdom of Israel after the revolt of the Israelite tribes against Rehoboam that put an end to the United Monarchy.

*Joan.* See *Pope Joan.*

*Jordan.* The River Jordan, biblical site of the baptism of Jesus.

*Lazar.* Lazarus, from the biblical story of Lazarus and the rich man (Luke 16:14–31).

*Lennox, Duke of.* Stuart, Esmé, third duke of Lennox (1579?–1624), nobleman, brother of the Duke of Richmond, patron of Ben Jonson; here seen in a vision by George Wither.

*Litchfield, John.* With William Turner, printer to the University of Oxford from 1623–43, here identified as the printers for John Taylor's poem.

*Lucan.* Marcus Annaeus Lucanus (39–65), Roman poet best known for his martial epic, *Pharsalia.*

*Lucina.* In Roman mythology, the goddess who presided over childbirth, sometimes identified with Juno or with Diana; hence, a midwife.

*Makerness.* Possibly the curate of the parish church at Childerly (c. 1625) in Cambridgeshire; here praised by George Wither for tending his congregation with care during a plague visitation.

*Mammon.* Inordinate desire for wealth or possessions, personified as a devil or demonic agent.

*Manilius, Marcus (fl.* 1st century CE). Roman didactic poet, author of *Astronomica.*

*Marybourne.* For many years the largest and wealthiest parish in London with public gardens, also called Marylebone.

*Massilia.* Marseille, France.

*Memphis.* Once the capital of ancient Egypt, it became a city of ruins.

*Millicent, John.* Sergeant Porter to the King, identified only by John Taylor the Water Poet in dedicatory verse of iambic pentameter.

*Nabal.* A churlish shepherd who would not assist David in protecting his flocks (1 Samuel 25).

*Nesis.* Nisida, a small once-volcanic island in the Bay of Naples.

***Nicks, J.*** Bookseller located at the *Hat and Star* in St. Paul's Churchyard, here identified as one of the places to buy William Pitt's poem; see also J. Bateman.

***Nottingham, Earl of.*** Charles Howard second Baron Howard of Effingham and first earl of Nottingham (1536–1624), naval commander; here appearing in George Wither's dream vision.

***Nylus.*** The River Nile.

***Okes, Nicholas.*** Well-established printer in London 1606–39, here identified as the printer for Richard Milton's poem.

***Oxford, Earl of.*** Henry de Vere, eighteenth earl of Oxford (1593–1625), nobleman and soldier; here appearing in George Wither's dream vision.

***Paul's.*** St. Paul's Cathedral.

***Palamede.*** In Greek mythology, said to have invented counting, currency, weights and measures, jokes, dice and a forerunner of chess as well as military ranks.

***Pelions.*** A mountain in Thessaly; figuratively, a difficult challenge.

***Percy, Algernon*** (1602–1668). 10th earl of Northumberland and son of Henry Percy, the 9th Earl, and Dorothy *née* Devereux, sister of Robert Devereux, Earl of Essex, a favorite of Queen Elizabeth's executed for treason; here the subject of a dedicatory by John Davies.

***Percy, Dorothy*** (1598–1659). Sister to Algernon and Lucy Percy, she would become Dorothy Sidney, wife of Robert Sidney, 2nd Earl of Leicester; here the subject of a dedicatory by John Davies.

***Percy, Lucy*** (1599–1660). Sister to Algernon and Dorothy Percy, she would become Lucy Hay, Countess of Carlisle and play a prominent role in the English Civil War; here the subject of a dedicatory by John Davies.

***Phayer, Thomas*** (1510?–1560). Translator and physician, the first Englishman to attempt to translate Virgil's *Aenied*.

***Phoebus.*** Apollo, classical god of light and the sun; truth and prophecy; medicine, healing, and plague; music, poetry, and the arts.

***Pope Joan.*** Legendary female Pope who supposedly reigned for a few years in the ninth century C.E.

***Puckham.*** Puckham Woods, near Cheltenham, in Gloucestershire, on the edge of the Cotswolds in the South-West region of England.

***Purslowe, Elizabeth*** (*fl.* 1633–46). London printer, widow of printer George Purslowe (d. 1632).

***Pygmalion.*** In Greek mythology, a sculptor who fell in love with his statue.

***Reading.*** Forty miles west of London in the county of *Berkshire*, an alternative location for the English courts when prohibited in London due to plague.

*Vesuvius.* Volcanic mountain in Naples, Italy.

*Vitellius.* Roman emperor for eight months until his position was disputed; considered in stories as a gluttonous heavy drinker.

*Westminster.* Palace of Westminster, location of the Houses of Parliament.

*White Hall.* The Palace of White Hall, primary London residence of English monarchs.

*Winchester, Bishop of.* Lancelot Andrewes (1555–1626), clergyman and scholar; here appearing Wither's dream vision.

*Whitsun King.* Person presiding at a parish festival formerly held at Whitsuntide (or Whit Sunday), the seventh Sunday after Easter, to commemorate Pentecost.

*Zouch.* Edward la Zouche, 11th Baron Zouche, 12th Baron St. Maur (1556–1625), an English diplomat, noted in Wither's dream vision.

# Bibliography

**Primary Sources**

Austin, William. *A joyous welcome to the most serene, and most illustrious queen of brides Catherine.* 1662.
———. *Atlas under Olympus, or The heroic poems of William Austin of Grays-Inn, Esq.* 1664.
———. *Epiloimia epē or The Anatomy of the Pestilence.* 1666.
———. *Triumphus Hymenaeus, a panegyric to the king and queen's most sacred majesties.* 1662.
Blackmore, Sir Richard. *A paraphrase on the book of Job.* 1700.
———. *Creation: A Philosophical Poem in Seven Books in Poetical Works.* 1729.
———. *A discourse upon the plague, with a preparatory account of malignant fevers.* 1721.
Brewer, Thomas. *A dialogue betwixt a citizen, and a poor country-man and his wife, in the country, where the citizen remaineth now in this time of sickness.* 1636.
———. *The Weeping Lady: Or London Like Nineveh in Sack-Cloth.* 1603.
Cary, Elizaeth. *The History of the Life, Reign and Death of Edward II.* 1680.
———. *The Tragedy of Miriam.* 1613.
Church of England. *A Form to be used in Common Prayer.* 1563.
Cibber, Theophilus. *The Lives of the Poets of Great Britain and Ireland.* 1753.
Clark, Thomas. *Meditations in my Confinement.* 1666.
Cogan, Thomas. *The haven of health.* 1584.
Cooper, Thomas. *Thesaurus linguae Romanœ & Britannicœ.* 1565.
Cowley, Abraham. *Davideis.* 1656.
Davies, John. *Microcosmos: The discovery of the little world.* 1603.
———. *The Triumph of Death.* 1609.
Defoe, Daniel. *A Journal of the Plague Year.* In Backscheider. 1-248.
Dekker, Thomas. *The wonderful year.* 1603.
Dekker, Thomas and Thomas Middleton. *News from Graves-end.* 1604.
Dod, John. *Four godly and fruitful sermons.* 1611.
Dryden, John. *Annus mirabilis, The year of wonders.* 1667.
Du Bartas, Guillaume de Salluste. *Bartas: his divine weeks and works translated: & dedicated to the King's most excellent Majesty, by Joshua Sylvester.* 1605.
Elyot, Sir Thomas. *The castle of health.* 1539.
Fracastoro, Girolamo. *Syphilis, or, A poetical history of the French disease written in Latin by Fracastorius; and now attempted in English by N. Tate.* 1686.
Fuller, Thomas. *A sermon intended for Paul's Crosse ...Upon the late decrease and withdrawing of God's heavy visitation of the plague of pestilence from the said city.* 1626.

Garth, Samuel. *The Dispensary.* 1699.

Holland, Abraham. *A Description of the Great, Fearful and Prodigious Plague, 1625.*1626.

Holland, Henry. *Spiritual preservatives against the pestilence.* 1593.

Holland, Philemon. *Regimen sanitatis Salerni.* 1617.

———. *The history of the world.* 1601.

Hunter, Josiah. *The dreadfulness of the plague.* 1666.

I. D. Preacher of God's Word. *Salomon's pest-house, or tower-royal.* 1630, 1636.

Lucan, *Lucan's Pharsalia: containing the civil wars between Cæsar and Pompey. Written in Latin heroical verse by M. Annæus Lucanus. Translated into English verse by Sir Arthur Gorges Knight.* 1614.

———. *Lucretius: De Rerum Natura,* translated by. W.H.D. Rouse, rev. M.F. Smith. The Loeb Classical Library. Cambridge, Mass. and London: Harvard University Press, 1975.

Manilius. *The sphere of Marcus Manilius made an English poem.*1675.

Markham, Gervase. *The English Housewife: Containing the Inward and Outward Virtues Which Out to Be in a Complete Woman,*edited by Michael R. Best. Toronto: McGill-Queen's University Press, 1998.

Milton, John. *Of Education.* In *John Milton: The Complete Poems and Essential Prose,* edited by William Kerrigan, John Rumrich, and Stephen M. Fallon. New York: Random House, 2007. 971–981.

———. *Paradise Lost.* In Kerrigan, Rumrich, and Fallon. 293–630.

———. *Paradise Regained.* In Kerrigan, Rumrich, and Fallon. 293–630.

———. *Reason of Church Government.* In Kerrigan, Rumrich, and Fallon. 835–44.

Milton, Richard. *London's Misery.* 1626.

Muggins, William. *London's Mourning Garment.* 1603.

Oxinden, Henry. *Jobus Triumphans.* 1656.

Phayer, Thomas. *The nyne fyrst bookes of the Eneidos of Virgil conuerted into Englishe vearse by Thomas Phaer Doctour of Phisike.* 1562.

Pitt, Christopher. *Aenied.* In *The Works of Virgil in Latin and English,* ed. Joseph Warton. 1753.

———. *The Plague of Marseilles.* 1721.

Pitt, Robert. *The craft and frauds of physic expos'd.* 1703.

Price, Sampson. *London's Remembrancer: for the staying of the contagious sickness of the plague.* 1626.

Quarles, Francis. *Job Militant.* 1624.

Quarles, John. *London's disease, and cure.* 1665.

———. *The Citizen's Flight.* 1665.

———. *The rape of Lucrece, committed by Tarquin the Sixth; and the remarkable judgments that befell him for it.* 1655.

Reynolds, Edward. *A sermon preached before the peers in the Abbey Church at Westminster.* 1666.

Sidney, Philip. *The Apology for Poetry,* edited by Robert W. Maslen. Manchester: Manchester University Press, 2002.

Sprat, Thomas. *History of the Royal Society of London*. 1667.

―――. *The Plague of Athens*. 1659.

Tabor, John. *Seasonable Thoughts in Sad Times*. 1667.

Taylor, John. *Against Swearing*. 1626.

―――. *Christian admonitions against the two fearful sins of cursing and swearing*. 1630.

―――. Taylor, *The Fearful Summer*. 1625.

Thucydides. *History of the Peloponnesian War*. Vol. 1. Translated by C. F. Smith. Loeb Classical Library. London, W. Heinemann; New York, G. P. Putnam's sons, 1919–23.Cambridge, MA: Harvard University Press, 1991.

Virgil. *Aenied*. In *Virgil in Two Volumes: I Eclogoues Georgics Aenied I-VI,* ed. H. Rushton Fairclough, The Loeb Classical Library (Cambridge and London: Harvard University Press, 1942. 240–571.

―――. *Georgics*. In*Virgil in Two Volumes: I Eclogoues Georgics Aenied I-VI,* ed. H. Rushton Fairclough, The Loeb Classical Library. Cambridge and London: Harvard University Press, 1942. 2–77.

―――. *The nyne fyrst bookes of the Eneidos of Virgil conuerted into Englishe vearse by Thomas Phaer Doctour of Phisike*. 1562.

Warton, Joseph, ed. *The Works of Virgil in Latin and English*. 1753.

William Winstanley, *The lives of the most famous English poets*. 1687.

Wither, George. *A memorandum to London*. 1665.

―――. *Britain's Remembrancer*. 1628.

―――. *History of the pestilence*. MS 1999. Pepys Library, Magdalene College, Cambridge.

―――. *Juvenilia, A collection of those poems heretofore imprinted, and written by George Wither* (1633);

―――. *Mr. Wither his prophesy of our present calamity, and (except we repent) future misery. Written by him in the year 1628*. 1643.


## Secondary Sources

Anselment, Raymond A. *The Realms of Apollo: Literature and Healing in Seventeenth-Century England*. Newark: University of Delaware Press and London: Associated University Presses, 1995.

Backscheider, Paula R. *Eighteenth-Century Women Poets and their Poetry: Inventing Agency, Inventing Genre*. Baltimore: The Johns Hopkins University Press, 2007.

―――, ed., *Daniel Defoe, A Journal of the Plague Year,* A Norton Critical Reader (New York and London: W. W. Norton & Company, 1992.

Belozerskaya, Marina. *The Medici Giraffe*. New York: Little, Brown, and Company, 2006.

Benson, Larry Dean. *The Riverside Chaucer*. Oxford and New York: Oxford University Press, 2008.

Biow, Douglas. *Doctors, Ambassadors, Secretaries: Humanism and Professions in Renaissance Italy*. Chicago: University of Chicago, 2002.

Blickman, Daniel R. "The Role of the Plague in the *Iliad.*" *Classical Antiquity* 6.1 (1987): 1–10.

Borris, Kenneth. *Allegory and Epic in English Renaissance Literature: Heroic Form in Sidney, Spenser, and Milton*. Cambridge and New York: Cambridge University Press, 2000.

Brady, Andrea. *English Funerary Elegy in the Seventeenth Century: Laws in Mourning*. Basingstoke: Palgrave Macmillan, 2006.

Capp, Bernard. "Taylor, John (1578–1653)." *Oxford Dictionary of National Biography*. Oxford University Press, 2004 (http://www.oxforddnb.com/view/article/27044, accessed 13 March 2010).

Chahoud, Anna. "Pitt, Christopher (1699–1748)." *Oxford Dictionary of National Biography*. Oxford University Press, 2004 (http://www.oxforddnb.com/view/article/22327, accessed 24 Feb 2011).

Colie, Rosalie. *The Resources of Kind: Genre-Theory in the Renaissance*. Berkeley, London, and New York: University of California Press, 1973.

Creighton, Charles. *History of Epidemics in Britain: From AD 664 to the Extinction of the Plague*. 2 vols. Cambridge: Cambridge University Press, 1891–94.

Cressy, David "National Memory in Early Modern England." In *Commemorations: The Politics of National Identity,* edited by John R. Gillis. Princeton: Princeton University Press, 1994. 61–73.

Dalzell, Alexander. *The Criticism of Didactic Poetry: Essays on Lucretius, Virgil, and Ovid*. Toronto: University of Toronto Press, 1996.

DeWall, Nichole. "'Sweet recreation barred': The Case for Playgoing in Plague-Time." In Totaro and Gilman. 133-49.

Donno, Elizabeth Story. *Elizabethan Minor Epics*. New York: Columbia University Press, 1963.

DuRocher, Richard J. *Milton among the Romans: The Pedagogy and Influence of Milton's Latin Curriculum*. Medieval & Renaissance Literary Studies. Pittsburgh: Duquesne University Press, 2001.

Eatough, Geoffrey. *Fracastoro's Syphilis: Introduction, Text, Translation and Notes with a Computer-generated Word Index*. ARCA: Classical and Medieval Texts, Papers and Monographs 12. Liverpool: Francis Cairns, 1984.

Finkelpearl, P.J. "Davies, John (1564/5–1618)." *Oxford Dictionary of National Biography*, Oxford University Press, 2004 (http://www.oxforddnb.com/view/article/7244, accessed 13 March 2010).

Gale, Monica, ed. *Latin Epic and Didactic Poetry: Genre, Tradition and Individuality*. Swansea: The Classical Press of Wales, 2004.

Gale, Monia. *Lucretius and the Didactic Epic*. London: Bristol Classical Press, 2001.

———. *Virgil on the Nature of Things: The Georgics, Lucretius and the Didactic Tradition*. Cambridge: Cambridge University Press, 2000.

Gillespie, Stuart. "Lucretius in the English Renaissance." In *The Cambridge Companion to Lucretius,* edited by Stuart Gillespie and Philip Hardie. Cambridge and New York: Cambridge University Press, 2007. 242–53.

Gilman, Ernest. "Afterword: Plague and Metaphor." In Totaro and Gilman. 219–36.

———. *Plague Writing in Early Modern England.* Chicago: University of Chicago Press, 2009.

Glaisyer, Natasha and Sara Pennell. Introduction to *Didactic Literature in England, 1500-1800: Expertise Constructed,* edited by Glaisyer and Pennell. Aldershot, England; Ashgate, 2003. 4–18.

Goldberg, Jonathan. *The Seeds of Things: Theorizing Sexuality and Materiality in Renaissance Representations.* New York: Fordham University Press, 2009.

Gould, Stephen Jay. *I Have Landed: The End of a Beginning in Natural History.* New York: Turbo, Inc., 2003.

Green, Ian. *Humanism and Protestantism in Early Modern English Education.* Farnham: Ashgate Publishing Ltd, 2009.

Greenblatt, Stephen. *The Swerve: How the World Became Modern.* New York: W. W. Norton, 2011.

Gregory, Tobias. *From Many Gods to One: Divine Action in Renaissance Epic.* Chicago: University of Chicago Press, 2006.

Hammond, Jeffry A. *The American Puritan Elegy, Cambridge Studies in American Literature and Culture.* Cambridge and New York: Cambridge University Press, 2000.

Hardie, Philip. "Cosmology and National Epic in the Georgics 2.458–3.48." In Volk. 161–81.

———. *Lucretian Receptions: History, the Sublime, Knowledge.* Cambridge and New York: Cambridge University Press, 2009.

Harris, Jonathan Gil. Sick Economies: Drama, Mercantilism, and Disease in Shakespeare's England. Philadelphia: University of Pennsylvania, 2003.

Healy, Margaret. *Fictions of Disease in Early Modern England: Bodies, Plagues and Politics.* Houndmills, UK and New York: Palgrave, 2002.

Higgins, Alison I. T. *Secular Heroic Epic Poetry of the Caroline Period,* Schweizer Anglistische Arbeiten 31. Bern: A. Francke, 1953.

Hodges, William Bridges. *A Milton Encyclopedia.* Volume. 8. New York: Associated University Presses, 1979 .

Horrox, Rosemary. *The Black Death,* Manchester Medieval Sources Series. Manchester and New York: Manchester University Press, 1994.

Houlebrook, Ralph. *Death, Religion, and the Family in England, 1480-1750.* Oxford Studies in Social History. Oxford and New York: Oxford University Press, 1998.

Howard, W. Scott. "'Mine Own Breaking': Resistance, Gender, and Temporality in Seventeenth-Century English Elegies and Jonson's 'Eupheme.'" In *Grief and Gender, 700–1700,* edited by Jennifer C. Vaught and Lynne Dickson Bruckner. New York: Palgrave Macmillan Ltd., 2003. 215–30.

Hulse, S. Clark. "Elizabethan Minor Epic: Toward a Definition of Genre" *Studies in Philology*, Vol. 73, No. 3 (Jul., 1976), pp. 302–319;

———. *The Metamorphic Verse: The Elizabethan Minor Epic.* Princeton: Princeton University Press, 1983.

Kelly, Van. "Introduction: Criteria for the Epic: Borders, Diversity, and Expansion." In *Epic and Epoch: Essays on the Interpretation and History of a Genre,* edited by Steven M. Oberhelman, Van Kelly, and Richard J. Golsan. *Studies in Comparative Literature* 24. Lubbock, Texas: Texas Tech University Press, 1994. 1–24.

Kenney, E. J. "Lucretian Texture: Style, Metre and Rhetoric in the *De rerum natura.*" *The Cambridge Companion to Lucretius,* edited by Stuart Gillespie and Philip Hardie. Cambridge and New York: Cambridge University Press, 2007. 92–110.

Kerwin, William. "Writing the Plague in English Prose Satire." In Totaro and Gilman. 37–53.

Kurth, Burton O. *Milton and Christian Heroism: Biblical Epic Themes and Forms in Seventeenth-Century England.* Hamden: Archon Books, 1966.

Lares, Jameela. *Milton and the Preaching Arts.* Medieval & Renaissance Literary Studies. Pittsburgh: Duquesne University Press, 2001.

Lee, M. Owen. *Virgil as Orpheus: A Study of the Georgics.* Albany: State University of New York Press, 1996.

Lee, Sidney. "Austin, William (*b.* 1627/8, *d.* in or before 1677)." Rev. Sarah Ross, *Oxford Dictionary of National Biography*, Oxford University Press, 2004 ; online edn, Jan 2008 (http://www.oxforddnb.com/view/article/918, accessed 24 Feb 2011).

Lewalski, Barbara Kiefer. "The Genres of *Paradise Lost*: Literary Genre as a Means of Accommodation." *Milton Studies.* Pittsburgh, PA: University of Pittsburgh Press, 1983. 75–103.

———. *The Life of John Milton: A Critical Biography.* Blackwell Critical Biographies. Malden, MA; Oxford: Blackwell, 2000.

———. *Milton's Brief Epic: The Genre, Meaning, and Art of* Paradise Regained. Providence: Brown University Press, 1966.

———. *Paradise Lost and the Rhetoric of Literary Forms.* Princeton: Princeton University Press, 1985.

Lilly, Marie Loretto, *The Georgic: A Contribution to the Study of the Vergilian Type of Didactic Poetry.* Baltimore: The Johns Hopkins Press, 1919.

Llewellyn, Nigel. *Funeral Monuments in Post-Reformation England.* Cambridge and New York: Cambridge University Press, 2000.

Low, Anthony. "New Science and the Georgic Revolution in Seventeenth Century English Literature." *English Literary Renaissance* 13 (1983): 231–59

———. *The Georgic Revolution* (Princeton: Princeton University Press, 1985).

Machacek, Gregory. *Milton and Homer: "Written to Aftertimes."* Medieval & Renaissance Literary Studies. Pittsburgh: Duquesne University Press, 2011. 76–81.

Manley, Lawrence. *Literature and Culture in Early Modern London.* Cambridge and New York: Cambridge University Press, 2000.

Mardock, James. *"The Spirit and the Muse:* The Anxiety of Religious Positioning in John *Taylor's* Prewar Polemics." *The Seventeenth Century* 14 (1999): 1–14.

———. 'Thinking to pass unknown': *Measure for Measure,* the Plague, and the Assession of King James I." In Totaro and Gilman. 113–130.

Marshall, Peter. *Beliefs and the Dead in Reformation England.* New York and Oxford: Oxford University Press, 2002.

Maslen, R. W. "The Healing Dialogues of Doctor Bullein, *The Yearbook of English Studies* 38.1 (2008): 119–135.

———. Introduction to *News from Gravesend: Sent to Nobody* (London, 1603). In *Thomas Middleton: The Collected Works,* edited by Gary Taylor and John Lavagnino. Oxford: Oxford University Press, 2007.

McKerrow, R.B., editor. *A Dictionary of Printers and Booksellers in England, Scotland and Ireland, and of Foreign Printers of English Books 1557–1640.* London: Blades, East & Blades, 1910.

Miller, Paul W. "The Elizabethan Minor Epic." *Studies in Philology.* 55.1 (1958): 31–8.

———. *Seven Minor Epics of the English Renaissance (1596–1624).* Gainesville: Scholars' Facsimiles and Reprints, 1967.

Mullett, Charles. *The Bubonic Plague and England: An Essay in the History of Preventative Medicine.* Lexington: University of Kentucky, 1956.

Munkhoff, Richelle. "Contagious Figurations: Plague and the Impenetrable Nation after the Death of Elizabeth." In *Representing the Plague in Early Modern England,* edited by Rebecca Totaro and Ernest B. Gilman. Routledge Studies in Renaissance Literature and Culture. New York and London: Routledge, 2011. 97–112.

O'Callaghan, Michelle. "Wither, George (1588–1667)." *Oxford Dictionary of National Biography*, Oxford University Press, 2004 [http://www.oxforddnb.com/view/article/29804, accessed 16 March 2010].

O'Meara, Jennifer. *Alchemists, Epics, and Heroes: The Rhetorical Construction of the Seventeenth Century Experimental Philosopher*. Dissertation. University of Illinois at Urbana-Champaign, 2007.

Oberhelman, Steven M., Van Kelly, and Richard J. Golsan, eds. "Epic and Epoch: Essays on the Interpretation and History of a Genre." *Studies in Comparative Literature* 24. Lubbock, Texas: Texas Tech University Press, 1994.

Oldenburg, Scott. "*London's Mourning Garment*: An Epidemiology of Class." Paper presentation. *Renaissance Society of America* conference (25 March 2006), http://www.rsa.org/resource/resmgr/annual_meeting/2006programsfrancisco.pdf.

Passannante, Gerard. "The Art of Reading Earthquakes: On Harvey's Wit, Ramus's Method, and the Renaissance of Lucretius." *Renaissance Quarterly* 61 (2008): 792–832.

———. "Homer Atomized: Francis Bacon and the Matter of Tradition." *English Literary History* 76.4 (2009): 1015–1047.

————. *The Lucretian Renaissance: The Philology and the Afterlife of Tradition*. Chicago: University of Chicago Press, 2011.

Paster, Gail Kern. *Humoring the Body: Emotions and the Shakespearean Stage*. Chicago: University of Chicago Press, 2004.

Pender, Stephen. "Rhetoric, Grief, and the Imagination in Early Modern England," *Philosophy and Rhetorica* 43.1 (2000): 54–81.

Perkinson, Richard H. "The Epic in Five Acts." *Studies in Philology* 43.3 (1946): 465–81.

Phillippy, Patricia. "London's Mourning Garment: Maternity, Mourning and Succession in Shakespeare's *Richard III*." In *Women, Death, and Literature in Post-Reformation England*. Cambridge and New York: Cambridge University Press, 2002. 109–138;

Phillips, Phillip Edward. *John Milton's Epic Invocations: Converting the Muse*, Renaissance and Baroque Studies and Texts 26. New York: Peter Lang, 2000.

Pigman, G.W. *Grief and English Renaissance Elegy*. Cambridge and New York: Cambridge University Press, 1985.

Plomer, Henry Robert, editor. *A Dictionary of the Booksellers and Printers Who Were at Work in England, Scotland and Ireland from 1641 to 1667*. London: Blades, East & Blades,1907.

Prescott, Anne Lake. "The Reception of Du Bartas in England." *Studies in the Renaissance* 15 (1968): 144–73.

Quint, David. *Epic and Empire: Politics and Generic Form from Virgil to Milton*. Princeton, NJ : Princeton University Press, 1993.

Revard, Stella P. *Pindar and the Renaissance Hymn-Ode: 1450–1700*. Tempe: Arizona Center for Medieval and Renaissance Studies, 2001.

Rogers, John. *The Matter of Revolution: Science, Poetry, and Politics in the Age of Milton*. Ithaca: Cornell University Press, 1998.

Scodel, Joshua. *Excess and the Mean in Early Modern English Literature*. Princeton: Princeton University Press, 2002.

Schwartz, Louis. *Milton and Maternal Mortality*. Cambridge and New York: Cambridge University Press, 2009.

Shawcross, John T. "Milton and Epic Revisionism." In *Epic and Epoch: Essays on the Interpretation and History of a Genre*, edited by Steven M. Oberhelman, Van Kelly, and Richard J. Golsan. Studies in Comparative Literature 24. Lubbock, Texas: Texas Tech University Press, 1994. 186–207.

————. John Milton: The Critical Heritage Volume 2 1732–1801. New York: Routledge, 1995.

Sherlock, Peter. *Monuments and Memory in Early Modern England*. Aldershot and Burlington: Ashgate, 2008.

Shuttleton, David E. *Smallpox and the Literary Imagination, 1660–1820*. Cambridge and New York: Cambridge University Press, 2007.

Slack, Paul. *The Impact of Plague in Tudor and Stuart England*. London and Boston: Routledge & Kegan Paul, 1985; reprinted with corrections, Oxford: Clarendon Press, 1985; New York: Oxford University Press, 2000.

Smythe, Adam. *Autobiography in Early Modern England.* Cambridge and New York: Cambridge University Press, 2010.

Stanwood, P.G. "Consolatory Grief in the Funeral Sermons of Donne and Taylor." In Swiss and Kent. 197–216.

Starr, George A. *Defoe and Spiritual Autobiography.* 1965; Princeton: Princeton University Press, 1971.

Steadman, John M. *Milton and the Paradoxes of Renaissance Heroism* Louisiana: Louisiana State University Press, 1987.

———. *Epic and Tragic Structure in* Paradise Lost. Chicago: University of Chicago, 1976.

Sullivan, Erin. "Physical and Spiritual Illness: Narrative Appropriations of the Bills of Mortality." In Totaro and Gilman. 76–94.

Suzuki, Mihoko. *Subordinate Subjects: Gender, the Political Nation, and Literary Form, 1588-1688.* Women and Gender in the Early Modern World. Aldershot and Burlington: Ashgate, 2003.

Swiss, Margo and David A. Kent, eds. *Speaking Grief in English Literary Culture: Shakespeare to Milton.* Medieval & Renaissance Literary Studies. Pittsburgh: Duquesne University Press, 2002.

Taylor, Gary and John Lavagnino, eds. *Thomas Middleton: The Collected Works.* Oxford: Oxford University Press, 2007.

Terry, Richard. *Mock-Heroic from Butler to Cowper: An English Genre and Discourse.* Aldershot and Burlington: Ashgate 2005.

Thackeray, Mark. "Christopher Pitt, Joseph Warton, and Virgil." *The Review of English Studies* 43.171 (1992): 329–46.

Thomas, Richard F. "Prose into Poetry: Tradition and Meaning in Virgil's Georgics." In Volk. 43–80.

Thorpe, Peter. *Eighteenth Century English Poetry.* Chicago: Nelson-Hall, 1975.

Toohey, Peter. *Epic Lessons and Introduction to Ancient Didactic Poetry.* New York: Routledge, 1996.

Totaro, Rebecca. "Chicken Soup (and Orange Juice) for the Plague-Time Soul?: Francis Bacon's Utopian Prescription." *English Language Notes* 47.2 (Fall/Winter 2009): 25–33.

———. "Mother London and the *Madonna Lactans* in England's Plague Epic." In *Rhetorics of Lactation in Late Medieval and Early Modern Europe,* edited by Jutta Sperling. In review.

———. *The Plague in Print: Essential Elizabethan Sources, 1558–1603.* Medieval & Renaissance Literary Studies. Pittsburgh: Duquesne University Press, 2010.

———. "'Revolving This Will Teach Thee How to Curse': Lessons in Sublunary Exhalation." In *Rhetorics of Bodily Disease and Health in Medieval and Early Modern England,* edited by Jennifer C. Vaught Aldershot and Burlington: Ashgate, 2010. 135–51.

———. *Suffering in Paradise: The Bubonic Plague in English Literature from More to Milton.* Medieval & Renaissance Literary Studies. Pittsburgh: Duquesne University Press, 2005.

Totaro, Rebecca and Ernest B. Gilman, editors. *Representing the Plague in Early Modern England. Routledge Studies in Renaissance Literature and Culture.* New York: Routledge, 2011.

Traister, Barbara. "'A plague on both your houses': Sites of Comfort and Terror in Early Modern Drama." In Totaro and Gilman. 169–182.

Tudeau-Clayton, Margaret. *Jonson, Shakespeare and Early Modern Virgil.* Cambridge and New York: Cambridge University Press, 1998.

Vickers, Brian. Shakespeare, *'A Lover's Complaint', and John Davies of Hereford.* Cambridge and New York: Cambridge University Press, 2007.

Volk, Katharina, ed. *Oxford Readings in Vergil's Georgics.* Oxford and New York: Oxford University Press, 2008.

———. *The Poetics of Latin Didactic: Lucretius, Vergil, Ovid, and Manilius.* Oxford and New York: Oxford University Press, 2002.

Weinfield, Henry. *The Poet without a Name: Gray's Elegy and the Problem of History.* Carbonville: Southern Illinois University Press, 1991.

West, David. "Two Plagues: Virgil, Georgics 3.478–566 and Lucretius 6.1090–1286." In *Creative Imitation and Latin Literature,* edited by David West and Tony Woodman. Cambridge: Cambridge University Press, 1979. 71–88.

# Index